Surgical Approaches to the Spine

Second Edition

Springer-Science+Business Media, LLC

Robert G. Watkins, MD

Professor of Clinical Orthopedic Surgery,
University of Southern California
Co-Director of the Los Angeles Spine Surgery Institute at
   St. Vincent's Hospital
Los Angeles, California

Surgical Approaches to the Spine

Second Edition

With 457 Illustrations, 341 in Full Color

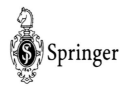 Springer

Robert G. Watkins, MD
Professor of Clinical Orthopedic Surgery
University of Southern California
Co-Director of the Los Angeles Spine Surgery Institute
   at St. Vincent's Hospital
Los Angeles, CA 90057
USA
spinergw@earthlink.net

Library of Congress Cataloging-in-Publication Data
Watkins, Robert G.
    Surgical approaches to the spine / Robert G. Watkins.—2nd ed.
      p. ; cm.
    Includes bibliographical references and index.
    ISBN 978-1-4612-6508-5   ISBN 978-1-4613-0009-0 (eBook)
    DOI 10.1007/978-1-4613-0009-0
    1. Spine—Surgery—Atlases. I. Title.
    [DNLM: 1. Spine—surgery—Atlases. WE 17 W335s 2003]
    RD533.W34 2003
    617.5'6059—dc21   2002036560

ISBN 978-1-4612-6508-5

9 8 7 6 5 4 3 2 1   SPIN 10568262

www.springer-ny.com

Preface to the Second Edition

In the years since publication of the first edition of *Surgical Approaches to the Spine*, a revolution has taken place in spinal surgery. Spinal technology has exploded, thereby increasing the need for multiple access sites to the spine. The book was originally written because the spinal surgeon sometimes lacked the ability to approach the spine with the ideal procedure. As a result, spinal problems were often handled with a posterior approach when the treatment theories and biomechanical considerations of the spine dictated an anterior approach. Then John O'Brien and other anterior surgeons began to emphasize the need to perfect the approach so that the ideal operation was provided for each individual patient. Through our work over the last 20 years, with surgeons such as Salvador Brau, a spinal access surgeon, surgeons are now dedicated to providing a safe, pain-free approach to the spine. This will ultimately be to the patient's great advantage. Advances in intradiscal devices, prostheses, and fusion techniques have mandated a safe and effective anterior approach to the spine. An operation to relieve spinal pain cannot exist if the approach produces more pain than the original problem.

This second edition contains chapters on very complicated operations, such as the approaches to the sacrum and pelvis, the total vertebrectomy, transclavicular cervicothoracic approach, and anterior approach to the clivus of C1–C2. It is these major operations that put the patient's life in jeopardy and require expertise in the approach. The text also discusses minimally invasive approaches, such as the laparoscopic fusion. Minimally invasive surgery is the future of spinal surgery and represents a major advance in protection of the patient, with lower morbidity than that associated with the minimally invasive approaches. The challenge of the next decade will be adapting minimally invasive computer-assisted, image-guided approaches to the patient's pathology and perfecting the available technology for solving that pathology.

The first edition of *Surgical Approaches to the Spine* was appreciated by its audience for its simple step-by-step, how-to method of presenting the surgical approach. The emphasis on how to avoid complications, what specific steps to take, and what specific tools to use was a distinct advantage over publications with the more broad-stroke type of "expose the spine." The use of color illustrations and photographs and the emphasis on a clear-cut presentation in a step-by-step fashion have been preserved.

This book is intended for all spinal surgeons and for the newer category of spinal access surgeon. Certainly, some spinal surgeons are very confident in performing their own surgical approaches to the spine. As the expertise of spinal access surgeons increases, the spinal surgeon may find this, as we have, to be a distinct advantage in producing a safe, effective operation. The secondary market for this text is for all professionals involved in treating the spine. Decision making in spinal surgery depends on a risk–benefit ratio. Everyone participating needs to understand the approach to the spine to determine if surgery is a viable option or not.

I would like to acknowledge Katherine Williams for her tireless work on this project. Her contribution began in 1983 and has continued through this edition. Her dedication to this project is indicative of her dedication to health and proper care of all spinal patients. Surgeons and patients owe a debt of gratitude to her for the effort in this book and other similar publications.

Robert G. Watkins, MD

Preface to the First Edition

This volume is designed to meet the need for a practical, well-illustrated guide to the normal anatomy of surgical approaches to the spine—the most fundamental information for spinal surgery. Most of the basic approaches, anterior and posterior, are covered for each level of the spine. The specific pathology and the operative procedure indicated for any particular patient will naturally influence the choice of approach. While we have illustrated only normal anatomy as seen through the surgical incision, we hope to have given the reader a sound basis for choosing the most appropriate surgical approach for various clinical conditions.

The illustrations are accompanied by a methodical description of operative technique for spinal exposure, emphasizing the critical anatomical landmarks. The bibliography accompanying each chapter is not comprehensive, nor does it necessarily cite the original reports of each technique: rather, we have chosen to include good descriptive reports of each approach. It is our hope that an improved understanding of surgical anatomy and operative approaches will free the spinal surgeon to implement the optimal treatment plan for each patient.

Robert G. Watkins, MD

phasis on how to avoid complications, what specific steps to take, and what specific tools to use was a distinct advantage over publications with the more broad-stroke type of "expose the spine." The use of color illustrations and photographs and the emphasis on a clear-cut presentation in a step-by-step fashion have been preserved.

This book is intended for all spinal surgeons and for the newer category of spinal access surgeon. Certainly, some spinal surgeons are very confident in performing their own surgical approaches to the spine. As the expertise of spinal access surgeons increases, the spinal surgeon may find this, as we have, to be a distinct advantage in producing a safe, effective operation. The secondary market for this text is for all professionals involved in treating the spine. Decision making in spinal surgery depends on a risk–benefit ratio. Everyone participating needs to understand the approach to the spine to determine if surgery is a viable option or not.

I would like to acknowledge Katherine Williams for her tireless work on this project. Her contribution began in 1983 and has continued through this edition. Her dedication to this project is indicative of her dedication to health and proper care of all spinal patients. Surgeons and patients owe a debt of gratitude to her for the effort in this book and other similar publications.

Robert G. Watkins, MD

Contents

†Deceased

Contributors

John A. Ameriks, MD
Michael L.J. Apuzzo, MD
Ranjeev Singh Bhangoo, MD
Salvador A. Brau, MD, FACS
†Roger C. Breslau, MD
H. Alan Crockard, FRCS
Peter Dyck, MD
Kevin T. Foley, MD
Sanjay Ghosh, MD
James M. Giuffre, BA
Masahiko Hata, MD
Yutaka Hiraizumi, MD, PhD
Bernard Jeanneret, MD
Frank T. Jordan, MD
Namir Katkhouda, MD
Norio Kawahara, MD, PhD

Frank Moore, MD
Hideki Murakami, MD
Y. Raja Rampersaud, MD, FRCSC
Srinath Samudrala, MD
Uttam K. Sinha, MD
Maurice M. Smith, MD
Alfred A. Steinberger, MD
Narayan Sundaresan, MD
John S. Thalgott, MD
Katsuro Tomita, MD, PhD
Hiroyuki Tsuchiya, MD, PhD
Robert G. Watkins, MD III
Robert G. Watkins, MD IV
Robert Warren Williams, MD
Paul H. Young, MD

Anterior Cervical Approaches to the Spine

The significant anatomical landmarks for differentiating the approaches to the cervical spine presented in Table 1.1 are the sternocleidomastoid muscle, the carotid sheath, and the longus coli muscle (Fig. 1A).[1-8] Categorization is based on the direction of approach relative to these specific structures, as demonstrated in the table. For example, approach no. 1 is medial to the sternocleidomastoid muscle (therefore, retracting it laterally) and medial to the carotid sheath (therefore, retracting it laterally as well). Approach no. 7 is directed lateral to the sternocleidomastoid muscle and lateral to the carotid sheath. A significant aspect of these approaches is whether to approach the carotid sheath medially or laterally. Approaching the carotid sheath medially and retracting laterally often requires sacrifice of vessels coursing from the carotid sheath to the medial musculovisceral column. Nerves running from lateral to medial also must be retracted. Approaching the carotid sheath laterally and retracting it medially, as in the anterolateral approaches,[1-5] produces a more avascular plane but may also result in a more limited exposure. Both the anteromedial and the anterolateral approaches have common points of dissection and anatomy.

The skin incision must be cosmetically acceptable but efficient (Fig. 1B). Superficial landmarks used to place the incision over the appropriate level of the spine are (1) C3–C4, which is 1 cm above the thyroid cartilage; and (2) C5–C6, which is at the cricoid cartilage.[6] Other superficial landmarks to be identified are the angle of the jaw, the sternocleidomastoid muscle, the hyoid bone, the cricoid cartilage, the superior border of the thyroid cartilage, and the insertion to the sternocleidomastoid to the clavicle. For best cosmesis, make a 3-cm transverse incision in a skin crease. A longer transverse incision from midline to anterior border of the sternocleidomastoid muscle will allow adequate exposure for three vertebral bodies and two disc levels. The exact pathology and the technical demands of the operation determine the size of the exposure and the structures that must be transected rather than retracted.

After the skin incision has been made, when a well-developed platysma muscle is visible, it is best to open the platysma muscle along the line of its fibers. The platysma muscle should be elevated with Adson pick-ups and opened carefully to, avoid damage to underlying veins and the sternocleidomastoid muscle.[6] (A well-

TABLE 1.1 Approaches to the Cervical Spine

	Sternocleidomastoid Muscle		Carotid Sheath		Longus Coli	
	Medial	Lateral	Medial	Lateral	Medial	Lateral
1. Anterior medial C1–C3[6–9]	X		X		X	
2. Anterior medial midcervical spine[6–9]	X		X		X	
3. Supraclavicular approach[4]		X		X		X
4. Anterolateral approach to C1–C3[2–5]		X		X	X	
5. Anterolateral approach to midcervical spine[2]	X		X			X
6. Lateral approach to midcervical spine[10]	X			X	X	
7. Lateral approach to midcervical spine[1]		X		X	X	

X = direction of the approach.

developed platysma muscle should be closed as one individual layer.) Under the platysma is the external jugular vein, which courses on the external surface of the sternocleidomastoid muscle, and the anterior jugular vein, which is in a more anteromedial location over the sternocleidomastoid–strap muscle interval or on the lateral aspect of the strap musculature. The anterior and external jugular veins must be divided and ligated when their presence interferes with the procedure. The sternocleidomastoid must be identified as the initial key to the approach; for anteromedial approaches, the medial border of the sternocleidomastoid; for the lateral approaches, the lateral border of the sternocleidomastoid. The second landmark, the carotid sheath, is first identified by finger palpation of the carotid pulse. The carotid sheath contains the carotid artery, internal jugular vein, the vagus nerve, and sometimes the sympathetic plexus.

The third landmark structure is the longus coli muscle, which must be identified under the prevertebral fascia over the spine. Palpate for the spine. Often the anterior tubercle of the transverse process is mistaken for the vertebral body. Inadvertent dissection in this more lateral area can damage the sympathetic plexus and cause bleeding from the longus coli. The more avascular area of the spine is the midline. Opening the prevertebral fascia in this area allows lateral retraction of the longus coli and causes less bleeding. Special note should be taken of the esophagus in any approach to the cervical spine; it is frequently a flat, ribbon-like structure lying over the anterior prevertebral fascia. A nasogastric tube aids in identification of the esophagus.

Retraction of Neurovascular Structures

Vessels may be either ligated or retracted, usually depending on their exact size and location. The retraction of nerves and arteries varies, but general guidelines can be used. For more cephalad exposures, retract the hypoglossal nerve, glossopharyngeal nerve, and the digastric muscle cephalad. The superior laryngeal nerve and superior thyroid artery and vein are often retracted caudad for C1–C3 approaches and cephalad for C4–C7 approaches. The middle thyroid vein is ligated. The inferior thyroid artery and vein are retracted caudally for C7 and above, often cephalad for levels distal to C7. In addition, the omohyoid muscle crosses above C6 and is divided or retracted for C5–C6 and below.

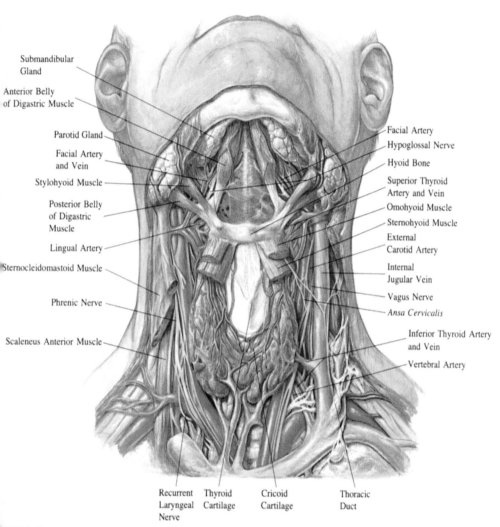

Submandibular Gland

Anterior Belly of Digastric Muscle

Parotid Gland

Facial Artery and Vein

Stylohyoid Muscle

Posterior Belly of Digastric Muscle

Lingual Artery

Sternocleidomastoid Muscle

Phrenic Nerve

Scaleneus Anterior Muscle

Facial Artery

Hypoglossal Nerve

Hyoid Bone

Superior Thyroid Artery and Vein

Omohyoid Muscle

Sternohyoid Muscle

External Carotid Artery

Internal Jugular Vein

Vagus Nerve

Ansa Cervicalis

Inferior Thyroid Artery and Vein

Vertebral Artery

Recurrent Laryngeal Nerve   Thyroid Cartilage   Cricoid Cartilage   Thoracic Duct

FIGURE 1A. The numerous soft tissue structures of the anterior neck. Note the relatively avascular area between the superior thyroid artery and the inferior thyroid artery. The standard approach to the anterior aspect of the spine is lateral to the thyroid gland and medial to the carotid artery.

Right or Left Approach?

To determine whether to approach the spine from the right or the left, consider the following. Approaches from the left in the supraclavicular area must beware of the point of entry of the thoracic duct into the jugular vein–subclavian vein junction (Fig. 1C). A large fatty meal the day before surgery in this area is an aid to identify the duct, but the majority of approaches will be well medial to this area and do not require definitive identification. Approaches from the right from C4 and below require identification of the right recurrent laryngeal nerve (Fig. 1C). This nerve passes from the area of the carotid sheath to the medial musculovisceral column in the C5–C7 area. As to whether

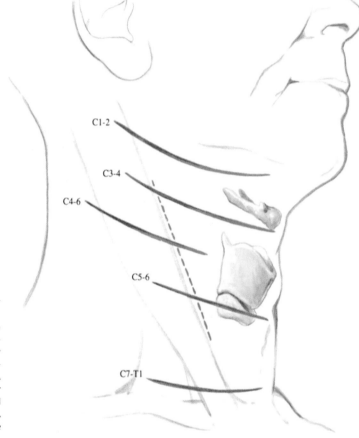

FIGURE 1B. The approximate skin areas for approaches to specific spinal levels are usually indicated by palpable subcutaneous structures. C1–C2 lies under the angle of the jaw, C3–C4 a centimeter above the thyroid cartilage in the region of the hyoid bone, C4–C6 at the level of thyroid cartilage, C5–C6 at the cricoid cartilage, and C7–T1 in the supraclavicular area. For best cosmesis, make a transverse skin incision. A transverse incision from midline to anterior border of the sternocleidomastoid muscle will allow adequate exposure for three vertebral bodies and two disc levels. A vertical incision along the anterior border of the sternocleidomastoid muscle, as seen on the *dotted line*, may be used for long exposures of the cervical spine.

the head should be turned with the approach, it is standard to rotate the head away from the side of the approach, but it is possible to perform most of the approaches described without rotating the head. This is especially true when the sternocleidomastoid muscle is taken down as in the anterolateral approach to C1, C3. In the original description of the operation, the head was rotated,[10] but its feasibility without rotating the head is now considered an indication for use of this approach.[5]

Traction During Surgery

Head halter traction is standard during the interbody grafting operations to allow distraction of the interspace and resulting compression after the bone graft has been placed. If the halter obscures the approach to the more cephalad levels of the cervical spine, tong traction must be used. Position the patient supine. An inflatable cervical pillow provides adequate immobilization of the neck during the surgery, or a roll of towels can be used. The head should rest on an occipital pad with head halter traction or tong immobilization as indicated.

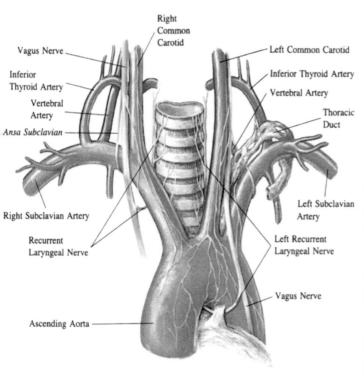

Right Common Carotid

Vagus Nerve

Inferior Thyroid Artery

Vertebral Artery

Ansa Subclavian

Right Subclavian Artery

Recurrent Laryngeal Nerve

Ascending Aorta

Left Common Carotid

Inferior Thyroid Artery

Vertebral Artery

Thoracic Duct

Left Subclavian Artery

Left Recurrent Laryngeal Nerve

Vagus Nerve

FIGURE 1C. Neurovascular structures of the base of the neck. In approaching the spine from the right side of the neck, the prominent recurrent laryngeal nerve must be identified in the area between the musculovisceral column medially and the carotid sheath laterally. When one is approaching the spine from the left side, the thoracic duct may be damaged at the base of the neck as it enters the subclavian vein. A large fatty meal the day before surgery may help with identification of the thoracic duct. Both vagus nerves seen here are in the carotid sheath.

Cervical Anatomy

Muscles and Anatomical Landmarks

The hyoid bone is situated at approximately C3 and serves as a dividing area for the musculature of the anterior neck (see Fig. 1A). The suprahyoid region is covered by the suprahyoid portion of external investing fascia. The musculature includes the digastric muscle that lies inferior to the mandible and extends from the mastoid process to the symphysis mente. The sling around the tendonous midportion of the digastric muscle separates its posterior from anterior belly. It holds the midportion of the muscle to the greater cornu of the hyoid bone. The digastric helps form the carotid triangle, which is bordered superiorly by the posterior belly of the digastric muscle, inferiorly by the omohyoid muscle, and posteriorly by the sternocleidomastoid muscle (see Figs. 4A, 4D). It is essentially through this triangle that the approach is made.

The stylohyoid muscle lies anterior and superior to the posterior belly of the digastric and rises from the styloid process passing to the hyoid bone. The stylohyoid ligament is a ligamentous band that passes with the stylohyoid muscle from the styloid process to the hyoid bone. The mylohyoid muscle and sternohyoid muscle run from the mandible to the hyoid bone. Structures coursing from the mastoid to the hyoid and from the mandible to the hyoid must be either retracted in a cephalad direction or severed. The sequential branches of the external carotid from caudad to cephalad are the superior thyroid artery, the lingual artery, and the facial artery. The external carotid artery continues coursing through the parotid gland and terminates as the superficial temporal artery (see Fig. 5E), the pulse of which can be felt just in front of the ear, and the maxillary artery, which crosses anteriorly through the parotid gland. The occipital artery arises from the posterior aspect of the carotid artery at the level of the facial artery. It crosses under the posterior belly of the digastric and stylohyoid muscles through the loop of the hypoglossal nerve and ascends in the interval between the transverse process of C1 and the mastoid process.

Nerves

In addition to the hypoglossal nerve, the superior laryngeal nerve also arises from the inferior ganglion of the vagus and crosses caudally and medially under the internal carotid artery to the superior border of the thyroid cartilage, where it joins the superior thyroid artery. The superior laryngeal nerve has external and internal branches; the external branch crosses at a more caudad level. The recurrent laryngeal nerve on the right side loops under the subclavian artery, passing dorsomedial to it to the side of the trachea and esophagus (see Fig. 1C). It is vulnerable to damage as it passes from the subclavian artery to the right tracheoesophageal groove.

On the left side, the recurrent laryngeal nerve loops under the arch of the aorta and is much more protected in the left tracheoesophageal groove. Both recurrent laryngeal nerves enter the larynx through the cricothyroid membrane with the inferior thyroid artery and therefore should not be present in more cephalad exposures. The seventh cranial nerve (facial nerve) emerges from the stylomastoid foramen and crosses anteriorly into the parotid gland across the external carotid artery (see Fig. 5E). Although this is in a very superior position in the dissection, care must be taken to avoid the facial nerve with any cephalad retraction. Important bony landmarks are the mastoid process and the smaller, more pointed, styloid process, which projects off the temporal bone just medial to the mastoid process. The styloid process is the origin of the stylohyoid muscle and ligament. The stylomastoid foramen is just medial to the styloid process and serves as the exit for the facial nerve. The jugular foramen lies between the occipital bone and the temporal bone and is the exit for the glossopharyngeal, vagus, and accessory nerves (see Fig. 5E). The hypoglossal canal in the occipital bone is the exit foramen for the hypoglossal nerve.

References

1. Hodgson AR: Approach to the cervical spine C3–C7. Clin Orthop 39:129–134, 1965.
2. Verbest H: Anterolateral operations for fractures and dislocations in the middle and lower parts of the cervical spine. J Bone Joint Surg 51A(8):1489–1530, 1969.
3. Verbest H: A lateral approach to the cervical spine: Technique and indications. J Neurosurg 28:191–203, 1968.
4. Nanson EM: The anterior approach to upper dorsal sympathectomy. Surg Gynecol Obstet 104:118–120, 1957.
5. Whitesides T Jr, McDonald AP: Lateral retropharyngeal approach to the upper cervical spine. Orthop Clin N Am 9(4):1115–1127, 1978.
6. Riley LH: Surgical approaches to the anterior structures of the cervical spine. Clin Orthop 91(16):10–20, 1973.
7. Robinson RA, Southwick WO: Surgical approaches to the cervical spine. In: American Academy of Orthopaedic Surgery: Instructional Course Lectures, Vol. XVII. St. Louis, Mosby, 1960, pp 299–330.
8. Robinson RA: Approaches to the cervical spine C1–T1. Chapter 22 in Schmidek HH, Sweet WH (eds): Current Techniques in Operative Neurosurgery. New York, Grune & Stratton, 1978, pp 205–302.
9. Cloward R: Ruptured Cervical Intervertebral Discs. Codman Signature Series 4. Codman and Shurtleff, 1974.
10. Henry AK: Extensive Exposure. Baltimore, Williams & Wilkins, 1959, pp 53–72.

Transoral Approach to C1–C2

1. Preoperative preparation of the patient should include oral and nasal cultures. Preoperative antiseptic gargles and tetracycline, which were used in the past,[1] are not needed. No special antibiotic coverage is used for normal oral flora.[2] Standard prophylactic antibiotics are used.

2. After intubation and anesthesia, perform a tracheostomy.[1] Insert the short cuff tube. Position the patient supine with the head slightly flexed on occipital pads. A more upright position can be used with certain precautions.

3. Insert the Boyle-Davis or McIver ENT retractor to allow depression of the tongue and self-retaining retraction of the mouth. Be certain there is adequate padding for the lips and teeth (Fig. 2A). Place a collagen sponge into the nasopharynx to control drainage. For adequate visualization of the posterior pharynx, usually the soft palate must be retracted first. Retract the soft palate with soft rubber tubes placed through the nasal cavity and out the oral cavity and tie with adequate padding on the lips (Fig. 2B).

4. If adequate soft palate retraction is not obtained, the soft palate is incised in a curvilinear incision around the uvula and the cut edges are retracted with stay sutures to the lateral walls of the oropharynx.[1,3]

5. Prep the oropharynx with Betadine solution and *reculture*.[2]

6. Inject the posterior pharyngeal tissue with a solution of lidocaine and epiphrine, which aids hemostasis.

7. After palpation and X-ray confirmation of the ring of C1, make a vertical incision from approximately 1 cm cephalad to the tip of the odontoid to 2 cm distal to the anterior tubercle of the ring of C1. Incise the four layers (posterior pharyngeal mucosa, superior constrictor muscle of the pharynx, the prevertebral fascia, and the anterior longitudinal ligaments) directly to bone (Fig. 2C).

8. Bluntly dissect the soft tissue off the body of C2 below the odontoid and off the anterior tubercle of C1 (Fig. 2D).

Caution: Venous bleeding may arise from the recesses just lateral to the base of the odontoid. The longus coli muscle inserts on the anterior tubercle of C1, and sharp dissection may be needed to remove it.

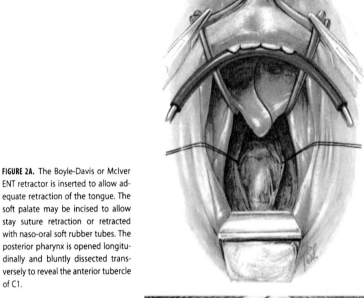

FIGURE 2A. The Boyle-Davis or McIver ENT retractor is inserted to allow adequate retraction of the tongue. The soft palate may be incised to allow stay suture retraction or retracted with naso-oral soft rubber tubes. The posterior pharynx is opened longitudinally and bluntly dissected transversely to reveal the anterior tubercle of C1.

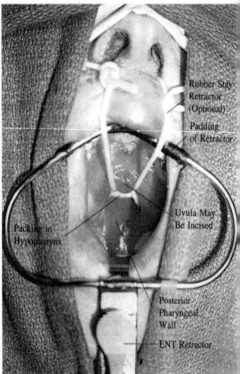

FIGURE 2B. The operative field showing the packing in the hypopharynx and the exposed posterior pharyngeal wall.

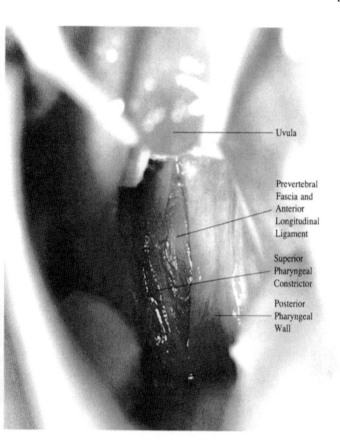

Uvula

Prevertebral
Fascia and
Anterior
Longitudinal
Ligament

Superior
Pharyngeal
Constrictor

Posterior
Pharyngeal
Wall

FIGURE 2C. Incise directly through the posterior pharyngeal wall, the pharyngeal constrictor muscle, and the prevertebral ligaments directly to the anterior tubercle of C1.

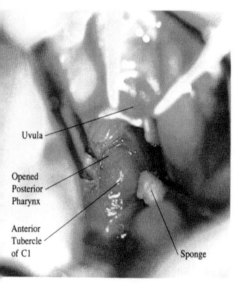

Uvula

Opened
Posterior
Pharynx

Anterior
Tubercle
of C1

Sponge

FIGURE 2D. Bluntly dissect the vertical incision laterally to expose the anterior tubercle of C1. The pharyngeal wall composite tissue may be retracted with special curved Homantype retractors or stay sutures.

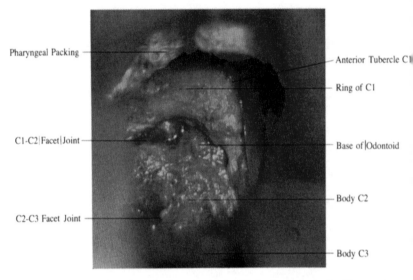

Pharyngeal Packing

Anterior Tubercle C1

Ring of C1

C1-C2|Facet|Joint

Base of |Odontoid

Body C2

C2-C3 Facet Joint

Body C3

FIGURE 2E. The base of the odontoid and anterior tubercle of C1 visualized in the depths of the wound after sufficient soft tissue dissection.

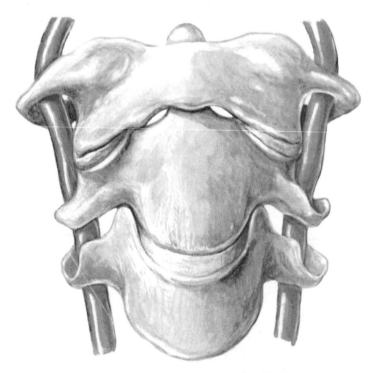

FIGURE 2F. Vertebral arteries lateral to the facet joints.

9. When needed, bluntly dissect the bone both transversely and vertically to expose the lateral masses of C1–C2 (Fig. 2E). Retract the cut edges of the wound with a blunt straight retractor to allow stay suturing or silver-clip attachment of the edges of the wound to the lateral pharynx. Self-retaining retractors may be used.[2]

Caution: Avoid plunging lateral to the facet joints (Fig. 2F). To avoid vertebral artery damage, do not pass a stay suture too deeply into the lateral pharyngeal wall.

10. Closure: After the bony work is completed and good hemostatis is obtained, close the posterior pharynx in a single layer with absorbable suture.

Remember:

1. Secure the head, pad the retractor, and do a tracheostomy.
2. Culture and reculture.
3. Palpation of the anterior tubercle of C1 may be deceptive. Have an X-ray cassette set up.
4. Stay on the bone. Bleeding may be encountered cephalad to C1, lateral to the facet, and in the recesses beside the odontoid.
5. Be careful with retractor tips and stay suture location.

2B

Transoral–Transpharyngeal Approach to the Cervical Spine

Uttam K. Sinha • *Srinath Samudrala*

1. Preoperative otolaryngologic evaluation of upper airway anatomy and velopharyngeal competence using a flexible nasopharyngoscope is obtained. Magnetic resonance imaging (MRI) and computerized tomography (CT) scanning of the craniocervical junction (CCJ) are done to define the location and extent of the lesion as well as cervicomedullary junction compression (Fig. 2G). Dynamic flexion and extension radiographs of the cervical spine are used to document preoperative instability. Vertebral artery angiograms are not performed routinely.

2. The patient is placed in a supine position on the operating table with a Mayfield headrest with the head slightly flexed. The electrodes for somatosensory evoked potential monitoring are attached to the patient. Orotracheal intubation is performed using an oral RAE tube, which is secured in the midline. Rarely, tracheotomy is performed if oral intubation cannot be done. Nasotracheal intubation under flexible endoscopic guidance is avoided, as the nasotracheal tube compromises surgical exposure.[4,5]

3. The face and neck are prepared in the usual sterile fashion. During draping no metal clamps are used because they may interfere with identification of the intervertebral spaces by intraoperative radiographic imaging. The oral cavity and oropharynx are rinsed with Peridex using a sterile toothbrush. A specially designed retractor (Spetzler/Sonntag Transoral System; Aesculap, San Francisco, CA) is used for this approach (Fig. 2H). The ball-and-socket joint of the assembly is secured to the bedrail, near the level of the neck–shoulder interface. The two-piece vertical bar from the fixation bar assembly is attached through the ball-and-socket joint. The horizontal bar is inserted into the vertical bar. The mouth gag with ratchet is carefully inserted into the oral cavity without causing injury to the mucosa, teeth, lips, or gum (Fig. 2I). A tongue blade of appropriate size is inserted into the mouth gag with the ratchet portion of the blade interfacing with the ratchet portion of the mouth gag. The endotracheal tube is placed in the groove of the tongue blade. The tongue blade is released every half-hour during the entire procedure to prevent ischemia and edema of the tongue. Patients receive

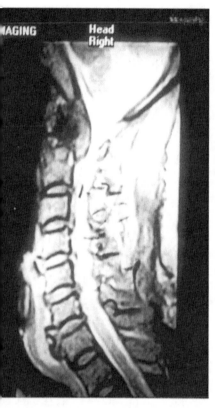

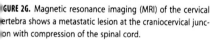

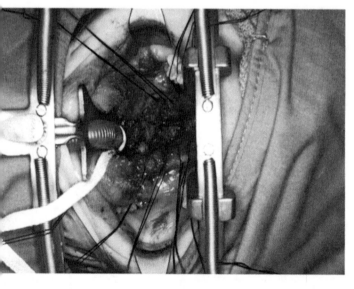

FIGURE 2H. Spetzler/Sonntag Transoral System. *1* = Mouth gag with ratchet (2); *3* = tongue blade; *4* = a pair of adjustable, low-profile pharyngeal retractors; *5* = clamps on the mouth gag for holding the pharyngeal retractors in position; *6* = a portion of the mouth gag that is attached to the fixation bar (not shown) using quick-connect coupling.

FIGURE 2G. Magnetic resonance imaging (MRI) of the cervical vertebra shows a metastatic lesion at the craniocervical junction with compression of the spinal cord.

FIGURE 2I. The mouth gag with ratchet is carefully inserted into the oral cavity without causing injury to the mucosa, teeth, lips, or gum.

perioperative antibiotics and decadron to reduce the chances of oropharyngeal edema. If the transoral system is not available, a Dingman mouth gag can be used for adequate exposure.

4. The soft palate, posterior portion of the hard palate, and the posterior pharyngeal wall are infiltrated with 1% lidocaine with 1:100,000 epinephrine. Using a scalpel, the soft palate is divided in its midline extending from the hard palate to the base of the uvula, and then deviating to one side of the uvula (Fig. 2J1). Bleeding is controlled by using bipolar cautery. Alternatively, splitting of the soft palate is done by using bipolar scissors (Ethicon; Johnson & Johnson, Somerville, NJ).[6] Unipolar cautery is never used to split the palate as this may interfere with restoration of palatal function and may increase the chance of wound dehiscence. The split soft palate is then retracted laterally using 2-0 silk stay sutures, exposing the posterior pharyngeal wall widely.

5. The openings of both eustachian tubes in the lateral pharyngeal walls are identified. Using a #15 blade on a long handle, an "H" incision is made on the posterior pharyngeal wall (Fig. 2J2). Care is taken not to injure the eustachian tubes. The vertical limbs of the H incision are placed as far lateral as possible. These limbs are not parallel, because the upper part of the posterior pharyngeal wall at the level of the Eustachian tube openings is narrower. The horizontal limb of the H incision is placed at the level of the soft palate. The incisions are then carried through all the layers of the pharyngeal wall. Two broad-based pharyngeal myomucosal flaps are then elevated superiorly and inferiorly (Fig. 2J3). The upper flap is elevated up to the pharyngeal tubercle in the midportion of the clivus. The inferior flap is elevated up to the level of the inferior border of the body of C3. Meticulous hemostasis is achieved with bipolar cautery and irrigation. The upper flap is isolated from the surgical field in the nasopharynx with two silk stay sutures, which are brought out with red rubber catheter through the nostrils and tied lightly against the anterior nasal septum. The lower flap is protected under the tongue blade (Fig. 2J4).

6. The fixation bar joints of the transoral system are now loosened to allow repositioning for alignment to the coupler on the mouth gag. The mouth gag is then assembled to the fixation bar using the quick-connect coupling (Fig. 2I). Care is taken not to press the patient's chest with the mouth gag. The fixation bar joints are tightened for stable fixation of the head. The adjustable, low-profile pharyngeal retractor are placed in the mouth, and the length is adjusted by turning the set screw at the proximal end of the retractor. The retractors are positioned to retract the cheeks and lateral pharyngeal walls.[7,8]

7. Positions of the intervertebral spaces are identified and confirmed by radiographic imaging after placement of spinal needles in these spaces (Fig. 2K). Under the operating microscope, attachment of the longus coli muscle and the anterior longitudinal ligament is released by blunt and sharp dissection. The dissection is continued until the inferior clivus, lateral masses of C1–C2, and body and transverse processes of C3 are exposed.

8. The pharyngeal arms of the transoral system are repositioned to retract the prevertebral soft tissue. All bleeding sites (particularly venous bleeding from the lateral recesses just lateral to the base of the odontoid) are meticulously cauterized using bipolar cautery and irrigation. Drilling of the arch of the atlas and the odontoid process is performed with an ultrapower diamond burr and continuous irrigation. Soft tissue or tumor, as indicated, is removed by sharp and blunt dissection until decompression of the CCJ is complete. If the dura is opened, primary closure is performed, followed by placement of fascia and fibrin glue deep to the myomucosal closure.

9. Both the upper and lower myomucosal pharyngeal flaps are released from the nasopharynx and retractor, respectively. The horizontal limb of the H incision is closed first in a watertight fashion using interrupted absorbable sutures followed by the vertical limbs.

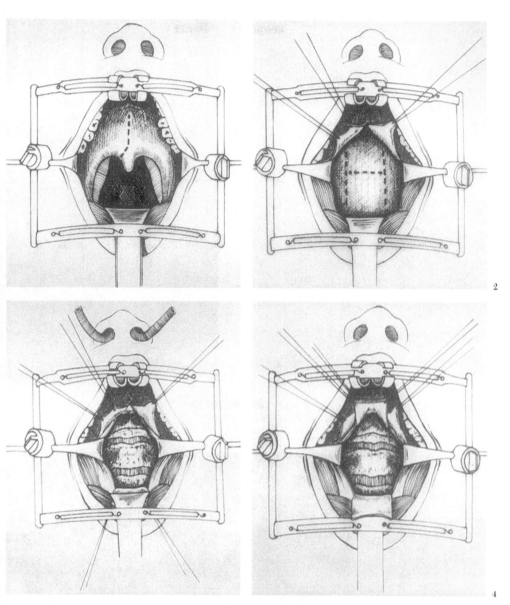

FIGURE 2J. Schematic diagram shows the steps of the modified transoral-transpharyngeal approach to the craniocervical junction. *1* = midline curvilinear incision through the soft palate; *2* = "H" incision in the posterior pharyngeal wall with the horizontal limb at the level of the soft palate; *3* = inferiorly and superiorly based myomucosal flaps are elevated to expose the craniocervical junction; *4* = the flaps are isolated in the nasopharynx and under the tongue blade.

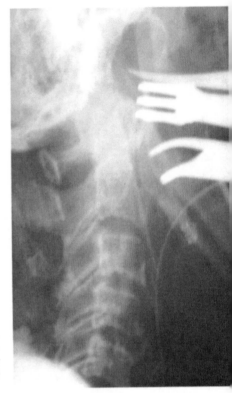

FIGURE 2K. Positions of the intervertebral spaces are identified and confirmed by radiographic imaging after placement of spinal needles in these spaces.

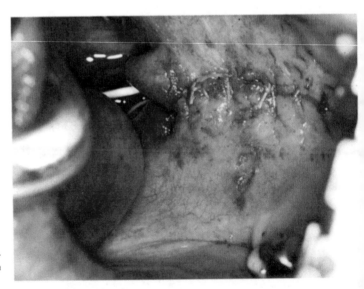

FIGURE 2L. The soft palate is approximated carefully in three layers, and a nasogastric tube is carefully placed.

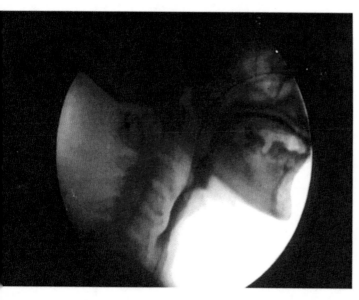

FIGURE 2M. Postoperative modified barium swallow study shows no evidence of velopharyngeal incompetence or aspiration.

10. The soft palate is approximated carefully in three layers. The mucosa of the naso- and oropharyngeal surfaces and the muscles are sutured by interrupted absorbable stitches (Fig. 2L). Fibrin glue is applied to the pharyngeal suture lines. A feeding tube is carefully introduced nasally under direct visualization through the area of the closed incisions.

11. On the basis of assessment of airway edema, the patient is either extubated in the operating room or transported to the intensive care unit, with subsequent extubation when deemed appropriate. Neurologic function and airway are observed in the intensive care unit. Intravenous antibiotics are given for 24 hours after surgery, and nasogastric nutritional support is started the morning of the first postoperative day.

12. Head immobilization, if necessary, is achieved with a hard or soft cervical collar or halo. Postoperative stability is later assessed by flexion-extension radiologic studies. A staged posterior stabilization, if indicated, is planned accordingly. If the likelihood of postoperative instability is high, the posterior stabilization is performed immediately after completion of the anterior approach with the patient under the same anesthetic.

13. Speech pathology evaluation and modified barium swallow studies are performed to assess velopharyngeal competence 1 week after surgery (Fig. 2M). Oral feeding is resumed if these studies do not show velopharyngeal insufficiency or aspiration.

References

1. Fang HSY, Ong BG: Direct anterior approach to the upper cervical spine. J Bone Joint Surg 44A(8):1588–1606, 1962.
2. Apuzzo MLJ, Weiss MH, Hyden JS: Transoral exposure of the atlantoaxial joint. J Neurosurg 3(2):201–207, 1978.
3. Hodgson AR, Rau ACM: Anterior approach to the spinal column. Rec Adv Orthop IX:289–326, 1969.
4. Di Lorenzo N. Transoral approach to extradural lesions of the lower clivus and upper cervical spine: an experience of 19 cases. Neurosurgery 24:37–42, 1989.

5. Merwin GE, Post JC, Sypert GW: Transoral approach to the upper cervical spine. Laryngoscope 101:780–784, 1991.
6. Kingdom TT, Nockels RP, Kaplan MJ: Transoral–transpharyngeal approach to the craniocervical junction. Otolaryngol Head Neck Surg 113:393–400, 1995.
7. Bennett E, Sinha UK, Samudrala S, Kempler D: Modified transoral-transpharyngeal approach to the craniocervical junction. Presented at the 1999 Western Triological Section Meeting, January 8–10, 1999, Denver, CO.
8. Bennett E, Sinha UK, Kempler D, Samudrala S: Transoral transpharyngeal approach to craniocervical junction. Presented at the Second Annual Southern California Resident Research Symposium, April 25, 1998, San Diego, CA.

3

Ventral Approaches to the Clivus, C1, and C2

Ranjeev Singh Bhangoo • *H. Alan Crockard*

Lesions placed anterior to the neuraxis are best approached anteriorly to minimize traction and further trauma on what may well be an already compromized structure. Although this concept is applied regularly in most spinal pathology, there has been understandable reluctance to apply this principle to pathology of the clivus, craniocervical junction, and upper two cervical vertebrae. The advent of microsurgical techniques, instruments designed specifically for transoral approaches (in particular), improvements in critical care and anesthesia, and perhaps most important, modern imaging have facilitated an anterior approach.

This chapter briefly discusses the relevant anatomy, appropriate investigation, and anterior approaches in general. The majority of the discussion centers on transoral surgical techniques, the approach most frequently used for the ventral midline pathology referred to this unit.

Surgical Anatomy

A thorough knowledge of the anatomy of the craniocervical junction and its variations is vital to operative success in this area, and the reader is urged to study some of the many detailed anatomical reviews available in the literature.[1-4]

The craniocervical junction is bounded by the ventral rim of the foramen magnum, the occipital condyles, the arch of C1, the odontoid peg, and the base of the second cervical vertebra (Fig. 3A). At the arch of C1, the vertebral artery is 24 mm from the midline, whereas at the C2–C3 disc and the ventral rim of the foramen magnum it lies 11 mm from the midline. The distance between the foramen magnum and the base of C2 is about 40 mm and that between the lateral masses of C1 is 27 mm. The wedge-shaped clivus is 38–42 mm long, 22 mm wide, and 4 mm thick at the foramen magnum

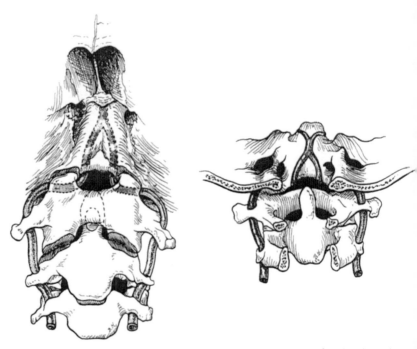

FIGURE 3A. Surgical anatomy of the craniocervical junction. If there is no rotation or significant lateral mass destruction, a direct midline approach will not encounter major hazards.

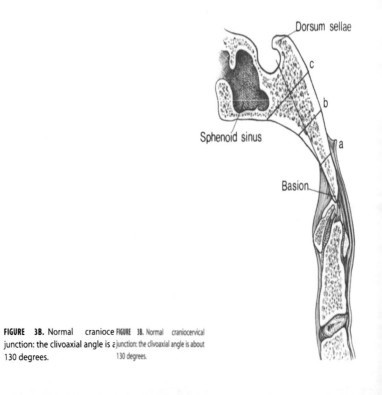

FIGURE 3B. Normal craniocervical junction: the clivoaxial angle is a 130 degrees.

FIGURE 3B. Normal craniocervical junction: the clivoaxial angle is about 130 degrees.

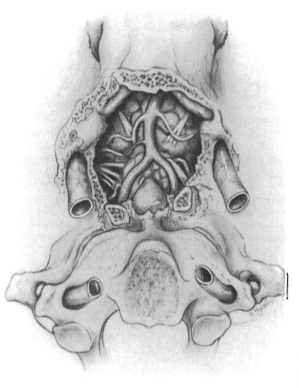

FIGURE 3C. Dissection of the craniocervical junction. The anterior arch of the atlas and most of the clivus and dura have been removed. The close relationship of the vertebrobasilar system, the lower cranial nerves, and the carotid arteries can clearly be seen.

nd 20 mm thick dorsal to the pituitary fossa (Fig. 3B). Rostrally, the unprotected knuckle" of the carotid as it leaves the petrous canal to enter the cavernous sinus is 11 nm from the midline arch of C1 (Fig. 3C). To this are attached the longus coli mus les and the anterior longitudinal ligament. A midline raphe can be seen extending to he tubercle. Above this are attached the longus capitis and rectus capitis anterior mus les; dorsal to them lies the pharyngobasilar fascia. The vertebral arteries run about 14 nm on each side lateral to the tubercle. Deep to the bones are the tectorial membrane, ne posterior longitudinal ligament, and the dura, which is often attached to the ven ral rim of the foramen magnum. Within this exposure, *provided that there is no rota on of C1*, there are no major neural or vascular structures that cross the operative field t should be noted, however, that venous bleeding can be encountered from the dural narginal sinus and bony diploic channels in the clivus).

Basic Indication

Details of each surgical procedure are discussed later, but broad definitions follow. In ne absence of basilar invagination, a transoral approach with elevation of the soft palate ill allow access to the arch of C1 and the odontoid peg. A midline split of the soft alate will gain the access to the anterior aspect of the foramen magnum. A division of ne hard and soft palate will gain access to the lower half of the clivus but has such lim ed lateral extension because of the upper teeth that it is now used very little. The ex nded "open door" maxillotomy (a combination of the Le Fort 1 osteotomy and a mid ne palatal split) will provide access from the sphenoid down to C3; this surgical procedure was developed in response to the challenge posed by basilar invagination. A transmandibular, transglottic approach is combined with a posterior approach for 360-degree eradicational surgery for tumors of the upper cervical spine.

Radiologic Investigations

Plain lateral films of the craniocervical junction in flexion and extension (Fig. 3D), together with an anteroposterior view (including a good view of the peg), allow for assessment of the bony limitations of the surgical field and provide a baseline for subsequent rapid office assessment. Magnetic resonance imaging (MRI) provides exquisite soft tissue images (Fig. 3E), but computed tomography (CT) and particularly computed myelography[5] still provide the most accurate means of identifying bony abnormalities and also provide absolute measurements of the structures involved. These methods also afford easy assessment of the craniocervical angles and the angle of the neuraxis. New software packages now allow the generation of sophisticated three-dimensional surface rendering images that can be evaluated from any angle. Vertebral angiography is required to outline tumor circulation or as part of a trial vertebral artery occlusion by balloon.

Preoperative Assessment for Transoral Surgery

The Mouth

Paramount to success in transoral surgery is the careful preoperative assessment of the oral cavity and its contents. The most important of these factors is the amount of mouth opening; if the interdental distance is less than 25 mm with the patient's mouth

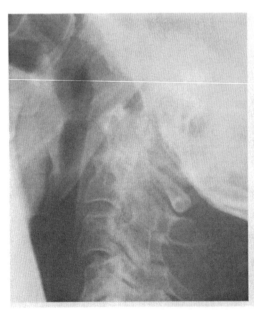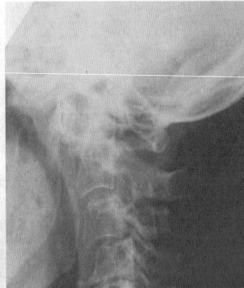

FIGURE 3D. Plain lateral radiographs of the cervical spine in a patient with rheumatoid arthritis show atlantoaxial subluxation and a step at the C2–C3 junction.

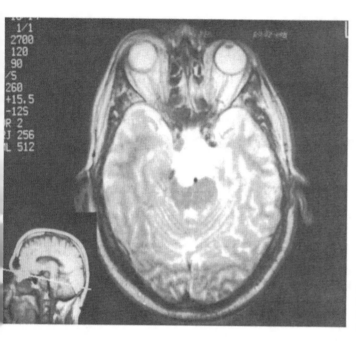

FIGURE 3E. Axial T$_2$ weighted magnetic resonance imaging (MRI) shows a skull base chordoma compressing the brainstem.

as wide open as possible, then a conventional transoral procedure is unlikely to be successful. In such a case, transoral surgery may be accomplished by splitting the symphysis of the mandible in the midline and laterally retracting the two parts of the mandible to allow inferior retraction of the tongue. An alternative is bilateral division of the mandibular ramus and subsequent titanium plate fixation. The patient's dentition is a potential source of sepsis, a situation analogous to cardiac valve surgery, and a preoperative referral for dental assessment and treatment is often required, particularly in the case of patients with rheumatoid arthritis.

Before surgery, bacteriologic swabs of the nasal and oropharyngeal cavity are taken. Should an unusual organism be identified or postoperative infection occur, the results of these swabs are used for initial guidance. In the absence of such an event, this unit's policy is to administer Cefuroxime and Metronidazole with the induction of anesthesia and for 48 hours postoperatively. Long-term pre- or postoperative antibiotic use increases the risk of fungal and bacterial superinfection and should be avoided. The problem posed by the edentulous patient is discussed later.

General Physical Evaluation

Many of the patients presenting for surgery have multiorgan disease (particularly those with rheumatoid arthritis), and a detailed assessment of their general condition is important. Pulmonary function may be impaired by direct pressure on the brainstem or the effects of the disease or its treatment directly on the lung parenchyma. For this reason, we routinely assess the vital capacity, arterial blood gases, and oxygen saturation of our patients. Sleep studies are often performed. In general terms, those patients with a vital capacity less than 1.2 L may have problems coming off artificial ventilation postoperatively. Cardiac and renal function also require careful assessment, and again the possible effect of the patient's medication on these organ systems is stressed, for example, steroids and cytotoxic agents in rheumatoid arthritis.

Electrical Studies

Somatosensory evoked potentials (SSEP) and motor evoked potentials (MEP) have been performed on some patients, but generally very large changes have not been seen in central conduction time despite marked radiologic compression and striking postoperative recovery of function. Perioperative assessment remains difficult and of more value in posterior upper cervical spine surgery.

Anesthesia

Airway

The key to success in managing the airway during and after a transoral procedure is the development of a policy that reflects local experience and best practice. Although nearly 100% of this unit's early transoral cases underwent a tracheostomy, this figure is now closer to 15%. The Phoenix group consistently use an orotracheal tube,[6] but our own preference is a nasotracheal airway.[7] The main objection to orotracheal intubation is not obstruction of the operative field but rather the need to remove it postoperatively because it causes extreme discomfort in the conscious patient; we remain unhappy about changing from one form of airway to another in the immediate postoperative period. With any instability of the craniocervical junction, fiberoptic nasotracheal intubation is employed in the awake patient. A tracheostomy is used only in those patients for whom long-term ventilatory problems are expected or in those for whom an extended maxillotomy is planned.

Ventilation

Tidal volume, respiratory rate, oxygen saturation, and end-tidal CO_2 have proved to be the most immediate indices of brainstem compression. Thus, during critical anterior and posterior surgical maneuvers muscle relaxation is reversed and the patient is allowed to breathe spontaneously.

Diversion of Gastric Contents

A nasogastric tube is inserted preoperatively, first because it is easier to do so before pharyngeal surgery and second to allow emptying of the stomach in the immediate postoperative period to prevent gastric contents from soiling the wound. In the extended "open door" maxillotomy, a pharyngogastric tube has been used in place of the nasogastric tube; it is passed into the stomach in the usual way and a stab incision made into the lateral fauces to one side through which the tube is pulled. More recently, we have used a per entral gastrotomy tube (PEG) passed 2 to 3 days before the operation.

Surgery

Positioning and Instrumentation

The lateral position with the head held in a Mayfield retractor[8] confers several advantages. Blood and washings drain away from the operative site, the operator may be seated and comfortable for an exacting procedure, and it is possible to perform an anterior decompression and a posterior fixation with the patient fixed in one position, minimizing risks to the neuraxis. This position does require some "relearning" of the anatomy, and it may be advisable to evaluate any doubtful anatomy with the patient supine and the aid of needle markers. If the head can be placed in slight extension, this will make the craniocervical junction slightly more accessible in patients with complex congenital malformations or tumor.

An integrated transoral system of gags and retractors (Codman and Shurtleff, Randolph, MA) with bayoneted instruments of the appropriate length has allowed the procedure to become routine in many centers. The advantages conferred by the use of an operating microscope (coaxial lighting and stereoscopic vision) are essential for all but the simplest transoral procedures.

Transoral Odontoidectomy

The mouth is cleaned with an aqueous solution of chlorhexidine. Hydrocortisone ointment (1%) is applied liberally to the mouth and lips to prevent postoperative swelling; following this the transoral retractor is inserted with a tongue blade of suitable length. If the patient's dentition is deficient in the upper jaw (or loose teeth are present), a gum guard made from flexible dental cement may be fashioned to fit over the teeth. The edentulous patient with mandibular resorption is a difficult problem in that the retractor may keep slipping; in these cases placing packing under the handle of the tongue blade may help. It is important to ensure that the tongue is not caught between the lower teeth and the tongue retractor and that the mouth is opened as far as possible. The soft palate is now "hooked up" on its nondependent aspect (the patient is in the lateral position) using the curved soft palate retractor, which is in turn firmly attached to the transoral retractor with a locking nut. The other soft palate retractor (modified specially to a right angle) is used to retract the nasotracheal and nasogastric tube out of the operative field into the dependent tonsillar fauces.

The surgical key to this area is the *tubercle on the anterior surface of C1.* If difficulty is encountered in defining this structure by its surface landmarks, the surgeon should not hesitate to request intraoperative radiography. The area to be incised is infiltrated with lidocaine and a 1:200,000 solution of adrenaline to reduce mucosal bleeding and separate out the tissue planes. A midline incision centering on the tubercle of C1 is now made and the edges of the incision separated with the pharyngeal retractor, converting the slit into a hexagon (Fig. 3F). It can now be seen that the two blades of the pharyngeal retractor, the tongue blade, and the soft palate blades form a "ring of steel" to protect the pharyngeal mucosa from inadvertent injury during surgery; undamaged pharyngeal mucosa remains the key to good postoperative healing. Using the cutting monopolar diathermy or the Nd-Yag laser, the longus coli muscles and the anterior longitudinal ligament are separated from their attachments to the arch of C1. An angled, high-speed air drill with a 3- to 4-mm cutting burr is used to remove cancellous bone, switching to a diamond burr when cortical bone appears. To expose the odontoid peg, 12 to 15 mm of the anterior arch of C1 is removed; if the pathology is below C1 or the odontoid peg is deficient, then the arch of C1 may be left intact to prevent lateral displacement of the C1 lateral masses and subsequent craniocervical instability. Even if the arch of C1 is removed, the transverse ligament can be maintained as a "tie beam" to hold the ring together and thus avoid lateral displacement of the lateral masses.

With the arch removed, the odontoid peg is now defined and removed by first hollowing it out until "transparent" and then using the 1- and 2-mm Kerrison upcuts to remove the rest of the thinned-out bone (Fig. 3G). If the posterior ligamentous structures are exposed too early, soft tissues may herniate through the dura, distended epidural veins may bleed, and there is risk of a dural tear. If there is only slight translocation, excision of some of the rim of the foramen magnum may not be necessary; head extension may allow presentation of the tip of the dens. Alternatively, the peg may be divided at its base, grasped with specially designed forceps, and pulled down into the operative field out of the foramen magnum; these forceps are also used to hold the unstable dens while it is being drilled out. The apical and alar ligaments are stretched and divided because they are attached to the tip of the dens. Bony decompression may be

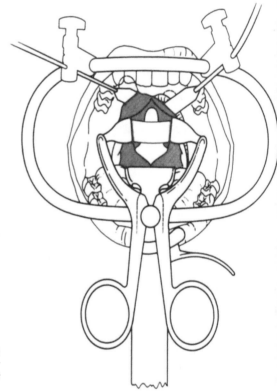

FIGURE 3F. Transoral incision showing the structures exposed and the protective "ring of steel" provided by the retractor system.

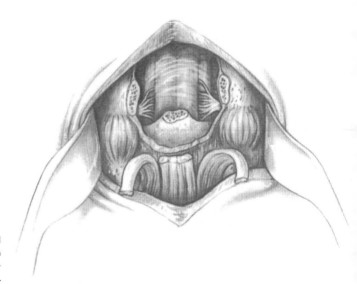

FIGURE 3G. Excision of the odontoid peg following division of the insertion of longus coli and the anterior longitudinal ligament into the C1 tubercle.

continued down to the C2–C3 disc space; if this space is entered, the disc must be removed and cortical bone exposed on the upper surface of C3. It is important to note that at this level of dissection the vertebral artery is at risk of injury.

In general terms, a reasonable decompression has been effected when the surgeon can see around the "equator" of the dural sac on both sides. The tectorial membrane and the posterior longitudinal ligament are removed if they are thickened and distorting the dura, although if good dural pulsations are seen after the bony decompression, they are left intact. Extradural tumor is removed piecemeal using suction, bayoneted curettes (Carlin), and the angled dissector (Crockard). The laser has a role to play in excision and hemostasis, but the currently available ultrasonic dissectors remain too bulky to be of use in this area. Closure below the foramen magnum is with two layers of interrupted Vicryl sutures, one for the muscle layer (the superior constrictor and the pharyngobasilar fascia) and the other for the mucosa. An incision into the midline raphe of the soft palate, sparing the uvula to one side, will allow good exposure of the anterior rim of the foramen magnum. This incision should be carefully closed in two layers.

Extended "Open Door" Maxillotomy

The extended "open door" maxillotomy was designed for access to the most severe examples of basilar invagination and for radical excisions of tumors of the clivus and upper cervical spine (Fig. 3H). A Le Fort 1 horizontal mucoperiosteal incision is made in

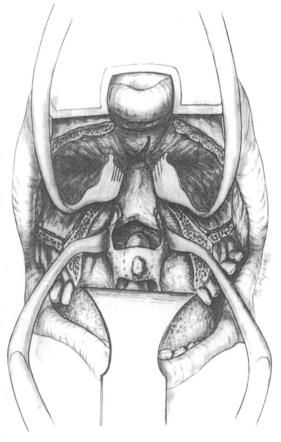

FIGURE 3H. View of the craniocervical junction following an extended maxillotomy.

the upper gingival margin to expose the maxillary buttress and the bone above the dental apices; this extends from the first molar tooth on each side. A preoperative orthopantomogram will accurately identify the dental roots. Titanium miniplates, held in position with titanium screws (Leibinger, Muhlheim-Stetten, Germany) are screwed into the maxillary buttress and the alveolar margin such that they avoid the dental apices. Two additional plates may be inserted posteriorly at the third molar buttress of bone. The plates are then removed and a saw cut made along the line described. The upper alveolar margin and palate are downfractured into the mouth, the vomer divided, and the inferior turbinates incised and reflected laterally or, if particularly large, removed. The two halves of the palate survive on blood supply derived from the mucosa and the alveolar branches of the maxillary artery on both sides; retraction on the palatal flaps is released from time to time to ensure vascular perfusion. As much mucosa as possible is preserved to act as cover in the postoperative period. The oscillating saw is used to divide the hard palate in the midline between the upper two medial incisors. The hard palate retractor is now inserted and the maxillotomy plate applied to the transoral upper gum guard, allowing it to act as countertraction on the cut surface of the maxilla, with the tongue retractor pulling down on the tongue and lower jaw. The pharyngeal retractors are inserted to hold apart he soft palate and the pharyngeal incision. The mucosa over the clivus is divided, separated laterally, and protected behind the hard palate and pharyngeal retractors to ensure that there is adequate tissue for closure. The angled high-speed air drill and Kerrison upcuts are used as was described for removal of the dens to thin down the clivus and expose the dura. Diploic channels may be encountered, leading to brisk bleeding that can be controlled with bone wax.

The mucosa is apposed in a single layer of interrupted absorbable sutures above the foramen magnum and in two layers below it. The palate is now repositioned and held in place with the titanium miniplates. The two portions of the posterior hard palate are wired together, and further compression achieved by wiring the upper medial incisor teeth. The soft palate is closed in two layers and the mucosa over the hard palate is one layer.

Transmandibular Transglottic Approach

Occasionally, a transmandibular approach (splitting the mandible at its symphysis), often used in combination with a transglottic approach, is required to gain access to tumor at C1 or C2 (Fig. 3I). Division of the tongue in the midline with cutting diathermy controls the blood loss that would otherwise considerably obscure the operator's view of the operative field. In combination with a posterior approach, this technique allows a total vertebrectomy for tumor of the upper cervical spine.

Technical Problems

Bleeding

Epidural bleeding, bleeding from venous sinuses, and bleeding from any cut bone surface can be troublesome. Rapid and widespread exposure of the area will take the pressure off these veins and allow them to be coagulated by diathermy or laser. Bleeding may also be controlled with bone wax, the use of the diamond burr and Surgicel when appropriate. Bleeding from inadvertent straying into the vertebral artery can be a major problem, but control can be achieved in the vertebral foramen with bone wax and Surgicel. Ultimately, an endovascular balloon occlusion may also be necessary. Intradural bleeding is extremely difficult to control and is to be avoided at all possible.

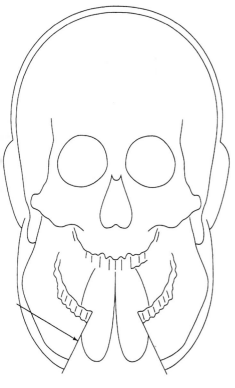

FIGURE 31. Transmandibular transglottic approach.

Intradural Surgery

Cerebrospinal fluid (CSF) leakage may occur, particularly in the severely translo-
cated odontoid peg, which may have transgressed the dura or, in the case of a tumor, may exhibit some element of intradural extension. If there is a possibility of a
breach of the dura, it is advisable to insert a wide-bore lumbar drain after the induction of anesthesia (after a CSF leak the catheter may be very difficult to insert).
Lumbar drainage is continued for up to 5 days if a leak occurs (10–20 mL/h), primarily to reduce the hydrostatic pressure on the wound and second to remove blood
and surgical debris.[10,11] If there is a very large hole in the dura, the drain is con-
verted into a shunt about 1 week after surgery. The reduction of CSF pressure over
the period of 1 month is usually enough to produce permanent waterproof closure.
Dural closure is very important if meningitis is to be avoided but is difficult because
of the poor quality of the dura in the area of the rostral clivus, especially when
stretched or breached by tumor. Our unit has tried a variety of approaches,[12] and
the current policy is as follows: a multilayer closure with thrombin fibrin glue (Tis-
seal; Immuno, Austria), dermal fat, and fascia is first constructed. Over this multilayer closure, mucosal flaps carefully mobilized from the nasal septum are trimmed
and rotated to cover a denuded sphenoid sinus and the upper one-third to one-half
of the exposed clival area; the mucosal flaps are approximated over with Vicryl sutures and held in place with nasal packs. Elsewhere, the presence of good mucosal
layers allows the pharyngeal tissues to be closed in one or two layers over the dural
graft.

Accurate Replacement of the Upper Jaw

Accurate replacement of the upper jaw is critical if the patient is to be spared the considerable discomfort and distress that will result from dental malocclusion. This accuracy is achieved as a result of positioning the titanium miniplates before making the saw cut in the maxilla.

Craniocervical Stability

Postoperative stability remains an important question. In some cases, such as translocation in rheumatoid arthritis, it is obvious that the lesion is unstable at the time of the procedure; in such cases our practice is to perform a posterior fixation at the same time as the anterior decompression.[8] In other conditions where stability seems reasonable, such as some congenital malformations, the anterior procedure is performed and then after 2 or 3 weeks dynamic scanning is carried out to assess craniocervical junction stability. These examinations are repeated every 3 and 6 months in case there is late acquired instability.

Whether fixation or fixation and fusion is used remains controversial; anterior bone grafting and fusion is recommended by some authors.[13,14] In our experience little or none of the bone that has been grafted anteriorly is identifiable by computed tomography (CT) 1 year later. As a result, the policy is now to perform some form of posterior procedure. If the problem is atlantoaxial subluxation in an "end-stage" rheumatoid patient, then the occiput is included in the fixation that employs a Ransford loop (Surgicraft, Stoke on Trent, UK) or a Ti frame (Codman) (Figs. 3J, 3K), with sublaminar titanium wires around C1, C2, and perhaps C3 and through holes made in the occiput (this is safer than passing wires around the rim of the foramen magnum). In view of the high incidence of nonfusion of bone graft observed in these patients (even in posterior fusion), the additional trauma of harvesting the graft did not seem justifiable, and a policy of fixation without bone fusion has been pursued successfully in these patients

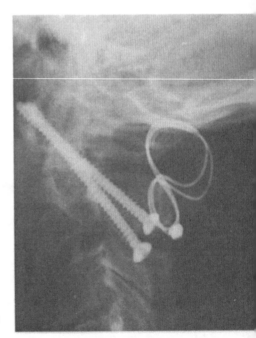

FIGURE 3J. Transarticular screws with interspinous wiring.

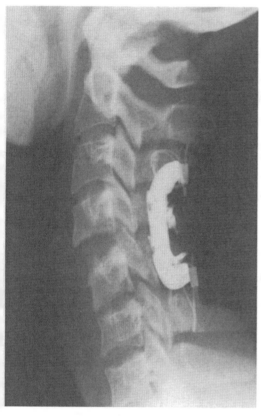

FIGURE 3K. A Ti frame used for post-operative stabilization of the cervical spine.

for more than 10 years.[8] In patients with a prognosis longer than 1 year, then bone grafting would be routinely used.

In patients with good quality bone posteriorly, a C1–C2 fixation using lateral mass/transarticular screws (combined with a Gallie fusion) or a Ti frame is commonly used. Occasionally, bone graft is inserted without instrumentation and the patient is placed in a halo body jacket for 3 months. Stiffness remains a major problem with the Ransford loop, although another problem posed by instrumentation, that of interference with follow-up on magnetic resonance imaging (MRI) may soon be overcome with the advent of titanium implants.

Dislocation of the Mandible

The mandible may become dislocated during the procedure, this problem should be checked at the end of the procedure when it is easily corrected, thus avoiding discomfort for the patient and the need for another general anesthetic.

Pharyngeal Function

Velopharyngeal dysfunction (VPD) manifesting as a hypernasal voice, nasal regurgitation, and dysphagia may be a significant problem. Although not well understood, this sequela is related at least in part to an increased pharyngeal dead space after tumor resection and also scarring of the soft palate and pharynx.[12,15] Many patients present with some degree of bulbar dysfunction caused by their underlying pathology; these should be investigated preoperatively with a video swallow as they may deteriorate significantly postoperatively and require a tracheostomy/gastrostomy for some months. Patients with significant VPD should be identified and treated early with velopharyngeal surgery or prostheses in an attempt to minimize long-term instability.

Postoperative Management

General Mouth and Nasal Care

Great care is taken with the mouth and nose. Hydrocortisone cream is applied at the end of the procedure and every 6 hours for the first 2 postoperative days. General mouth care is given every 4 hours; no food is given by mouth for 5 days, and gastric and tracheal secretions are diverted. Oronasal fistulae may occur, particularly at the junction of the hard and soft palate, but these heal well with regular applications of Whitehead's varnish. Any nasal packs should be left in place for 5 days.

The Airway

The airway is not removed if there is any problem with respiration or with tracheal secretions. The tube can usually be removed after 24 to 48 hours when a lateral cervical X-ray has confirmed the lack of posterior pharyngeal swelling.

Nasogastric/Pharyngogastric Tube

The tube is kept for at least 5 days for feeding and diversion of gastric contents; feeding is commenced on the resumption of bowel sounds.

Antibiotics

Cefuroxime and Metronidazole are continued for 2 days.

Antiemetics

Metoclopramide is administered every 6 hours for 2 days, and an H_2 antagonist is used to reduce gastric acidity.

Analgesia

An infusion pump is used to deliver a slow continuous morphine dose with a careful check on respiratory rate.

Physiotherapy

Chest physiotherapy and mobilization are most important, and the patient is usually sitting up out of bed within 48 hours.

Conclusion

Transoral procedures, although uncommon, have an important role in the treatment of craniocervical junction anomalies and are best performed by a team of surgeons and anesthetists who are familiar with this complex and demanding form of skull base surgery.

References

1. Olivera E, Rhoton AL, Peace D: Microsurgical anatomy of the region of the foramen magnum. Surg Neurol 24:293–352, 1985.
2. Lang J: Craniocervical region, surgical anatomy. Neuroorthopaedics 3:1–26, 1987.
3. Koksel T, Crockard HA: "Clivus" through the eyes of the transoral surgeon. Turk Neurosurg 1:146–150, 1990.
4. Crockard HA, Johnston F: Development of transoral approaches to lesions of the skull base and craniocervical junction. Neurosurg Q 3(2):61–82, 1993.
5. Hunter JV, Stevens J, Kendall BE, et al: Radiological assessment for transoral surgery in rheumatoid arthritis, using dynamic CT myelography. Neuroradiology 33(suppl):413–415, 1991.
6. Hadley MN, Spetzler RF, Sonntag VK: The transoral approach to the superior cervical spine: a review of 53 cases of extradural cervicomedullary compression. Neurosurgery 71:16–23, 1989.
7. Calder I: Anesthesia for transoral surgery and craniocervical surgery. In Jewkes D (ed): Balliere's Clinical Anaesthesiology. London, Saunders, 1987, pp 441–457.
8. Crockard HA, Calder I, Ransford AO: One stage transoral decompression and posterior fixation in rheumatoid atlantoaxial subluxation: a technical note. J Bone Joint Surg [Br] 72:682–685, 1990.
9. James D, Crockard HA: Surgical access to the base of the skull and upper cervical spine by extended maxillotomy. Neurosurgery 29:411–416, 1991.
10. Spetzler RF, Selman WR, Nash CL: Transoral microsurgical removal, odontoid resection and spinal cord monitoring. Spine 4:506–510, 1979.
11. Crockard HA: The transoral approach to the base of the brain and upper cervical cord. Ann R Coll Surg Engl 67:321–325, 1985.
12. Crockard HA: Transoral surgery: some lessons learned. Br J Neurosurg 9:283–293, 1995.
13. Louis R: Chirugia anteriore del rachide cervicale superiore. Chir Organi Mov 77:75–80, 1992.
14. Von Grumppenburg S, Harms J: Aketue Technische Konzepte in der Wirbelsaulenchirugie Indikation und Technik der Osteosynthese bei Halswirbelsaulenverletzungen. Chirurg 63:849–855, 1992.
15. Menzes AH: The anterior midline approach to the craniocervical junction in children. Pediatr Neurosurg 18:272–281, 1992.

4

Anterior Medial Approach to C1, C2, and C3

1. The standard approach is from the left side to avoid the recurrent laryngeal nerve. Rotate the head to the right and inflate the cervical pillow to support the head and neck. The necessity for intraoperative traction is determined by the pathologic lesion. When necessary, use Gardner Wells tong traction rather than the halter.

2. Make the skin incision transversely starting one fingerbreadth from the midline below the mandible and proceed laterally, curving around the angle of the mandible posteriorly across the mastoid process (Fig. 4A). For a pathologic process that extends to C3 or below, make the skin incision along the anterior border of the sternocleidomastoid muscle, extending it cephalad and curving in a similar manner across the mastoid process.

3. Incise the layer of the platysma muscle, inserting small spring retractors in the subcutaneous tissue. Open the platysma muscle along the line of the incision and retract it in a similar manner. The greater auricular nerve and anterior cervical nerve are branches of the ansa cervicalis that course around from the posterior edge of the sternocleidomastoid muscle, crossing the muscle for distribution to the auricular and mandibular skin. Preserve these nerves when possible.[1]

4. Identify the medial border of the sternocleidomastoid muscle. To facilitate this identification use scissors to incise the superficial investing fascia. To locate the carotid sheath, palpate the carotid pulse. Use finger dissection and blunt right-angle blade retraction to develop the incision medial to the sternocleidomastoid muscle and the carotid sheath and lateral to the musculovisceral column (strap muscles, esophagus, and trachea).

5. If needed for additional exposure, divide the anterior third of the insertion of the sternocleidomastoid muscle from the mastoid process. Leave sufficient fascial tissue to reattach the muscle when closing the wound.[2]

6. Palpate the carotid pulse and deepen the incision medial to the carotid sheath and the sternocleidomastoid muscle through the middle cervical fascia with blunt, longitudinal finger dissection and scissors.

7. The neurovascular structures crossing from lateral to medial are found in this layer.

8. Identify the superior thyroid artery and vein. The superior thyroid artery arises from the external carotid artery at approximately the level of the hyoid bone. It crosses through the carotid triangle, arches deep to the strap muscles, and enters the lateral

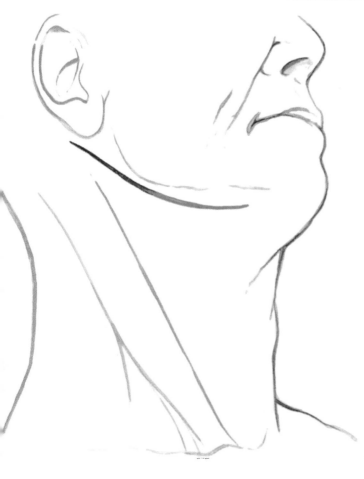

FIGURE 4A. The skin incision is made under the angle of the mandible from posterior sternocleidomastoid muscle toward the midline.

superior aspect of the thyroid gland. Retract the superior thyroid artery and vein inferiorly (Fig. 4B).

9. Identify and retract the hypoglossal nerve (Fig. 4C). The hypoglossal nerve is found passing from lateral to medial superficial to the external carotid, lingual, and facial arteries. The hypoglossal nerve exits the skull in close proximity to the vagus nerve and courses between the internal carotid artery and internal jugular vein, becoming superficial at the angle of the mandible. After its usual point of identification over the arteries, it passes deep to the tendon of the digastric muscle and stylohyoid muscle for distribution to the muscles of the tongue. The hypoglossal nerve is retracted cephalad, and the superior thyroid artery and vein are usually retracted caudad.

Caution: Be positive of the identification of the hypoglossal nerve before ligation of any structure. It is a superficial structure first coursing vertically and parallel to the carotid sheath, then horizontally, crossing medially over the carotid and its branches (Fig. 4D).

10. Identify the lingual artery. This artery arises from the external carotid. From the level of the hyoid it crosses under the digastric and stylohyoid muscles in its ascent to the oral pharynx. Ligate the lingual artery (Fig. 4D).

11. Identify and ligate the facial artery. The facial artery next leaves the external

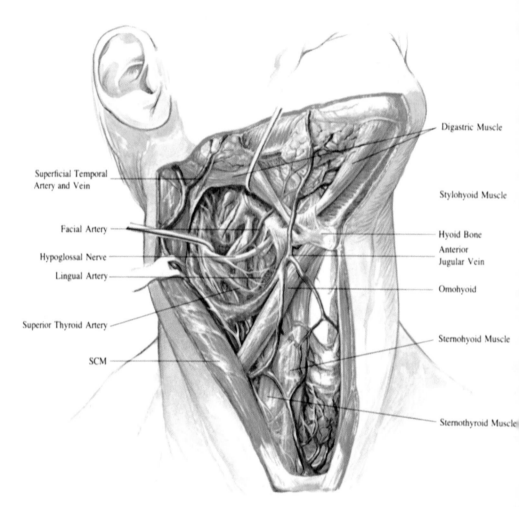

Superficial Temporal Artery and Vein

Facial Artery

Hypoglossal Nerve

Lingual Artery

Superior Thyroid Artery

SCM

Digastric Muscle

Stylohyoid Muscle

Hyoid Bone

Anterior Jugular Vein

Omohyoid

Sternohyoid Muscle

Sternothyroid Muscle

FIGURE 4B. Dissection of the cephalad portion of the anterior neck shows the carotid triangle area, which is bordered superiorly by the posterior belly of the digastric muscle, inferiorly by the omohyoid muscle, and posteriorly by the sternocleidomastoid muscle. The digastric muscle lies inferior to the mandible and extends from the mastoid process to the symphysis mente. The sling around the tendonous midportion of the digastric muscle separates its posterior from its anterior belly, and holds the midportion of the muscle of the cornu of the hyoid bone. The stylohyoid muscle (retracted by hook) lies anterior and superior to the posterior belly of the digastric, passing from the styloid process to the hyoid bone. Within the carotid triangle the lingual artery, the facial artery, and the hypoglossal nerve course from lateral to medial. The hypoglossal nerve is usually retracted cephalad, for the cephalad approach to C1–C2, and the lingual and facial arteries are sacrificed. *Caution:* Always identify the hypoglossal nerve before any ligation of structures in this area.

carotid artery, coursing under the ramus to the mandible within the carotid triangle. It passes deep into the digastric muscle and enters the face at the anterior edge of the mastoid after crossing on the submandibular gland.

12. Identify the digastric muscle (Figs. 4E, 4F). This muscle is easily retracted cephalad with the hypoglossal nerve. When necessary, divide the stylofascial band running from the stylohyoid process to the posterior pharynx.

13. Difficulties may be encountered with the superior laryngeal nerve, both external and internal branches, and the pharyngeal branches of the vagus nerve; these

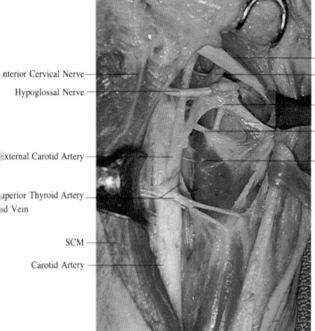

Anterior Cervical Nerve

Hypoglossal Nerve

External Carotid Artery

Superior Thyroid Artery
and Vein

SCM

Carotid Artery

Digastric Muscle

Facial Artery

Lingual Artery

Superior Laryngeal Nerve

Pharyngeal Muscle

FIGURE 4C. Dissected anatomy of the carotid triangle and area just below emphasizes the importance of identification of the hypoglossal nerve before ligation of the arterial structures in this area. The most common approach is cephalad to the superior thyroid artery and caudad to the digastric muscle, medial to the sternocleidomastoid muscle (SCM).

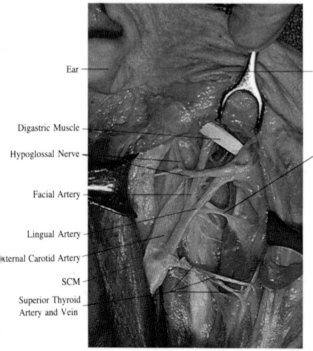

Ear

Digastric Muscle

Hypoglossal Nerve

Facial Artery

Lingual Artery

External Carotid Artery

SCM

Superior Thyroid
Artery and Vein

Mandible

Superior
Laryngeal Nerve

FIGURE 4D. Further retraction reveals the plane of dissection medial to the sternocleidomastoid muscle. Pharyngeal branches of the sympathetic plexus are frequently damaged by retraction without major consequence, Avoid damage to the superior laryngeal nerve and retract it with the superior thyroid artery. The fibrous tissue sling around the hypoglossal nerve may be divided to allow further retraction.

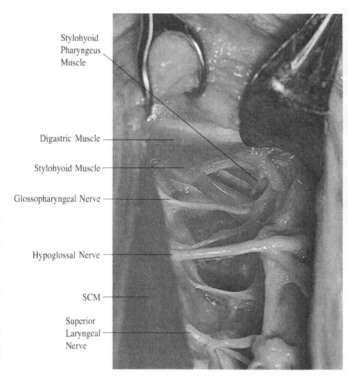

Stylohyoid
Pharyngeus
Muscle

Digastric Muscle

Stylohyoid Muscle

Glossopharyngeal Nerve

Hypoglossal Nerve

SCM

Superior
Laryngeal
Nerve

FIGURE 4E. A more detailed look at the structures of the carotid triangle running from lateral to medial shows the relationship of the digastric muscle, the stylohyoid pharyngeus muscle, and the stylohyoid muscle. The glossopharyngeal nerve, dissected free here, usually is not identified in approaches in this area. The hypoglossal nerve is again the predominate neural structure of the area and must be protected. Sternocleidomastoid muscle (SCM).

should be identified and retracted but frequently suffer from the retraction (Fig. 4D). Continue to use finger palpation to identify the spine and the carotid artery.

14. Retract the carotid sheath and the ligated stumps of lingual and facial arteries laterally and the musculovisceral column medially with deep right-angle, handheld blunt retractors.

15. Dissect bluntly with a Kitner dissector, slowly at this point, to identify the prevertebral fascia. Be sure the esophagus and pharynx have been retracted sufficiently with the medial column. Palpate and X-ray to confirm the midline of C2. Identify the prevertebral fascia in the midline to avoid unnecessary bleeding. Insert the long, deep smooth-tip bladed Cloward retractor under the carotid sheath laterally and the esophagus and pharynx medially. Insert a second Cloward retractor longitudinally to retract the hypoglossal nerve and digastric muscle cephalad and the superior thyroid artery and vein distally.

16. Elevate the fibers of the longus coli muscle and fascia off the vertebral body in a lateral and cephalad direction. Replace the retractor blades of the transverse Cloward retractor with the sharp claw blades and insert these under the longus coli muscle. The smooth-tipped blades can be used if firm fixation cannot be obtained under the longus coli.[3] Deep handheld retractors are also quite effective (Figs. 4G, 4H).

17. Cephalad exposure of the superior tip of the odontoid process is made by careful blunt dissection on the spine in the retropharyngeal space. The upper extent of the pharyngeal retraction is limited by the pharyngeal tubercle of the occiput to which the

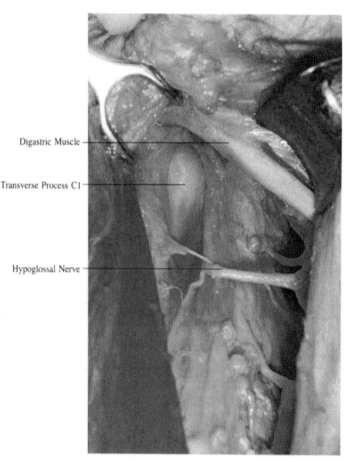

Digastric Muscle

Transverse Process C1

Hypoglossal Nerve

FIGURE 4F. Dissection of the soft tissue in the area to emphasize the point of entry caudal to the digastric muscle and hypoglossal nerve, medial to the transverse process of C1. The transverse process of C1 frequently can be palpated in the more lateral aspect of the anterior approach to this area.

pharynx is attached.[4] Incise the prevertebral tissue in the midline and dissect from the midline laterally (Fig. 4H).

18. Closure: The soft tissue falls together without deep sutures. Close the platysma muscle separately and always drain the wound with closed suction drains.

Remember:

1. Avoid the superficial cutaneous nerves on the sternocleidomastoid muscle.
2. Identify the medial edge of sternocleidomastoid.
3. Know where the carotid pulse is at all times.
4. Isolate the hypoglossal nerve before ligating any arteries.
5. Identify the superior laryngeal nerve and its internal and external branches.
6. Dissect carefully to retract the esophagus from the spine.
7. Incise the prevertebral fascia in the midline.
8. Dissect in a lateral cephalad direction to remove longus coli in this area.

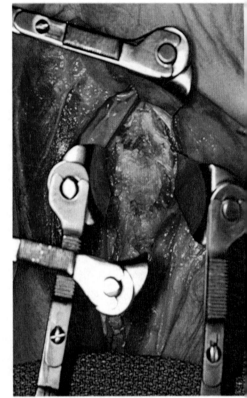

FIGURE 4G. Dissect the fibers of the longus coli muscle fascia off the vertebral body in a lateral and cephalad direction. Placement of the sharp blade claw of the transverse. Cloward retractors under the longus coli muscle produces firm fixation. Blunt-tip blades can be used. The cephalad exposure is enhanced by use of similarly placed Cloward retractors vertically.

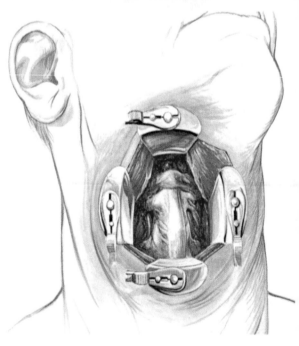

FIGURE 4H. Spine exposed with deep retractor blades.

References

1. Perry J: Surgical approaches to the spine. In Pierce D, Nichol V (eds): The Total Care of Spinal Cord Injuries. Boston, Little, Brown, 1977, pp. 53–79.
2. Henry AK: Extensive Exposure. Baltimore, Williams & Wilkins, 1959, pp. 53–72.
3. Cloward R: Ruptured Cervical Intervertebral Discs. Codman Signatures Series 4. Codman and Shurtlessf, 1974.
4. DeAndrade JR, MacNab I: Anterior occipito-cervical fusion using an extrapharyngeal exposure. J Bone Joint Surg 51A:1621–1626, 1969.

5

Anterior Lateral Approach
to the Upper Cervical Spine

The anterior lateral approach is medial to the sternocleidomastoid muscle and lateral to the carotid sheath. For approaches to C1, C2, and C3, in which the head should not be turned or rotated, and for surgeons who do not feel comfortable with the neurovascular structures medial to the carotid sheath, this approach offers a relatively bloodless field.

1. Position the patient supine. Use the neurosurgical head-holding frame with skeletal skull fixation for better exposure and stability.

2. Incise the skin and subcutaneous tissue beginning on the medial border of the sternocleidomastoid muscle at the superior edge of thyroid cartilage and extend this cephalad to the mastoid process and curve posteriorly across the process[1] (Fig. 5A).

3. Open the external investing fascia along the line of the incision. Place superficial spring retractors and obtain hemostasis. Avoid the cutaneous sensory nerves crossing the sternocleidomastoid muscle.

4. Palpate the transverse process of C1 and the mastoid process. Delineate the medial edge of the sternocleidomastoid muscle with scissors (Fig. 5B). Incise the fascia and sternocleidomastoid muscle at the insertion of the sternocleidomastoid and mastoid portion of the splenius capitus on the mastoid process. Leave a fascial edge suitable for reattachment. The splenius capitis is deep in the wound. Incise the superficial medial portion. Remember that the mastoid process is just posterior to the styloid process (Fig. 5C). Between the two is the stylomastoid foramen from which exits the facial nerve (Fig. 5D). The jugular bulb enters the skull anteromedial to the mastoid and stylohyoid processes. The jugular foramen from which exit cranial nerves XI (accessory), X (vagus nerve), IX (glossopharyngeal nerve), and XII (hypoglossal) is medial to the jugular bulb (Fig. 5C). The accessory nerve courses laterally under the internal jugular vein to reach the sternocleidomastoid muscle (Fig. 5E).

5. Identify the accessory nerve. It enters the sternocleidomastoid muscle two to three fingerbreadths below the mastoid tip.[1] Care must be taken to identify the accessory nerve and avoid the internal jugular vein in immediate medial proximity. Dissect the accessory nerve proximally to allow lateral retraction with the sternocleidomastoid muscle (Fig. 5F). For approach to only C1–C2, the accessory nerve may be retracted medially with the internal jugular vein and carotid.[2,3]

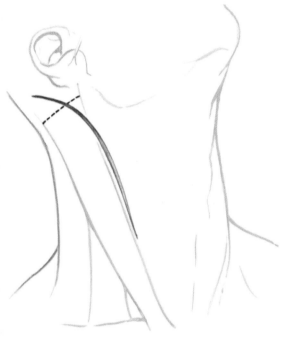

FIGURE 5A. With the ear lobe retracted medially by a stay suture, make a longitudinal incision along the anterior border of the sternocleidomastoid muscle, posteriorly curving across the mastoid process. The *dotted line* is the incision in the insertion of the sternocleidomastoid muscle

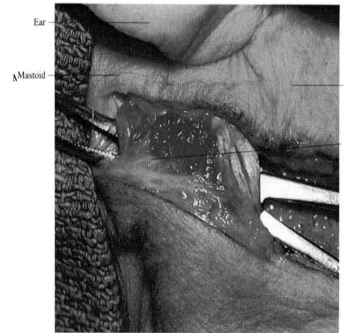

Ear

Mastoid

Mandible

Division of the Sternocleidomastoid Muscle *Splenius Capitis* Muscle

FIGURE 5B. After palpation of the transverse process of C1 and the mastoid process, delineate the medial and lateral edges of the sternocleidomastoid with scissors. Incise the fascia and the sternocleidomastoid muscle and the mastoid portion of the splenius capitis muscle on the mastoid process. Leave a fascial edge suitable for reattachment.

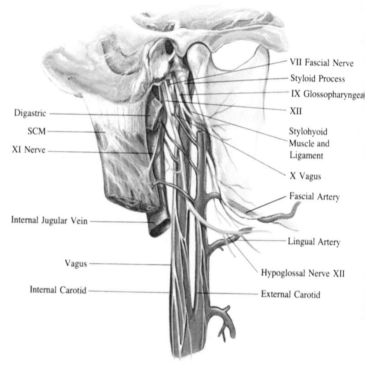

Digastric

SCM

XI Nerve

Internal Jugular Vein

Vagus

Internal Carotid

VII Fascial Nerve

Styloid Process

IX Glossopharyngeal

XII

Stylohyoid Muscle and Ligament

X Vagus

Fascial Artery

Lingual Artery

Hypoglossal Nerve XII

External Carotid

FIGURE 5C. The structures exiting the jugular bulb are the hypoglossal nerve, vagus nerve, spinal accessory nerve, and glossopharyngeal nerve. The jugular bulb is the entry point of the jugular vein and carotid artery. Cranial nerve VII exits from the stylomastoid foramen. Sternocleidomastoid muscle (SCM).

FIGURE 5D. After identification of the mastoid process, remember that just medial to the mastoid process is the styloid process. Between the two is the stylomastoid foramen, from which exits cranial nerve VII. Unneeded cephalad dissection or too vigorous retraction may damage cranial nerve VII at this point. The jugular bulb enters the skull anteromedial to the mastoid and stylohyoid processes. Medial to the jugular bulb is the jugular foramen from which exit cranial nerves XI (accessory), X (vagus nerve), XII (hypoglossal nerve), and IX (glossopharyngeal nerve). The accessory nerve courses laterally over the internal jugular vein to reach the sternocleidomastoid muscle. The other cranial nerves course medially in the medial musculovisceral column.

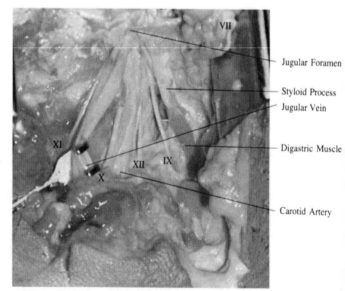

VII

Jugular Foramen

Styloid Process

Jugular Vein

Digastric Muscle

Carotid Artery

XI

XII   IX

X

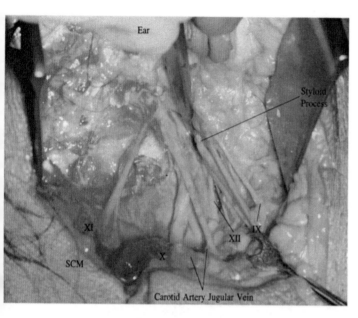

FIGURE 5E. The accessory nerve may be dissected medially toward the jugular foramen to allow greater freedom of retraction of the sternocleidomastoid muscle. The styloid process is prominent in the wound, with the stylohyoid ligament attached to its tip. The more medially placed IXth, Xth, and X11th cranial nerves should be retracted immediately and dissection carried posterior to these structures. Cranial nerve X is incorporated in the carotid sheath, and XII and IX course considerably more distally in the neck.

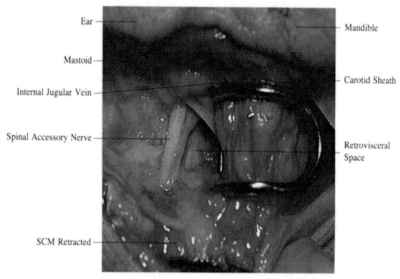

FIGURE 5F. After dividing the sternocleidomastoid insertion from the mastoid process, retract the sternocleidomastoid caudally and identify the spinal accessory nerve, which enters the muscle approximately two fingerbreadths from the mastoid process. Care must be taken to identify the spinal accessory nerve and to avoid injuring the internal jugular vein in immediate medial proximity. Dissect the accessory nerve proximally to allow lateral retraction of the sternocleidomastoid muscle (SCM).

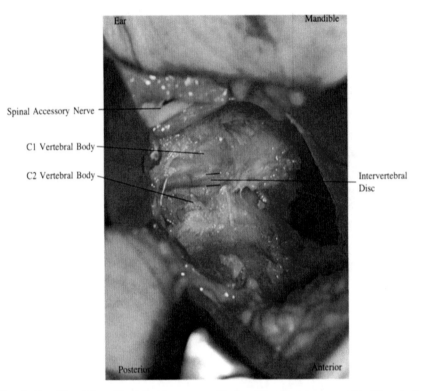

Ear
Mandible

Spinal Accessory Nerve

C1 Vertebral Body

C2 Vertebral Body

Intervertebral
Disc

Posterior
Anterior

FIGURE 5G. After retraction of the soft tissue, identify the transverse process of C1 as a large palpable bony prominence in the wound. By careful palpation distinguish the transverse process of C1, the transverse process of C2, and the anterior tubercle of C1. After iden-tification of these structures, more medial midline palpation reveals the intervertebral disc and vertebral bodies. The transverse process may be mistaken for the anterior aspect of the spine.

6. Identify the transverse process of C1 as a large, palpable bony prominence in the wound. By careful palpation distinguish the transverse process of C1, the transverse process of C2, and the anterior tubercle of C1 (Fig. 5G).

7. Retract the carotid sheath and musculovisceral column medially with a blunt, angled retractor (Fig. 5H). During medial retraction of the internal jugular vein and carotid sheath, remember the origin and location of the vagus and hypoglossal nerves. Although the vagus nerve enters the carotid sheath cephalad to C2 and should be re-tracted with the sheath, if it does appear to be a direct tether to medial retraction, dis-sect it distally from the sheath. The hypoglossal nerve may be exposed but should eas-ily retract medially. The internal jugular vein is in a vulnerable position with medial anterior retraction of the carotid sheath and should be protected in the approach.

8. Develop the retropharyngeal space anterior to the spine and behind by dis-secting the sagittal fibers connecting the visceral fascia to the prevertebral fascia.[1] Avoid dissection within the longus coli muscle and proceed to the midline disc and vertebral body. Palpate the anterior tubercle of C1.

9. Incise the prevertebral fascia and anterior longitudinal ligament in the mid-line. Although this approach begins far laterally, exposure of the spine is now aided with the double-curved Hodgson retractor placed on the right side of the spine.

10. Closure: Drain the wound; reattach the sternocleidomastoid muscle; and close the platysma muscle, subcutaneous tissue, and skin.

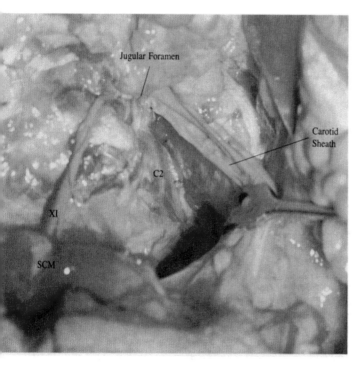

FIGURE 5H. The structures exiting from the jugular foramen are now retracted, the XIth nerve laterally and the IXth, Xth, and XIIth nerves along with the carotid sheath medially. After having developed the retropharyngeal space anterior to the spine and dissecting the sagittal fibers connecting the visceral fascia to the prevertebral fascia, open the longus coli muscle in the midline for dissection of longus coli muscle and proceed to the anterior midline aspect of the prevertebral body and disc. Palpate the anterior tubercle of C1. Incise the prevertebral fascia and anterior longitudinal ligament in the midline and dissect the spine free of soft tissue.

Remember:

1. Remove the sternocleidomastoid and a portion of the splenius capitus muscles from the mastoid process, but leave enough for reattachment.
2. Beware of the facial nerve in the cephalad portion of the wound.
3. Identify the accessory nerve, which enters the sternocleidomastoid muscle two fingerbreadths below its insertion.
4. The styloid process is superficial to the jugular foramen, from which exit cranial nerves X, XI, XII, and IX. Beware of damaging these nerves.
5. Retract the XIth cranial nerve laterally or dissect cephalad on the accessory nerve toward the jugular foramen to allow medial retraction of this nerve.
6. Retract the larynx, internal jugular vein, carotid artery, and cranial nerves IX, X, and XII anteromedially.
7. Open the prevertebral fascia in the midline when possible.

References

. Henry AK: Extensive Exposure, 2nd edn. Edinburgh, Livingstone, 1957, pp 53–80.
. Whitesides TE Jr, McDonald AP: Lateral retropharyngeal approach to the upper cervical spine. Orthop Clin N Am 9(4):1115–1127, 1978.
. Whitesides TE Jr, Kelly RP: Lateral approach to the upper cervical spine for anterior fusion. South Med J 59:879–883, 1966.

6

Anterior Medial Approach
to the Midcervical Spine

1. Position the patient supine on the operating table. Turn the head to the right.

2. Usually, the incision goes from the midline to the medial sternocleidomastoid muscle (SCM). After the transverse skin incision (Fig. 6A), at the appropriate level, dissect through subcutaneous tissue to the platysma muscle. Open the platysma muscle in the line of its fibers when possible. Elevate the platysma muscle with Adson pick-ups and open carefully. Beware of damage to veins and the sternocleidomastoid muscle.[1,2] Insert spring retractors.

3. Open the superficial, cervical fascia and identify the medial border of the sternocleidomastoid muscle.[3] "The first key to successful exposure is adequate identification of the medial border of the sternocleidomastoid so that may be retracted laterally."[4] With identification of this medial border, bluntly develop the interval between the sternocleidomastoid muscle and the sternohyoid and sternothyroid muscles (Figs. 6B, 6C). Retract the posterior cutaneous nerves. Bluntly dissect and spread the soft tissue vertically in this interval.

4. Retract the sternocleidomastoid laterally and the strap musculature medially with angled retractors. Identify the middle cervical fascia. The omohyoid muscle crosses from proximal medial to lateral distal through the middle cervical fascia at C6–C7 (Figs. 6C, 6D, 6E). (The omohyoid arises from the scapula. Its inferior belly crosses ventromedially through a sling of deep cervical fascia that attaches to the clavicle. The muscle passes under the sternocleidomastoid muscle close to the lateral border of the sternohyoid muscle and inserts into the body of the hyoid bone.) Retract the omohyoid, when necessary divide it laterally.

5. Maintain retraction with the angled retractors and incise and split vertically the middle cervical fascia just medial to the carotid sheath.[4] Use finger dissection, spreading vertically and horizontally.[5] Identify, ligate, and divide the inconstant middle thyroid vein crossing at approximately C5. Insert the right-angled retractors directly to the spine but beware of entering the tracheoesophageal groove (and thereby damaging the recurrent laryngeal nerve with the retractor tip).[6]

6. Distally retract the inferior thyroid artery and vein at the C6–C7 level and proximally retract the superior thyroid artery and vein with the superior laryngeal nerve at C3–C4 (Figs. 6D, 6F).

7. Identify the spine with a finger. Palpate the anterior surface of the vertebral body.

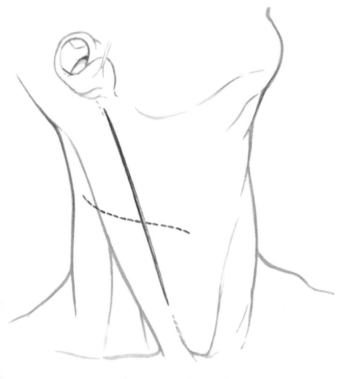

FIGURE 6A. The more cosmetically suitable transverse incision is made at the appropriate level and should allow exposure of as many as two discs and three vertebrae. A vertical incision can be used for an even greater exposure.

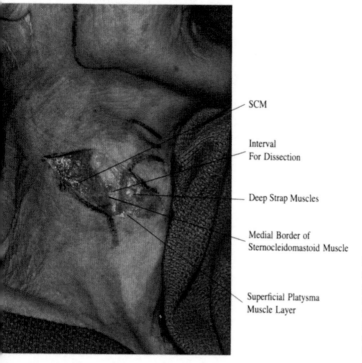

SCM

Interval
For Dissection

Deep Strap Muscles

Medial Border of
Sternocleidomastoid Muscle

Superficial Platysma
Muscle Layer

FIGURE 6B. After the skin incision, dissect through subcutaneous tissue to platysma muscle, which in this specimen is very thin. Open the platysma muscle carefully in line with its fibers. Beware of damage to veins and the sternocleidomastoid muscle (SCM). Insert spring retractors.

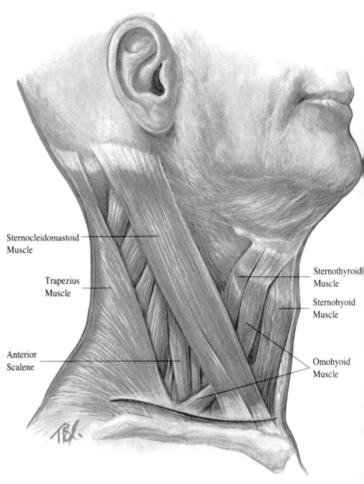

Sternocleidomastoid
Muscle

Trapezius
Muscle

Anterior
Scalene

Sternothyroid
Muscle

Sternohyoid
Muscle

Omohyoid
Muscle

FIGURE 6C. The key to the dissection at this point is to identify the medial border of the sternocleidomastoid muscle. With lateral retraction of the sternocleidomastoid, the interval between this muscle and the medial strap muscles is delineated.

Caution: Do not mistake the transverse process for the anterior surface of the vertebral body, as an incision deep in this area will damage the longus coli muscle, the sympathetic chain, and possibly the vertebral artery. An incision into the longus colli muscle produces bleeding.

8. Palpate a disc in the midline of the spine and open the prevertebral fascia with a small dissector longitudinally until the disc can be identified. The empty esophagus is only a soft, flat, ribbon-like structure simulating the musculature over the anterior portion of the spine. Always use either an esophageal stethoscope or a nasotracheal tube to help identify the esophagus.

9. Insert a needle for lateral X-ray confirmation of the level.

10. Retract the esophagus, trachea, and anterior strap muscles medially and the carotid sheath and sternocleidomastoid muscle laterally.

11. Incise the prevertebral tissue in the midline on the disc and dissect with a sharp periosteal elevator in a lateral direction. With the Cloward deep self-retaining re-

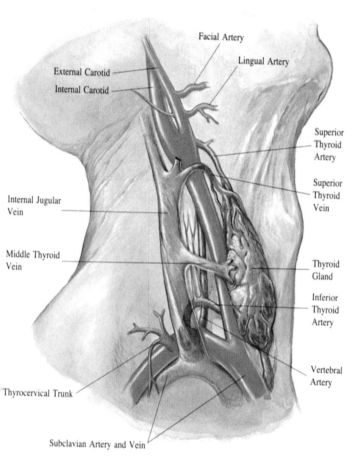

FIGURE 6D. After retracting the sternocleidomastoid muscle laterally and the strap musculature medially, the arteriovenous structures of the middle cervical fascial layer must be identified. Palpate the carotid pulse. Open the midline cervical fascia medial to the carotid artery. Ligate and tie the medial thyroid vein. Retract the superior thyroid artery cephalad and the inferior thyroid artery caudad to expose the midcervical spine.

actor, the clawed blades are inserted into the longus coli on both sides of the spine. se the blunt-tipped Cloward vertically if needed to expose the desired disc.[5] (Fig. 6G).

12. Closure: After hemostasis has been achieved, the deep wound closes with removal of retractors. Close the platysma muscle very carefully to prevent superficial scarng of subcutaneous and skin layers. Use subcuticular skin closure and always use a osed suction wound drainage system.

emember:

Plan skin incision for proper spine level.
Open platysma muscle along the line of its fibers and close carefully for cosmesis.
Identify medial border of sternocleidomastoid muscle.
Ligate middle thyroid vein.
Retract and do not damage the superior thyroid artery and vein cephalad and the inferior thyroid artery and vein caudad.
Palpate carotid pulse and the spine.
Dissect bluntly to the spine.
Open prevertebral fascia in midline.

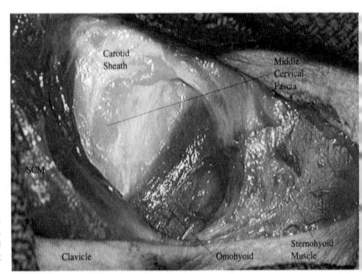

FIGURE 6E. The midcervical fascia layer. The omohyoid muscle crosses from proximal medial to lateral distal through the middle cervical fascia at C6–C7.

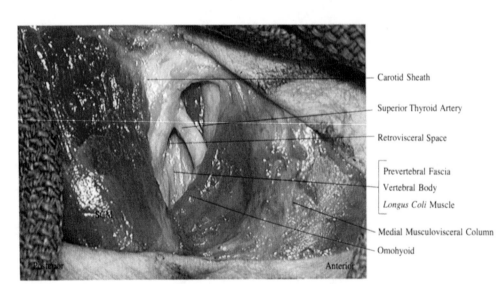

FIGURE 6F. For the approach to C5–C6 enter the retropharyngeal space cephalad to the omohyoid. Retract the superior thyroid artery cephalad. After retracting the sternocleidomastoid muscle and carotid sheath laterally and the medial musculovisceral column medially, locate the spine with finger palpation. Palpate the anterior surface of the vertebral body. Open the prevertebral fascia with a smal dissector longitudinally until the disc can be seen. Blunt dissectio and finger palpation will allow the esophagus to move easily wit the medial musculovisceral column. Insert angle retractors to the fu depth of the wound before vigorous medial retraction.

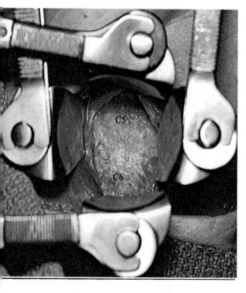

FIGURE 6G. Incise the prevertebral tissue in the midline on the disc and dissect with a sharp periosteal elevator in a lateral direction. Insert the Cloward self-retaining retractor with the clawed blades into the longus coli on both sides of the spine. Use the blunt-tipped Cloward vertically if needed to expose the desired disc space. Remember that the disc spaces are the prominent raised areas of the spine and the vertebral bodies the more sunken areas. Passing the needle tip into the area after it is fully exposed often helps delineate the extent of the disc space, differentiating it from the vertebral body.

References

1. Bailey RW, Bagley CD: Stabilization of the cervical spine by anterior fusion. Am J Bone Joint Surg 42:565, 1960.
2. Riley L: Surgical approaches to the cervical spine. Clin Orthop 91:16, 1973.
3. Robinson RA, Southwick WO: AAOS Instructional Course Lectures. Surgical Approaches to the Cervical Spine, Vol XVII. St. Louis, Mosby, 1960, pp 299–330.
4. Robinson RA: The Craft of Surgery, 2nd edn. Boston, Little, Brown, 1873, 1971.
5. Cloward R: Ruptured Cervical Intervertebral Discs. Codman Signature Series 4. Codman and Shurtleff, 1974.
6. Perry J: Surgical approaches to the spine. In Pierce D, Nichol V (eds): The Total Care of Spinal Cord Injuries. Boston, Little, Brown, 1977, pp 53–79.

7

Lateral Approach to the Cervical Spine (Verbiest)

This lateral approach is a direct approach to the spinal nerve and the vertebral artery in the intervertebral foramen.[1]

1. Position the patient supine with a slight roll under the shoulders. The head is not rotated.

2. Incise the skin with a transverse collar-type incision for one- or two-level disease and with a longitudinal incision along the medial border sternocleidomastoid for multilevel disease. With retraction of the skin and subcutaneous tissue, the platysma muscle is divided longitudinally in line with its fibers. The superficial layers of the investing cervical fascia are opened to identify the medial border of the sternocleidomastoid muscle and the interval between sternocleidomastoid and the medial strap muscles. Angled retractors are used by the assistant to open this interval.

3. Identify the great auricular nerve and the anterior cutaneous nerve. These cutaneous branches of the cervical plexus penetrate the deep fascia on the posterior surface of the sternocleidomastoid muscle at approximately midbelly. The great auricular nerve crosses in a cephalad direction on the surface of the sternocleidomastoid muscle toward the ear. The anterior branch of the greater auricular nerve innervates the skin over the face in the area of the parotid gland. The anterior cutaneous nerve takes a more horizontal course across the sternocleidomastoid before dividing into ascending and descending branches. The ascending branch of the anterior cutaneous nerve pierces the platysma muscle and is distributed to the skin overlying the mandible. Loss of sensation from damage to this nerve can result in decreased sensation over the mandible.[2]

4. Retract the sternocleidomastoid muscle laterally. When retraction is difficult, the sternocleidomastoid muscle is separated from its attachment to the mastoid process. In any separation of the proximal mastoid, cranial nerve XI must be identified entering the sternocleidomastoid two to three fingerbreadths below the mastoid tip and the proximal third of the muscle. The spinal accessory nerve exits the muscle obliquely caudally, passing across the posterior triangle of the neck to the ventral border of the trapezius.

5. With lateral retraction of the sternocleidomastoid muscle, identify by finger palpation the carotid sheath. Open the middle cervical fascia with Metzenbaum scissors and dissect longitudinally with fingertips to expand the interval between the sternocleidomastoid muscle and the carotid sheath laterally and musculovisceral column medially. Retract the medial structures with a blunt-angled retractor, and palpate the carotid pulse and the anterior tubercle of the transverse process. Ligate and divide any tethering vessel. Divide the omohyoid muscle, if needed.

6. Identify the anterior tubercle of the transverse process (Figs. 7A, 7B). This prominent process is suitable for insertion of longus coli, longus capitis, and anterior scalene muscles, and is the key to dissection.[1,3,4] Palpation of the spine under the prevertebral fascia reveals the disc spaces, the anterior tubercle of the transverse process, and, medial to the tubercle, the longitudinal groove of the costotransverse lamellae (Figs. 7A, 7B). It is approximately the size of a small fingernail, joins the anterior tubercle to the vertebral body, and is the roof of the foramen transversarium covering the vertebral artery.[3] The prominent Chassaignac's tubercle, the anterior tubercle of C6, is a relatively consistent landmark, but every level should be identified with X-ray control after exposure of the anterior tubercle of the transverse process.

7. Open the prevertebral fascia with scissors and extend it longitudinally. Visualize the longus coli and longus capitis muscles on the spine. The longus coli muscle, a three-belly muscle broad in the middle and narrow at the end running from C2 to T3, consists of a vertical and an oblique portion. The vertical portion arises and inserts on the anterior surface of the vertebral bodies. The oblique portion inserts with the longus capitis predominantly on the anterior tubercles of the transverse processes. The sympathetic chain is anterior to the transverse process; it is either embedded in the posterior carotid sheath or lies on the connective tissue between the sheaths and longus coli. The superior cervical ganglion at C1 and the middle cervical ganglion at C6 should be

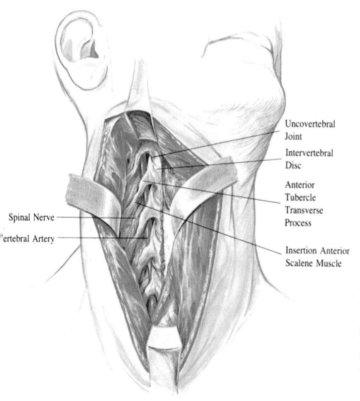

Spinal Nerve

Vertebral Artery

Uncovertebral Joint

Intervertebral Disc

Anterior Tubercle Transverse Process

Insertion Anterior Scalene Muscle

FIGURE 7A. A large expansile approach of the anterolateral aspect of the cervical spine with soft tissue removal to reveal the vertebral artery passing through each foramen transversarium. The anterior tubercle of the transverse processes with its muscular attachment and the costotransverse lamellae are a protective covering over the vertebral artery and nerve. Note the relationship of the vertebral artery anterior to the spinal nerve at each level.

Posterior Tubercle   Anterior Tubercle   C5 Vertebral Body

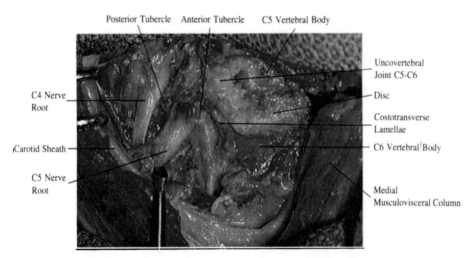

C4 Nerve
Root

Carotid Sheath

C5 Nerve
Root

Uncovertebral
Joint C5-C6

Disc

Costotransverse
Lamellae

C6 Vertebral Body

Medial
Musculovisceral Column

FIGURE 7B. After exposure of the anterior tubercle of the transverse process at the desired level, palpate medially and identify the prominent disc space and the depressed area of the vertebral body at the level above and below. The bony covering between the transverse process and the vertebral body is the costotransverse lamella. This bony curved depression is approximately the size of the tip of the index finger.

included with the sympathetic chain as it is retracted from lateral to medial together with the longus coli muscle.

8. Remove the muscular insertions on the anterior tubercle and dissect sharply to bone, carefully avoiding the nerve root laterally and the vertebral artery medially. The vertebral artery is in an exposed position medially in the areas between the bony grooves on each vertebra (Figs. 7A, 7C, 7D). Dissection of the longus coli off the bone in this area will produce bleeding. Control bleeding with electrocautery and hemostatic gauze. Strip the longus coli muscle above in a superiorly directed motion while inferior to C4–C5 and in an inferiorly directed motion when superior to C4–C5.[3] Remove the bone of the anterior tubercle with a needle-nose rongeur; delineate the cephalad and caudad margins of the bony groove of the costotransverse lamellae with a curette or dissector (Fig. 7E). The vertebral artery need not be exposed above and below the involved costotransverse lamellae (Fig. 7F). If the venous plexus surrounding the vertebral artery or the vertebral artery itself is damaged, direct fingertip pressure usually allows adequate hemostasis for control of the vessels. Control by ligature pressure at the levels above and below the lesion may be necessary in the event of a major transection of the vertebral artery.

9. Remove the bone of the costotransverse lamellae and the anterior wall of the foramen transversarium. The nerve root lies posterior to the vertebral artery at the level of the foramen transversarium and intervertebral foramen (Fig. 7G). At the superior medial position of the costotransverse lamellae is the joint of Luschka and the lateralmost extent of the intervertebral disc. Remember that the main vertebral veins draining the vertebral body and the spinal cord are attached to bone in the foramen transversarium.[2,3] Removing this bone without damaging the veins is usually impossible. Again, obtain hemostasis with hemostatic gauze and direct pressure packing. It is through this interval that the vertebral artery is gently moved laterally only a few millimeters and the spinal nerve root is identified medially along with the lateral aspect of the disc space.

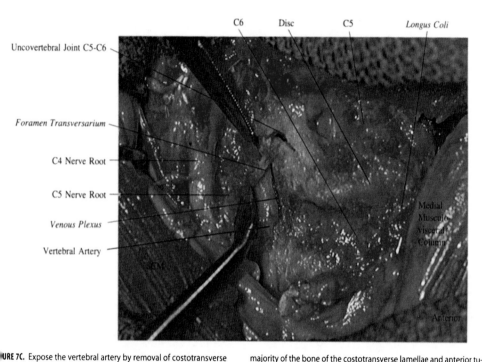

C6   Disc   C5   *Longus Coli*

Uncovertebral Joint C5-C6

Foramen Transversarium

C4 Nerve Root

C5 Nerve Root

Venous Plexus

Vertebral Artery

Medial
Muscul
Viscera
Column

Anterior

URE 7C. Expose the vertebral artery by removal of costotransverse
mellae and the anterior tubercle of the transverse process. Remove
bone of the anterior tubercle with a needle-nose ronguer and
lineate the cephalad and caudad margins of the costotransverse
mellae with a dissector. If the venous plexus surrounding the ver-
ral artery or the vertebral artery itself is damaged, direct finger-
pressure usually allows adequate hemostasis for control of the
ssels. The vertebral artery need not be routinely isolated above
d below the involved costotransversectomy, but control by liga-
e pressure at the levels above and below the lesion could be nec-
ary in the face of a major transection of the vertebral artery. The
majority of the bone of the costotransverse lamellae and anterior tubercle has been removed. The nerve root lies posterior of the vertebral artery at the level of the foramen transversarium and intervertebral foramen. Remember that the main vertebral veins draining
the vertebral body and the spinal cord are attached to bone in the
foramen transversarium. Removing this bony wall of the foramen
transversarium without damaging the veins is usually impossible.
The vertebral artery is gently moved laterally a few millimeters and
the spinal nerve identified adjacent to the disc space in the intervertebral foramen. Vigorous retraction and major mobilization of the
vertebral artery are dangerous.

Caution: Bleeding is caused by fully mobilizing and retracting the vertebral artery.
otect the radicular artery leaving the vertebral artery just inferior to the nerve.[4]

10. Closure: Remove retractors, drain the wound, and close skin and subcutaneous
sue.

member:

Approach medial to the sternocleidomastoid muscle and carotid sheath.
Identify and expose the anterior tubercle of the transverse process and the costo-
transverse lamellae.
Remove the anterior tubercle and expose the vertebral artery with its venous plexus.
Approach the spinal nerve, which is posterior to the vertebral artery, medially.
Avoid venous bleeding by pressure, hemostatic gauze, and minimal vertebral artery
retraction.

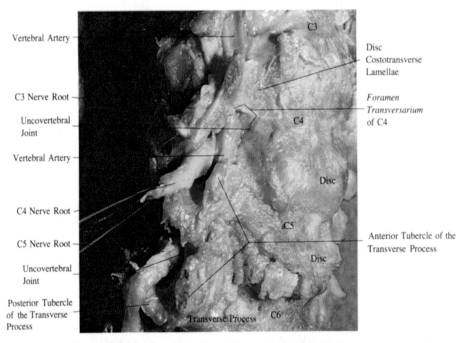

FIGURE 7D. A dissected specimen demonstrating presence of vertebral artery above and below the foramen transversarium of C4, the costotransverse lamellae, the anterior and posterior tubercles of the transverse processes, and the nerve roots exiting at each level.

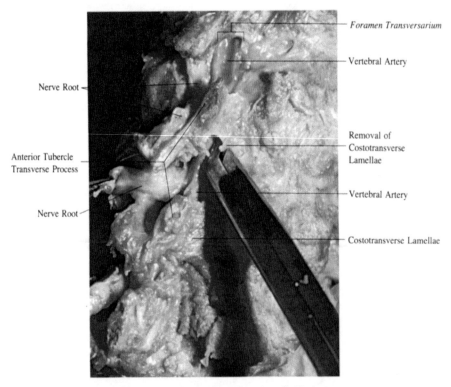

FIGURE 7E. Removal of the costotransverse lamellae and anterior wall of the foramen transversarium.

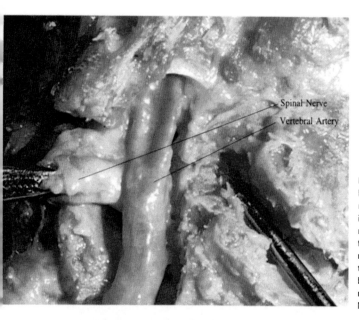

Spinal Nerve
Vertebral Artery

FIGURE 7F. The vertebral artery has been exposed. The prominent venous plexus is not visible in this specimen, but venous bleeding follows removal of the bone of the wall of the foramen transversarium. The spinal nerve is posterior to the vertebral artery, and there are often dense fibrous adhesions between the spinal nerve and the vertebral artery at each level.

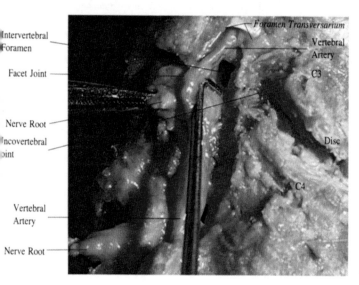

Intervertebral Foramen

Facet Joint

Nerve Root

Uncovertebral Joint

Vertebral Artery

Nerve Root

Foramen Transversarium

Vertebral Artery

C3

Disc

C4

FIGURE 7G. Gentle lateral retraction of only a few millimeters of the vertebral artery will expose the spinal nerve in the intervertebral foramen and the impingement of the uncovertebral joint on the spinal nerve.

References

. Verbiest H: Anterolateral operations for fractures and dislocations in the middle and lower parts of the cervical spine. J Bone J Surg 51A(8):1489–1530, 1969.
. Louis E, Ruge D: Lateral approach to the cervical spine. In Wiltse LL, Ruge D (eds): Spinal Disorders. London, Henry Kimpton, 1977, pp 132–136.
. Henry AK: Extensive Exposure. Baltimore, Williams & Wilkins, 1959, pp 53–72.
. Verbiest H: A lateral approach to the cervical spine: technique and indications. J Neurosurg 28:191–203, 1968.

8

Lateral Approach to the Cervical Spine (Hodgson)

The lateral approach to the cervical spine, when combined with the more proximal detachment of the sternocleidomastoid muscle, as in the anterolateral C1–C3 approach, and with the more distal partial detachment of sternocleidomastoid muscle from the clavicle, as in the Nanson supraclavicular approach, allows good exposure from C1 to T2. The standard midcervical approach to the lateral spine C3–C7 as described by Hodgson is lateral to the sternocleidomastoid muscle and lateral to the carotid sheath. The approach is in a relatively avascular plane avoiding the medial neurovascular structures but is more restrictive in its exposure.

1. Position the patient with the head turned to the left. Make a transverse incision in a skin crease at an appropriate level in the neck to correspond with the level of the spine. The approach is from the right side and extends from the posterior border of sternocleidomastoid approximately 4 inches toward the midline[1] (Fig. 8A).

2. Divide subcutaneous tissue and platysma muscle. Ligate any large branches of the external jugular vein present in the wound and retract cutaneous nerves when possible.

3. Identify the medial and lateral borders of the sternocleidomastoid muscle and retract its lateral border medially (Fig. 8B). If there is an impediment to retraction, the sternocleidomastoid can be wholly or partially divided.

4. Identify the fat pad of the posterior triangle[1] (Fig. 8C). Blunt dissection and finger palpation should follow the fat pad through the posterior triangle to the spine.

5. Beware of the supraclavicular nerve, which is out of view in the lower portion of the field. The brachial plexus is not seen, as the dissection is anterior to the anterior scalene muscle (Fig. 8C).

6. Identify and avoid the sympathetic plexus on the lateral portion of the prevertebral musculature.[1] Direct palpation will identify the transverse process. Blunt soft tissue dissection should be carried to the anterior aspect of the spine.

Caution: The vertebral artery enters the foramen transversarium of C6. Chassaignac's tubercle is the anterior tubercle of the transverse process of C6. The anterior scalene and longus coli muscles insert on the transverse process. Stay superficial to these

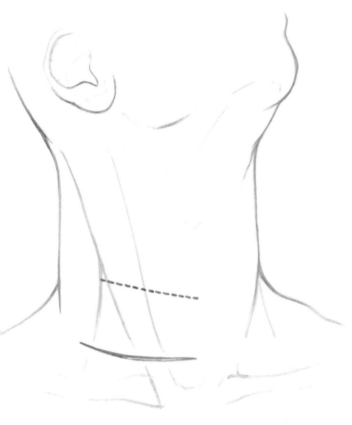

FIGURE 8A. The lateral approach to the cervical spine can be used for C3–C7. The transverse incision is made at the appropriate level, and dissection is carried through the skin and platysma muscle as in any of the standard approaches to this area.

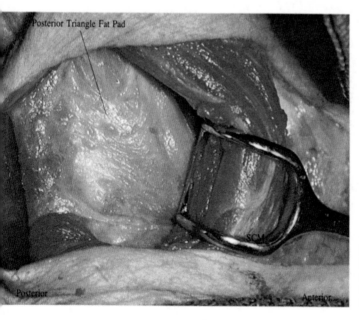

FIGURE 8B. Identify the medial and lateral borders of the sternocleidomastoid muscle and retract its lateral border medially. If there is an impediment to retraction, the sternocleidomastoid can be wholly or partially divided. Identify the fat pad of the posterior triangle.

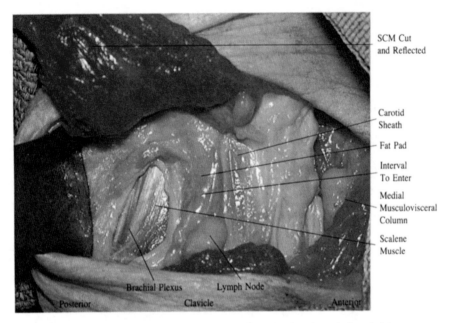

FIGURE 8C. In the lateral portion of the wound are the scalene muscles and brachial plexus, the fat pad of the posterior triangle, and, medially, the carotid sheath and medial musculovisceral column. Sternocleidomastoid muscle (SCM).

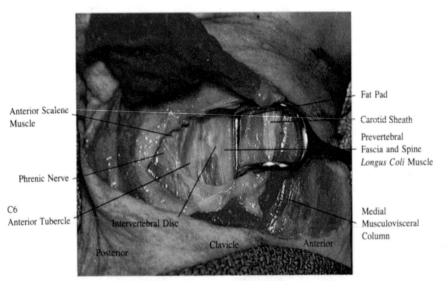

FIGURE 8D. Blunt dissection and finger palpation through the area of the posterior fat pad with medial retraction of the fat pad and carotid sheath leads to the prevertebral fascia and longus coli muscle covering the spine. Avoid damaging the sympathetic plexus on the lateral prevertebral musculature. First palpate the transverse process. The anterior tubercle transverse process of C6 is the prominent Chas- saignac's tubercle. It serves as the insertion of the anterior scalene and longus coli muscles and is the entry point for the vertebral artery into the spine. Stay superficial to these structures and bluntly dissect medially to the midline. Palpate the midline for the interver tebral disc.

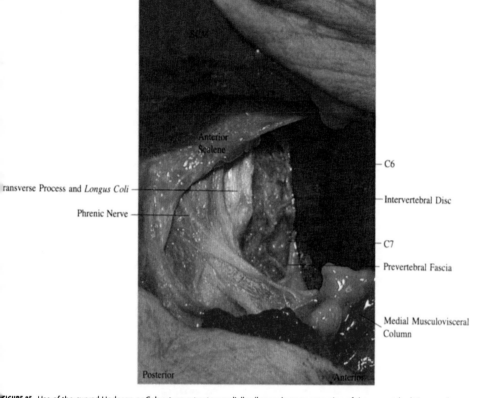

FIGURE 8E. Use of the curved Hodgson or Cobra-type retractor medially allows adequate retraction of the prevertebral tissue and medial musculovisceral column and allows adequate exposure for work on intervertebral discs and vertebrae.

insertions and to the anterior tubercle of the transverse process to avoid damaging the vertebral artery or the nerve root.

7. At this point, the approach is still somewhat lateral. Bluntly dissect with a sponge-covered elevator across to the left side of the spine (Fig. 8D). *Carefully* insert a curved Hodgson retractor or Cobra-type curved retractor on the medial left side of the spine and retract the carotid sheath. Retract the remaining portion of sternocleidomastoid muscle and the musculovisceral column medially.

8. Obtain a marker film to identify the level.

9. Make a direct midline incision on the disc itself. Bluntly dissect the prevertebral fascia and longus coli muscle off the spine from the midline laterally (Fig. 8E).

10. The recurrent laryngeal nerve need not be identified with this medial retraction of the carotid sheath and musculovisceral column, but it is in a vulnerable position as it enters the tracheoesophageal groove on the right.

11. Closure: Drain the wound and close subcutaneous tissue and skin.

Remember:

1. Identify the lateral border of the sternocleidomastoid muscle.

2. Identify the fat pad of the posterior triangle.

3. Stay superficial and anterior to the anterior tubercle of the transverse process.
4. Identify the sympathetic plexus.
5. Make a midline prevertebral incision and dissect the longus coli muscle medial to lateral.

Reference

1. Hodgson AR: Approach to the cervical spine C3–C7. Clin Orthop 39:129–134, 1965.

9

Supraclavicular Approach

1. Position the patient supine. Slightly hyperextend the neck, rotated away from the side of the approach. Use the inflatable cervical pillow for support; a small roll under the shoulder often helps to extend the neck. Location of the thoracic duct and recurrent laryngeal nerve becomes even more important at this level. Approaches from the left for C6 through T2 are directly in the vicinity of the thoracic duct. Identify the thoracic duct when possible and protect it. A large fatty meal the day before surgery will help. If the thoracic duct is inadvertently divided, double ligate both ends well. The approach to the right should definitely identify the recurrent laryngeal nerve and protect it. We recommend the right supraclavicular approach with identification of the recurrent laryngeal nerve.

2. Make a transverse incision approximately one fingerbreadth above the clavicle from the midline to the posterior border of the sternocleidomastoid muscle (see Fig. 8A). After division of the skin and subcutaneous tissue and the placement of small skin self-retaining retractors, incise the platysma muscle in the line of the incision. As with the higher approaches, identification of the medial border of the sternocleidomastoid is imperative.

3. In addition, identify and define the anterior and posterior borders of the sternocleidomastoid muscle. The external jugular vein, although somewhat variable, is usually directly in the operative field and the anterior jugular vein is positioned more medially. Divide if necessary.

4. Incise the external investing fascia. Pass a probe or finger laterally from the medial border of the sternocleidomastoid to clear off the venous structures underneath the clavicular head of the sternocleidomastoid.

5. Divide the sternocleidomastoid laterally to medially, watching for the internal jugular vein.[1] If required for visualization, remove the sternal head of the sternocleidomastoid muscle in the same fashion. Eventual reattachment depends on suturing the fascial coverings of the muscle.

6. Retract the divided sternocleidomastoid in a cephalad–caudad direction with self-retaining blunt retractors. The floor of the incision, at this point, consists of the middle cervical fascia, which contains the omohyoid and the sternohyoid muscles (see Fig. 6C).

7. Enter the middle cervical fascia lateral to the carotid sheath. Bluntly dissect to the surface of the anterior scalene muscle (Fig. 9A). The superficial surfaces of the anterior scalene are composed of the outer layer of the prevertebral fascia, the third and deepest of the fascial layers addressed in this approach. Lying on the surface of the anterior scalene is the phrenic nerve. The phrenic nerve crosses lateral to medial, cephalad to caudal (Figs. 9B, 9C). Retract the phrenic nerve medially after freeing it from the surface of the anterior scalene muscle. Identify the large internal jugular vein medially and feel the carotid pulse (Fig. 9D). Although there are standard approaches to retract the carotid sheath laterally[2] (Fig. 9E), attempt to retract the internal jugular vein and carotid sheaths medially (Figs. 9A, 9F). Retract the phrenic nerve to obtain good visualization of the anterior scalene muscle. The brachial plexus courses under the anterior scalene, between it and the middle scalene. The brachial plexus and suprascapular nerves are more superficial at the lateral border of the anterior scalene (Fig. 9C).

8. Delineate the medial and lateral borders of the anterior scalene muscle. The fascia on the deep surface of the anterior scalene is Sibson's fascia, a continuation of the prevertebral fascia that encloses this muscle. The apex of the parietal pleura and lung form the undersurface of Sibson's fascia.

9. Retract the anterior scalene laterally (Fig. 9A). Bluntly dissect medially under the retracted carotid sheath. Stay on the prevertebral fascia to the spine.

10. If exposure is inadequate, carefully dissect under the anterior scalene without violating the major portions of Sibson's fascia and divide the anterior scalene muscle (Fig. 9D). Retract it cephalad–caudad with self-retaining blunt retractors. The wound now consists of Sibson's fascia in the floor of the wound, the large internal jugular vein

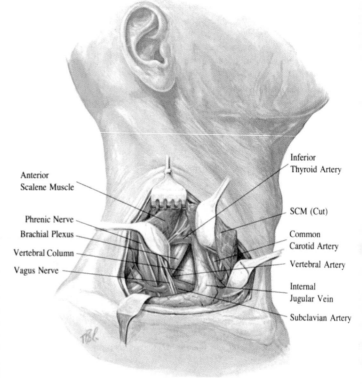

FIGURE 9A. After a transverse incision approximately one fingerbreadth above the clavicle from the midline to the posterior border of the sternocleidomastoid muscle, as described in Chapter 7, delineate the medial and lateral borders of the sternocleidomastoid muscle (SCM). Divide the sternocleidomastoid muscle, avoiding damage to the internal jugular vein and muscular venous branches under the sternocleidomastoid, by passing a peon or angled retractor medial to lateral under the muscle before cutting with electrocautery. This composite picture shows the cut and retracted sternocleidomastoid muscle, the laterally retracted anterior scalene muscle and phrenic nerve, and a medially retracted internal jugular vein.

Anterior Scalene Muscle

Phrenic Nerve

Brachial Plexus

Vertebral Column

Vagus Nerve

Inferior Thyroid Artery

SCM (Cut)

Common Carotid Artery

Vertebral Artery

Internal Jugular Vein

Subclavian Artery

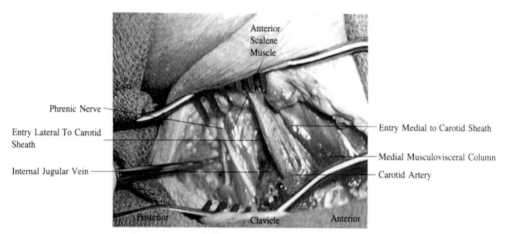

FIGURE 9B. After division and retraction of the sternocleidomastoid muscle, three basic areas of approach are seen. (1) By retracting the phrenic nerve and resecting the anterior scalene muscle approach from the most lateral direction medially, an approach standardly used for a sympathectomy. (2) Lateral to the carotid sheath and me- dial to the anterior scalene muscle is an approach that allows me- dial retraction of the internal jugular vein and carotid sheath. (3) A more conventional approach medial to the carotid sheath and in- ternal jugular vein may require division and ligation of the inferior thyroid artery as described in Chapters 6 and 10.

and the carotid sheath medially, the apex of the lung beneath Sibson's fascia in the floor of the wound, and laterally the brachial plexus as it courses superficial to the scalenus medius. The proximal portion of the anterior scalenus muscle may be dissected from the anterior tubercle of the transverse processes to allow greater exposure of the spine or brachial plexus.[3]

11. Incise Sibson's fascia at the transverse processes and bluntly retract inferiorly; this retracts the pleura of the lung, which is usually at the T1 level. The recurrent la-

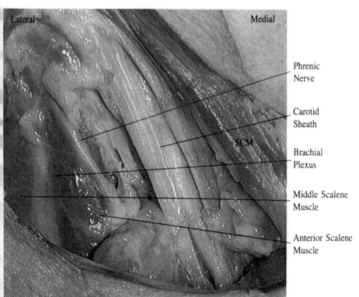

FIGURE 9C. The approach from lateral to the carotid sheath, as originally seen in Figure 9A.

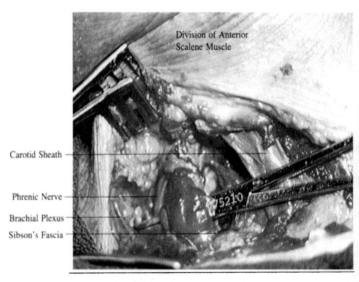

Carotid Sheath

Phrenic Nerve

Brachial Plexus

Sibson's Fascia

FIGURE 9D. Division of the anterior scalene muscle after retraction of the phrenic nerve. The anterior scalene muscle originates from the anterior tubercles of the transverse processes and inserts on the 1st rib. The phrenic nerve courses from cephalad lateral to caudad medial on the superficial surface of the anterior scalene muscle. The brachial plexus lies under the anterior scalene muscle, between it and the middle scalene. The brachial plexus and supraclavicular nerves are superficial at the lateral border of the anterior scalene. The fascia on the deep surface of the anterior scalene muscle is Sibson's fascia. Under Sibson's fascia is the apex of the lung. Protect the undersurface of the anterior scalene and divide it transversely at the level of the wound, or it may be resected from the transverse processes at multiple levels.

ryngeal nerve is mobilized medially with the carotid sheath and medial visceral column. The spine is exposed by opening the fascia in the midline over the body. Continue the caudal exposure of the transverse processes and rib heads.[4]

12. Dissect to the 2nd and 3rd rib heads, producing a rather lateral exposure of the spine from the rib heads that must be carried medially to enter the all-important retropharyngeal fascial cleft on the anterior surface of the spine without having to dissect the longus coli muscle.[4] The vertebral artery enters the spine at C6 and can be identified (Fig. 9G). The subclavian vein courses on the floor of the wound.

13. If the approach is done from the left, the junction of the internal jugular veins and the subclavian veins will contain the thoracic duct (Fig. 1C). Identify the thoracic duct. In case of damage, double-tie proximally and distally. Chylothorax can be prevented with proper ligation. Often a more judicious approach involves blunt dissection, progressing cephalad to caudad, as has been described for the transverse processes of C5, C6, and C7 to the rib head of the 1st rib down on the spine; this will sweep most of these structures cephalad to caudad. The danger, of course, lies in cutting restraining structures that cross the field. The sympathetic chain (stellate ganglion at C7) lies on the rib heads in a lateral position. Avoid damage by dissecting more medially.

14. Closure: Drain and suture sternocleidomastoid fascia, subcutaneous tissue, and skin.

Additional Anatomy[5]

1. The external investing fascia forms the anterior and posterior sheaths of the sternocleidomastoid muscle and the fascial covering of the visceral structures of the neck.

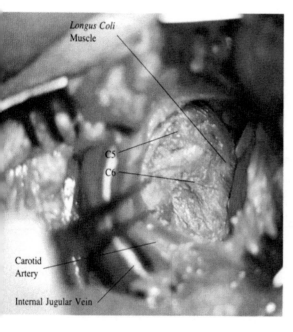

Longus Coli
Muscle

C5
C6

Carotid
Artery

Internal Jugular Vein

FIGURE 9E. The most medial supra-clavicular approach demonstrates a lateral retraction of the carotid sheath and internal jugular vein and the approach medial to these structures. The recurrent laryngeal nerve must be identified in this area. The longus coli muscle is opened in the midline and dissected from medial to lateral.

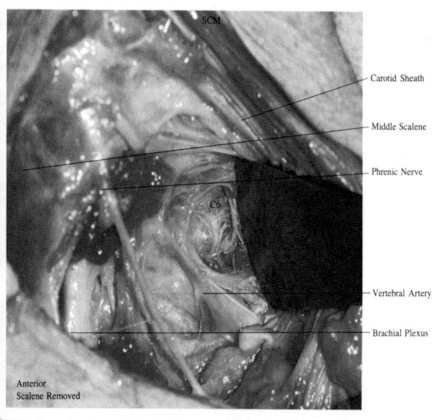

SCM

Carotid Sheath

Middle Scalene

Phrenic Nerve

C6

Vertebral Artery

Brachial Plexus

Anterior
Scalene Removed

FIGURE 9F. The anterior scalene muscle is removed, the phrenic nerve is lateral, and the carotid sheath and jugular vein are retracted medially.

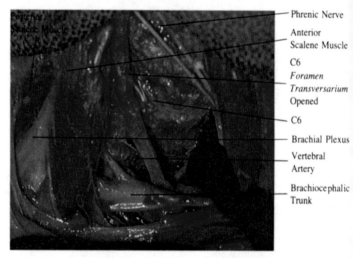

Posterior
Scalene Muscle

Phrenic Nerve

Anterior
Scalene Muscle

C6

*Foramen
Transversarium*
Opened

C6

Brachial Plexus

Vertebral
Artery

Brachiocephalic
Trunk

FIGURE 9G. The vertebral artery dissected free.

This investing layer of cervical fascia is attached inferiorly to the acromion, clavicle, and manubrium of the sternum in an outer and inner layer superiorly to the hyoid bone, posteriorly to the mandible and mastoid processes, and superior to the nuchal line. The interval between the two laminae of the external investing fascia is called the suprasternal space or the space of Burns.[5] This space contains the anterior jugular veins and sternal head of the sternocleidomastoid muscle. The lateral extension of the space, deep to the heads of the sternocleidomastoid, is referred to as the cul-de-sac of Bruger. Communication between the anterior and external jugular veins is channeled through this inner laminar area.

2. The middle cervical fascia attaches to the carotid sheath and joins the external investing fascia at the posterior border of the sternocleidomastoid muscle. Inferiorly the middle cervical fascia attaches to the posterior surface of the sternum, as do the muscles that they cover. It is the middle cervical fascia that attaches to the clavicle and forms the loop for the inferior belly of the omohyoid muscle.

3. The prevertebral fascia is continuous with the endothoracic fascia caudally and laterally covers the levator scapuli and splenius muscles. It extends posteriorly to attach to the spinous processes of the vertebrae. In the neck and throughout the spinal column it covers the longus coli and capitis muscles and is secured to the tips of the transverse processes.

4. The origin of the anterior scalene muscle rises from the anterior tubercles of the transverse processes of C3, C4, C5, and C6. It inserts into the scalene tubercle on the inner border of the 1st rib and into the ridge on the cranial surface of the rib ventral to the subclavian groove. The scalenus medius originates from the posterior tubercles of the transverse processes of the last six cervical vertebrae and inserts into the 1st rib.

5. The scalenus medius is a muscular reenforcement of Sibson's fascia. These fascial connections and the scalenus minimus connect the transverse processes of the seventh cervical vertebra to the 1st rib. Sibson's fascia, as a portion of the prevertebral fascia, becomes continuous with the endothoracic fascia on the inner surface of the 1st rib. Extending medially between the anterior scalene muscle and the spine is the all-important retropharyngeal fascial cleft. This is the space beneath the visceral structures, superficial to the prevertebral fascia, and it is in this space that retraction and work on the anterior portion of the spine take place.

6. Identify the thyrocervical trunk off the subclavian artery in the lateral aspect of this subanterior scalene plane (Fig. 9G). The thyrocervical trunk consists of the vertebral artery, which courses medially to enter the foramen transversarium at C6, the anterior cervical artery, which progresses cephalad lateral to the vertebral artery, and the transcervical artery, which courses posterior across the posterior cervical triangle. The inferior thyroid artery, usually a branch off the carotid at about C7–T1, in certain cases arises from the thyrocervical trunk. Although it passes at the level of the operative field, it usually need not be ligated.

Remember:

1. Identify the medial and lateral borders of the sternocleidomastoid muscle.
2. Protect the venous structures on the undersurface of the sternocleidomastoid and the internal jugular vein medially.
3. Identify the inferior thyroid artery and the vertebral artery.
4. Identify the phrenic nerve on the surface of the anterior scalene muscle.
5. Retract the internal jugular vein, phrenic nerve, and carotid sheath medially.
6. If the anterior scalene is divided, dissect cephalad to caudad Sibson's fascia and the apex of the lung.
7. Stay medial toward the spine and superficial to the sympathetic plexus and longus coli muscle as you approach the midline surface of the spine.

References

1. Henry AJ: Extensive Exposure. Baltimore, Williams & Wilkins, 1959, pp 53–72.
2. Robinson RA: Approaches to the cervical spine C1–T1. Chapter 22 in Schmidek HH, Sweet WH (eds): Current Techniques in Operative Neurosurgery. New York, Grune & Stratton, 1978, pp 205–302.
3. Riley L: Surgical approaches to the anterior structures of the cervical spine. Clin Orthop 91(16):10–20, 1973.
4. Nanson EM: The anterior approach to upper dorsal sympathectomy. Surg Gynecol Obstet 104:118–120, 1957.
5. Goss CM (ed): Gray's Anatomy of the Human Body, 29th edn. Philadelphia, Lea & Febiger, 1973.

10

Lincoln Highway Approach to the Cervical Spine

Occasionally the need arises for maximally expanded exposure of the cervical spine. For exposure of multilevel anterior cervical disease from C1 to T2;[1] Riley expanded the basic anterior medial Robinson approach. Various aspects of the approach, seen in Chapters 4, 6, and 9, are combined into one extensive exposure.

1. The skin incision is a modified Shoebringer incision described by Riley.[1] It begins under the mandible at the midline and extends posteriorly under the angle of the mandible to the tip of the occiput, down the posterior border of the sternocleidomastoid muscle, and swings anteriorly into a modified hemithyroid approach to the sternal notch (Fig. 10A).

2. Open the skin, subcutaneous tissue, and platysma muscle in line with the incision. Open the full extent of the wound through the superficial cervical fascia dissecting the flap lateral to medial.

3. Identify the anterior border of the sternocleidomastoid muscle (Fig. 10B). As with all the anterior medial approaches, this is the key to proper orientation at this level. Develop the interval between the medial border of sternocleidomastoid and the strap muscles (Fig. 10C). Spread longitudinally the entire length of the anterior sternocleidomastoid border. Beware of the mandibular branch of the facial nerve in the cephaladmost extent of the exposure.

4. After the borders of the sternocleidomastoid and strap musculatures have been delineated, palpate for the carotid pulse. Incise the middle cervical fascial layer medial to the carotid pulse in the midportion of the neck (Fig. 10D). Gently retract the carotid laterally and develop the interval between the medial musculovisceral column and the carotid artery. The middle thyroid vein should be identified, tied, and ligated. Continue to develop this interval, aided by deep digital palpation in the wound for the spine. It is important to attempt to dissect directly to the spine before placement of angled retractors, which could slip into the tracheal/esophageal groove and damage the recurrent laryngeal nerve. Bluntly spread longitudinally, dissection at this point should be caudad to the superior thyroid artery and cephalad to the inferior thyroid artery in the relatively avascular plane. The esophagus may be lying as a flat ribbon on the spine; this should be bluntly dissected off the prevertebral fascia with the musculovisceral column (Fig. 10E).

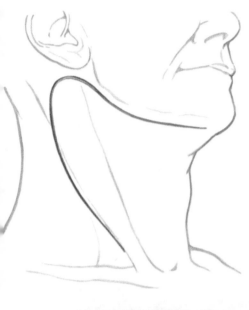

FIGURE 10A. Total exposure to the cervical spine from C1 to T2. A curvilinear incision producing a flap on the anterior lateral aspect of the neck may be used. Incise through the skin and subcutaneous tissue, divide the platysma muscle in line with the incision, and carefully retract the skin margins. When necessary, divide and ligate prominent external jugular veins.

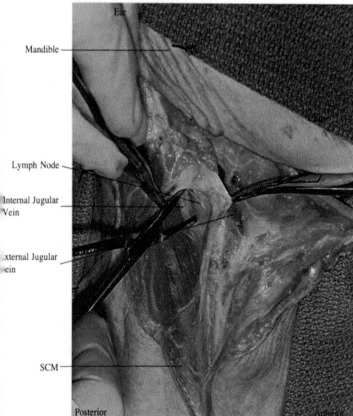

FIGURE 10B. As in the standard anteromedial approach to cervical spine (Chapter 6), identify the medial border of the sternocleidomastoid muscle (SCM), and delineate this border throughout the length of the incision.

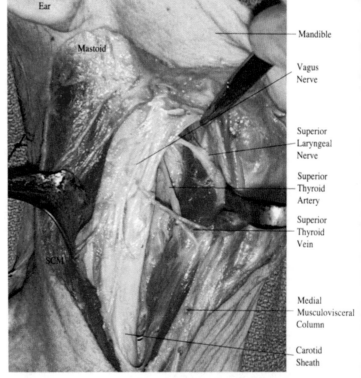

FIGURE 10C. Retract the sternocleido-mastoid muscle laterally and develop the plane between the carotid sheath and the medical musculovisceral column.

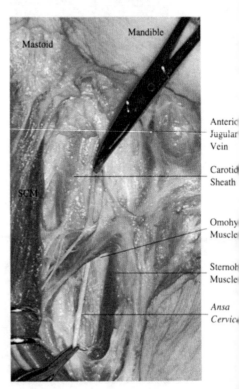

FIGURE 10D. The omohyoid muscle crosses the middle cervical fascial layer approximately at C6–C7. Fibers of the ansa cervicalis may course with the muscle. The omohyoid may be divided.

74

5. Angled blunt retractors should be used to allow identification of the longus coli muscle and the prevertebral fascia. Palpate for the disc surface, which is a raised, softer area of the spine, to allow a more midline exposure. Do not mistake the anterior tubercle of the transverse process for the midline anterior structures of the cervical spine. A Kitner dissector will allow blunt dissection for positive identification of an intervertebral disc.

6. Having reached the prevertebral plane of dissection in the midcervical spine, open the more superficial middle cervical fascia in a cephalad direction (Fig. 10F). The superior thyroid artery and vein should be the first major vascular structures encountered. Identify and dissect out sufficiently this artery and vein. Continue the cephalad dissection to identify five major structures: (1) the superior laryngeal nerve; (2) the hypoglossal nerve; (3) the facial artery; (4) the lingual artery; and (5) the digastric muscle. The superior laryngeal nerve should be preserved. Its more caudad external branch enters the medial musculovisceral column in close proximity with the superior thyroid artery. Isolate and preserve this nerve. Progressing in a cephalad direction, the hypoglossal nerve, described well in Chapter 4, courses superficially across the external carotid artery and its branches from lateral to medial. Identify and isolate the hypoglossal nerve before ligation of the lingual or facial arteries; this will prevent inadvertent transection of the hypoglossal nerve. With identification, ligation, and division of the lingual and facial arteries, the carotid can be laterally retracted with greater ease.

7. Use angled retractors in the cephalad portion of the wound to separate the carotid sheath and the medial musculovisceral column. The hypoglossal nerve and the

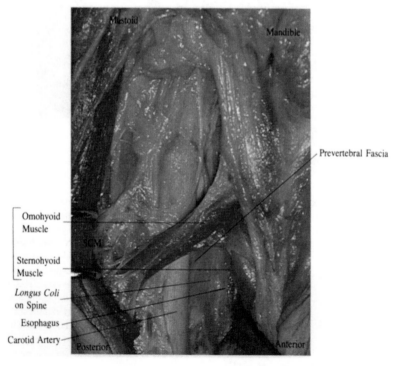

FIGURE 10E. The omohyoid muscle in place, blunt dissection in the caudal aspect of the wound deepens the appropriate interval between carotid sheath and medial musculovisceral column to the longus coli muscle on the spine. The esophagus, which may be only a flat ribbon of tissue on the spine, is retracted medially with the medial musculovisceral column. Make positive identification of the longus coli muscle before any incision.

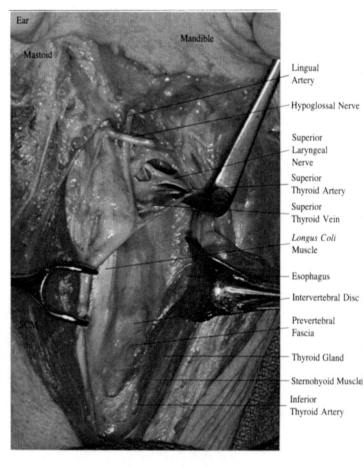

Ear

Mandible

Mastoid

Lingual Artery

Hypoglossal Nerve

Superior Laryngeal Nerve

Superior Thyroid Artery

Superior Thyroid Vein

Longus Coli Muscle

Esophagus

Intervertebral Disc

Prevertebral Fascia

Thyroid Gland

Sternohyoid Muscle

Inferior Thyroid Artery

SCM

FIGURE 10F. Visualize the midportion of the cervical spine, open the longus coli muscle in the midline, and dissect from medial to lateral. The approach to the more cephalad portion of the wound is described in Chapter 2. The approaches of Chapters 2, 6, and 8 may be combined here in this Lincoln Highway exposure of the entire cervical spine. This is an extension of the most useful standard Robinson anteromedial approach.

superior laryngeal nerve are preserved when crossing the wound. Maintain the depth of the dissection in the prevertebral area. Identify each intervertebral disc level as you progress cephalad (Fig. 10G).

8. A marker film for level of the spine should be obtained. The cephalad musculotendonous structures passing from lateral to medial are principally the digastric muscle, the stylohyoid ligament, and stylohyoid muscle. These may be divided in the midportion of the wound. The glossopharyngeal nerve is cephalad, under the digastric muscle and stylohyoid muscle. Care should be taken to avoid damaging this nerve. Palpate the tip of the styloid process to identify the stylohyoid ligament. Remember the facial nerve exits from the stylomastoid foramen. This dissection should be medial to the jugular foramen and the jugular bulb. Maintain the prevertebral tissue plane level.

9. It may be necessary to expand the exposure by closed dislocation of the temporal mandibular joint. A large submandibular gland may be resected, if necessary; this will allow an exposure of the clivus and tip of the odontoid process. With a standard approach to the base of the odontoid at the C1–C2 junction, it is not necessary to dislocate the mandible.

10. For the caudal extent of the wound, continue the dissection in the prevertebral plane to the inferior thyroid artery and vein. Identify, tie, and ligate.

11. The standard approach is from the left. If approached from the right because

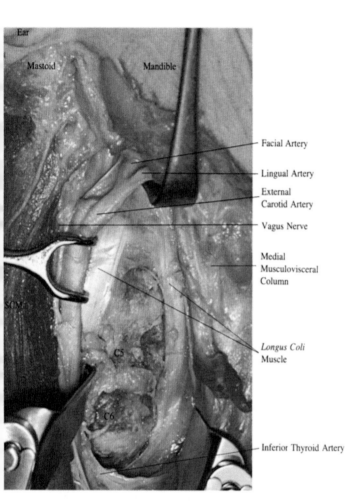

Ear

Mastoid

Mandible

Facial Artery

Lingual Artery

External
Carotid Artery

Vagus Nerve

Medial
Musculovisceral
Column

Longus Coli
Muscle

SCM

C5

C6

Inferior Thyroid Artery

FIGURE 10G. Good visualization of the medial portion of the spine reveals prominent disc spaces with retraction of soft tissue both medially and laterally.

of a particular aspect of the pathology, the recurrent laryngeal nerve must be identified as it courses from lateral to medial in the C7–T1 area.

12. Divide the mylohyoid muscle in its belly and retract the ends. Further exposure from this point may consist of division of the sternal and/or clavicular heads of the sternocleidomastoid and identification of the phrenic nerve and anterior scalene muscle. Total resection of the anterior scalene may be needed (see Chapter 9). Remember, the apex of the lung is medial under Simpson's fascia, under the anterior scalene muscle.

13. The vertebral artery enters the spine at C6. Maintain the prevertebral plane on the midline of the vertebral body and disc. Exposure of the entrance of the vertebral artery into the spine is not necessary, but with lateral dissection at the C7–T1 area such as in resection of the anterior scalene muscle, the vertebral artery must be identified. Osteotomy of the sternoclavicular joint may be needed to allow distal extension of the wound to easily include T3.

14. Closure: The muscular planes fall together with removal of the retractors. Drainage should be used with an incision this large. Close the platysma in a separate layer.

Remember:

1. Extend the incision laterally to the posterior border of the sternocleidomastoid muscle and distal medially to the sternal notch.
2. Avoid the mandibular branch of the facial nerve in the cephalad extent of the wound.
3. Expose the spine in the safer midcervical spine region.
4. Identify the superior laryngeal nerve and the hypoglossal nerve and isolate these structures before division of arteries and veins.
5. Do not include the glossopharyngeal nerve with any division of the digastric and stylohyoid muscles.
6. Dislocate the mandible and resect the submandibular gland, but only when needed for exposure.
7. Identify the inferior thyroid artery and vein and the recurrent laryngeal nerve on the right side.
8. Identify and protect the vertebral artery entering the spine at C6.
9. Avoid damage to the apex of the lung under Simpson's fascia.
10. Identify and protect the phrenic nerve and Simpson's fascia with any division of the anterior scalene muscle.
11. Osteotomize the sternoclavicular joint after adequate clearance of soft tissue, but only if necessary for distal exposure.

Reference

1. Riley L: Surgical approaches to anterior structures of the cervical spine. Clin Orthop 91:16–20, 1973.

Cervicothoracic Junction

he anteromedial approach is an extension of the Smith–Robinson approach. It is meal to the sternocleidomastoid muscle and medial to the carotid sheath. This method
lows exposure from C1 to T2[1] and can be combined with an osteotomy of the stern-
lavicular joint to allow a greater exposure at T2. The thoracic duct must be avoided
ith the left anteromedial approach. The recurrent laryngeal nerve should be identi-
ed with the right-side approach. The inferior thyroid artery and vein may need liga-
on, and the apex of the lung must be avoided.

The anterolateral approach to the cervicothoracic junction is an extension of the
odgson approach[2] combined with the Nanson supraclavicular approach,[3] in which the
ernocleidomastoid is removed from the clavicle. The spine is approached from the
ght side, lateral to the carotid sheath and vessels. With the carotid sheath and inter-
l jugular vein retracted medially, the anterior scalene muscle may be divided and the
renic nerve retracted for greater exposure.

The 3rd rib resection allows good exposure to T1–T3. When there is a thoracic
phosis deformity, exposure of C6–T3 is possible.[4] The morbidity associated with di-
ding the scapular muscle attachments can be significant. The operating space can be
hanced by removal of both the 2nd and 3rd ribs.

By cephalad extension of the posterior proximal limb of the 3rd rib incision, cut-
g the rhomboid and trapezial attachments to the scapula and sweeping the scapula
erally, the 1st, 2nd, 3rd, and 4th ribs can be removed for maximum exposure. One
, usually the 3rd, is left to support the scapula.[5]

Although the axillary approach has very limited exposure, it does allow biopsy of
e T1–T3 area and limited spinal work. The morbidity associated with dividing
e pectoralis major is less than that occurring when dividing the scapular muscle
tachments.

eferences

Riley L: Surgical approaches to the anterior structures of the cervical spine. Clin Orthop
91(16):10–20, 1973.

2. Hodgson AR, Yau ACMC: Anterior surgical approach to the spinal column. In Apley AG (ed): Recent Advances in Orthopaedics. Baltimore, Williams & Wilkins, 1964, pp 289–323.

3. Nanson EM: The anterior approach to upper dorsal sympathectomy. Surg Gynecol Obstet 104:118–120, 1957.

4. Perry J: Surgical approaches to the spine. In Pierce D, Nichol V (eds): The Total Care of Spinal Cord Injuries. Boston, Little, Brown, 1977, pp 53–79.

5. Dawson E: Personal communication.

Anterior Approach to the Cervicothoracic Spine

Salvador A. Brau

Anterior exposure of the cervicothoracic spine (C7 to T2) presents a significant challenge because of the limited access afforded by anatomical considerations. The junction of the cervical and thoracic spine not only represents the apex of two physiologic curvatures but is also crowded by important neurovascular structures, the trachea and the esophagus at the narrowed thoracic outlet. Median sternotomy as well as partial resection of the manubrium and part of the clavicle on one side have been described but may not be necessary for adequate exposure because of recent improvements in instrumentation and technique. In addition, the increasing familiarity of many surgeons with the anatomy of the area makes less radical approaches more desirable. We present a stepwise approach to the area that may obviate resection of the clavicle or the manubrium, depending on how much exposure can be obtained before proceeding with those steps.

  1. Under general endotracheal anesthesia, the patient is placed supine with a bolster between the scapulae with the head turned to the right and the neck slightly extended. A slight reverse Trendelenburg position may help reduce venous distension. The vocal cords should be evaluated by the anesthesiologist at the time of intubation to confirm their integrity, and a nasogastric tube is inserted to help localize the esophagus.

  2. An inverted L-shaped incision is marked off on the skin with the transverse limb 1 to 2 cm above the left clavicle, extending from the lateral border of the sternomastoid muscle to the midline just above the suprasternal notch. From there the vertical limb is marked in the midline extending to the bottom of the manubrium (Fig. 12A). The skin is initially incised only along the transverse plane, with the vertical portion reserved for use only if exposure is not adequate without resection of the clavicle and part of the manubrium. Subplatysmal flaps are then elevated. These flaps should be wide

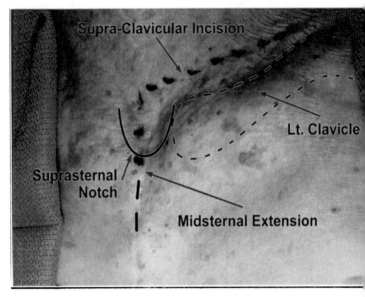

FIGURE 12A. The skin incision extension has been marked off with anatomical relationships highlighted. Incision extends from just lateral to the sternomastoid to the midline about 1 to 2 cm above the clavicle.

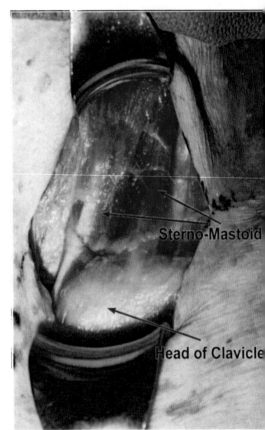

FIGURE 12B. Skin flaps have been elevated superiorly and inferiorly, exposing the distal one-third of the sternomastoid and the distal end of the clavicle.

enough to expose the lower one-third of the sternomastoid and strap muscles superiorly and extend inferiorly 3 to 4 cm below the clavicle (Fig. 12B).

3. Dissection between the medial border of the sternomastoid and the strap muscles is carried superiorly to the extent of the flap exposure and inferiorly to the insertion at the clavicle. Blunt dissection is then used to create a plane posterior to the sternoclavicular joint to expose the superior mediastinal fat pad. The dissection then mobilizes the sternomastoid muscle with the jugular vein laterally and the strap muscles medially to expose the avascular plane between the carotid sheath laterally and the trachea and esophagus medially (Fig. 12C). This plane is then developed down to the prevertebral fascia. Very careful dissection in this area is necessary to possibly identify the recurrent laryngeal nerve, which lies in the tracheoesophageal groove.

4. The plane between the esophagus and the prevertebral fascia is then developed to mobilize the trachea and esophagus to the right (Fig. 12D); this is a clear vascular plane, and careful finger dissection can be used to develop it as far inferiorly as possible. A spinal needle is then inserted into at least two of the disc spaces visualized at this point and an X-ray is taken to corroborate their identity. This step helps determine whether this exposure will be sufficient without proceeding to resection of the distal third of the clavicle or manubrium (Fig. 12E).

5. Further dissection to expose the anterior surface of the spine is then carried out with cautery and blunt dissection as far inferiorly and superiorly as possible. Self-retaining retractors are placed under the prevertebral muscles to complete the exposure. Depending on the pathology, this may provide sufficient visualization to carry out the necessary work (Fig. 12F).

6. If exposure is not adequate at this point, the next step would be to extend the skin incision along the vertical plane and resect the medial one-third of the clavicle. To do this, the sternal and clavicular heads of the sternomastoid muscle are detached from their insertions by cautery and retracted superiorly and laterally. The strap muscles (sternothyroid and sternohyoid) are sectioned just above the clavicle and sternal notch and retracted superiorly and medially. The sternal origin of the pectoralis major muscle is stripped laterally off the body of the sternum and the inferior border of the me-

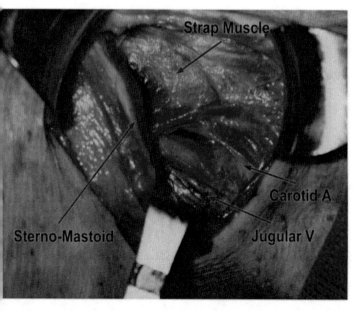

FIGURE 12C. The sternomastoid has been mobilized laterally and away from the strap muscles, which go medially. The carotid sheath is exposed and mobilized laterally with the internal jugular vein.

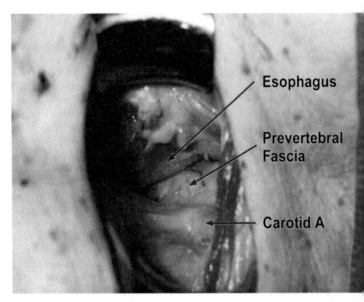

FIGURE 12D. Clear demonstration of the avascular plane anterior to the prevertebral fascia and the esophagus. Finger dissection superiorly and inferiorly is easy here and should be used to expose the anterior surface of the spine.

dial third of the clavicle. The clavicle is stripped subperiosteally and then sectioned using a Gigli saw (Fig. 12G). This segment of clavicle is then disarticulated from the manubrium and the joint here is resected with rongeurs. Great care must be exercised here to prevent injury to the innominate vein. This maneuver may now afford adequate exposure to the affected area by allowing wider lateral mobilization of the vessels and more medial mobilization of the esophagus and trachea (Fig. 12H).

7. If more room is needed, progressive resection of the manubrium can then be carried out using a power saw or drill to carve away as large a window as necessary. The

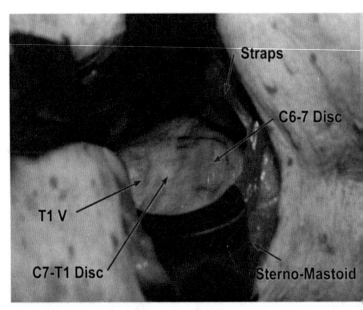

FIGURE 12E. Exposure before taking X-rays to verify the level.

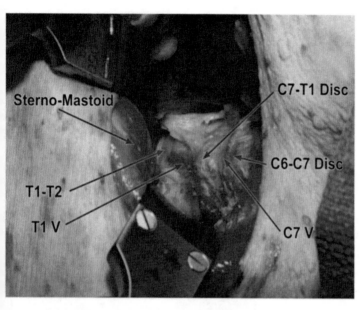

FIGURE 12F. After X-rays have documented the levels, the paravertebral muscles are elevated and further exposure carried out as far distally as necessary. Note that the T1–T2 disc space is accessible at this point without taking the clavicle or the manubrium.

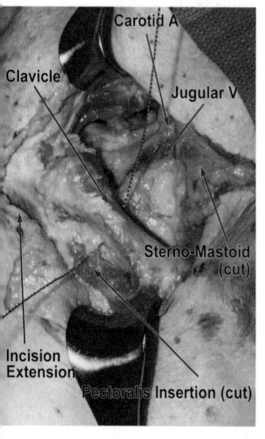

FIGURE 12G. Skin incision has been extended and preparation for resection of the clavicle is complete.

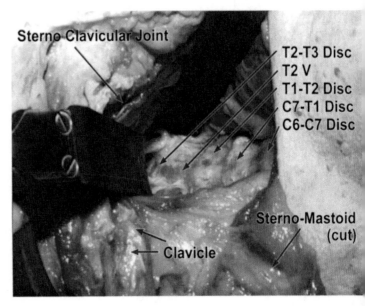

Sterno-Clavicular Joint

T2-T3 Disc
T2 V
T1-T2 Disc
C7-T1 Disc
C6-C7 Disc

Sterno-Mastoid (cut)

← Clavicle

FIGURE 12H. After resection of the clavicle, exposure can now be carried out to the T2–T3 level.

inferior thyroid vein can be ligated and the innominate vein mobilized inferiorly. The thymus and surrounding fat behind the manubrium can be dissected and mobilized to the right or resected if necessary.

8. We have been able to perform partial vertebrectomy and tumor resection at T2–T3, with fusion using a strut graft, without resection of either the clavicle or the manubrium. This procedure allows for much quicker recovery with less morbidity than if the bony structures must be resected.

9. Closure: Anatomical layers including the platysma can be approximated with running absorbable sutures. If the clavicle is transected, it can be replaced in situ if not used as a strut graft. The strap muscles should be reapproximated with running absorbable sutures, and the sternomastoid can be reattached to the periosteum in similar fashion. Suction drains may be used under the flaps as necessary, and the skin is closed with staples.

Remember:

1. Adequate exposure may be obtained through a transverse supraclavicular incision alone, but plan to extend vertically if necessary.
2. Try to identify the recurrent laryngeal nerve at the tracheoesophageal groove.
3. Watch out for the innominate vein beneath the manubrium.
4. Try to stay within the avascular plane between the prevertebral fascia and the esophagus.

Transsternal Approach to the Cervicothoracic Junction

Narayan Sundaresan • *Alfred A. Steinberger* • *Frank Moore*

The cervicothoracic junction represents one of the more complex areas of the spine because of the proximity of visceral and vascular structures at the thoracic inlet. With the introduction of magnetic resonance imaging (MRI), it is apparent that most tumors, infections, and degenerative processes result in compression of the cord from a ventral direction. Logically, therefore, direct anterior approaches offer the best exposure for direct decompression of the spinal cord. In the majority of cases, restoration of spinal stability by reconstruction of the resected segments represents an equally important goal of surgery. Such reconstruction should be carried out in conjunction with instrumentation to achieve rigid and immediate internal fixation.

In 1957, Cauchoix and Binet described a direct approach to the cervicothoracic region through median sternotomy.[1] In their classic approach, the skin incision included two parts: a cervical component along the anterior border of the sternomastoid muscle and a thoracic incision in the midline, carried down to the xyphoid process. The sternum was completely split and retracted. Although median sternotomy provides complete access to the cervicothoracic segments from C4 down to T4, complete median sternotomy is not always indicated for standard approaches. During the past decade, we and others have described a variety of modifications to this original operative procedure.[2–8]

Clinical indications for this operative exposure include not only lesions involving the spine but also tumors of the superior mediastinum (thymomas), as well as the management of vascular injuries involving the innominate artery.[7–9] For spinal lesions, this approach is indicated for tumors, tuberculosis involving the cervicothoracic junction, trauma with collapse of the upper thoracic vertebra, and the correction of cervicothoracic kyphosis.

Surgical Anatomy

The thoracic inlet is kidney shaped with an average anteroposterior diameter of 5 cm and a transverse diameter of 10 cm. It is bounded by the first thoracic vertebra posteriorly, the top of the manubrium anteriorly, and the 1st ribs on each side. Its plane slopes forward and downward, but there is considerable variation in the size, shape, and obliquity of the inlet. The sternomastoid muscle arises from the sternum and clavicle by two heads (Fig. 13A). The sternal head is a rounded fasciculus that is tendonous and arises from the upper part of the anterior surface of the manubrium. The clavicular head is more fleshy and arises from the superior border and anterior surface of the medial third of the clavicle. The infrahyoid strap muscles lie more posteriorly. The sternohyoid muscle arises from the posterior surface of the medial end of the clavicle, the posterior sternoclavicular ligament, and the posterior surface of the manubrium and medial end of the 1st rib. Important vascular structures in the superior mediastinum include the innominate, common carotid, and left subclavian arteries arising from the arch of the aorta. The innominate artery originates from the convexity of the aortic arch and passes obliquely upward, backward, and to the right. A high-riding arch with a more distal origin of the innominate artery may necessitate considerable retraction if a right-sided approach is used.

The vagus nerve and its branches are the most important nerves to identify in the neck (Fig. 13B). The vagus nerve is (1) motor to all smooth muscle, (2) secretory to all glands, and (3) afferent from all mucous surfaces in the following parts: the pharynx (lowest part), larynx, trachea, bronchi, and lungs; esophagus (entire), stomach, and gut down to the left colic flexure; liver, gallbladder, and bile passages; pancreas and pancreatic ducts; and perhaps spleen and kidney; (4) motor to all muscles

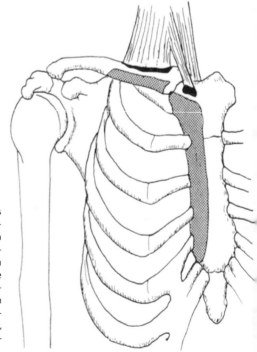

FIGURE 13A. Muscular and tendonous attachment of the origin of the sterno-cleidomastoid muscle is shown on the sternum and the clavicle. The sternal head is tendonous and arises from the anterior superior part of the manubrium. (From O'Shea J, Sundaresan N, Stein Berger A, Moore F. In Menezes A, Sonntag VKH (eds): Principles of Spinal Surgery. New York, McGraw-Hill, 1996, p 1254, with permission.)

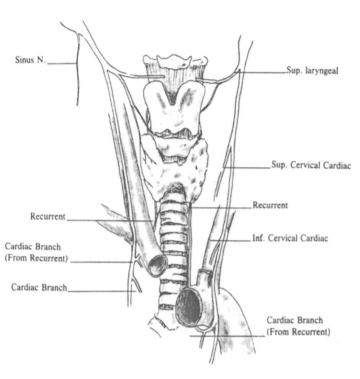

Sinus N.

Sup. laryngeal

Sup. Cervical Cardiac

Recurrent

Recurrent

Inf. Cervical Cardiac

Cardiac Branch
(From Recurrent)

Cardiac Branch

Cardiac Branch
(From Recurrent)

FIGURE 13B. The branches of the vagus nerve in the neck include the recurrent layngeal nerve, the superior clavicular nerve, the superior laryngeal nerve, and inferior cervical cardiac and cardiac branches from the recurrent laryngeal nerve. (From O'Shea J, Sundaresan N, Stein Berger A, Moore F. In Menezes A, Sonntag VKH (eds): Principles of Spinal Surgery. New York, McGraw-Hill, 1996, p 1255, with permission.)

of the larynx, all muscles of the pharynx (except the stylopharyngeus), and all the muscles of the palate (except the tensor veli palatini); (5) the conveyor of taste from the few taste buds about the epiglottis; (6) inhibitory to cardiac muscle; and (7) sensory to the outer surface of the eardrum, the external acoustic meatus, and the back of the auricle. In the neck, the vagus nerve gives (1) a pharyngeal branch to the superior and middle constrictors and muscles of the soft palate; (2) the superior laryngeal nerve, via the internal laryngeal nerve, is sensory to the larynx above the vocal cords and to the lowest part of the pharynx and, via the external laryngeal nerve, motor to the inferior constrictor and cricothyroid and (3) a twig (sinus nerve) to the carotid sinus, and (4) two cardiac branches.

The recurrent laryngeal nerve arises from the vagus and courses around the subclavian artery on the right and around the aortic arch on the left. It traverses the operative field obliquely at a higher level on the right; on the left side, it reaches the tracheoesophageal groove more caudally and is thus less liable to injury with a left-sided exposure. In addition, the recurrent laryngeal nerve may occasionally be nonrecurrent on the right side and take a more direct course. On the left side, no such anatomical variations are seen. For this reason, a left-sided approach to the cervicothoracic region is generally recommended.

Another important structure that is potentially vulnerable to injury is the thoracic duct (Fig. 13C). At this level, it usually lies to the left of the midline and empties at the junction of the internal jugular and subclavian veins posteriorly. Occasionally, it may divide into two branches, one emptying on the left side and the other into the right subclavian vein with the right lymphatic duct. The right lymphatic duct is much less prominent and should not be encountered during this dissection.

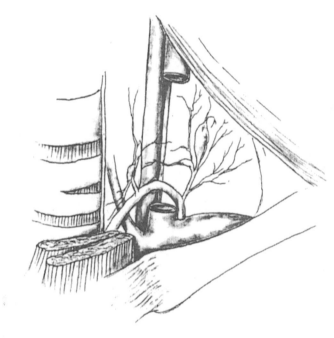

FIGURE 13C. The thoracic duct was to the left of the midline and empties into half the junction of the internal jugular subclavian veins posteriorly. (From O'Shea J, Sundaresan N, Steinberger A, Moore F. In Menezes A, Sonntag VKH (eds): Principles of Spinal Surgery. New York, McGraw-Hill, 1996, p 1255, with permission.)

Operative Approach

The operation is performed under general endotracheal anesthesia with the patient placed in the supine position. In patients with unstable spines, awake nasotracheal intubation may be performed at the discretion of the surgeon. Arterial lines and wide-bore intravenous lines are used, as well as compression stockings for the lower extremities. The neck is extended slightly using a folded sheet under the shoulders and a doughnut under the head. The range of extension and flexion of the neck is tested preoperatively with the patient awake. In patients with obvious instability, a halo traction device is applied and traction maintained intraoperatively. We currently monitor somatosensory evoked potentials (SSEP) routinely, as well as an image intensifier that is draped in place. Both arms are positioned by the sides, and traction bands are applied to both wrists to pull the arms down for lateral radiographic imaging during the procedure.

  1. Two different skin incisions may be used: a vertical incision along the medial aspect of the sternomastoid extending along the midline of the sternum down to the xyphoid, or a transverse incision 1 cm above the clavicle that is then extended in the shape of a T over the sternum (Figs. 13D1, 13D2).

  2. After the skin incision is made, it is deepened with cautery through the platysma, and subplatysmal flaps are elevated and retained by sutures (Figs. 13E1–13E3). Alternatively, the skin flaps may be retracted by fishhooks. Several veins (the anterior jugular veins and the jugular venous arch) and the medial supraclavicular nerve may cross the operative site and need to be sectioned and securely ligated with silk sutures.

  3. The sternal and clavicular heads of the sternomastoid are detached from their bony origins by cautery, as shown in Figure 13F1. Figures 13F2 and 13F3 demonstrates detaching the sternomastoid from the manubrium and left clavicle by cautery. This muscle is retracted superiorly and laterally. The strap muscles (sternohyoid and sternothyroid muscles) on the ipsilateral side are sectioned just above the clavicle and retracted

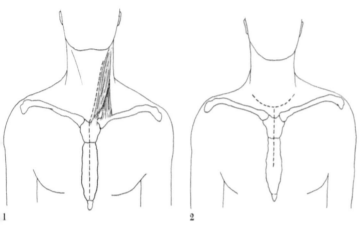

FIGURE 13D. (1) The vertical incision extends along the medial border of the sternocleidomastoid to the midline of the sternum extending down the xyphoid process. (2) The transverse incision is 1 cm above the clavicle and then is extended in the shape of a "T" over the sternum. (From O'Shea J, Sundaresan N, Stein Berger A, Moore F. In Menezes A, Sonntag VKH (eds): Principles of Spinal Surgery. New York, McGraw-Hill, 1996, p 1256, with permission.)

superiorly and medially (Fig. 13G). All fatty and areolar tissues in the suprasternal space are cleaned.

4. The clavicle should be stripped of its muscle attachments so that it can be removed; these muscles include the pectoralis major inferiorly, the subclavius posteriorly, and the trapezius laterally. The sternal origin of the pectoralis major muscle is stripped subperiosteally, as far laterally as possible. Great care should be taken to protect the undersurface of the clavicle to prevent injury to the subclavian vein (Fig. 13H). The medial half of the clavicle should then be resected. The lateral cut can be done with either a Gigli saw or a microsagittal saw (Figs. 13I1, 13I2). To free the medial end, the cartilage of the sternoclavicular joint must be removed piecemeal with rongeurs (Fig. 13I3). The resected clavicle (Fig. 13I4) can be fashioned into an excellent strut graft to replace the resected vertebral bodies. Resection of the clavicle enhances the overall exposure and allows vascular control of the innominate arteries of the ipsilateral side.

5. At this juncture, a decision must be made as to the necessity of sternal resection: the sternum can be removed partially (manubrium alone), or completely split (sternotomy). Manubrial resection may not always be necessary in thin patients with long necks, and others without kyphosis, in whom the second thoracic segment can be reached by the transcervical exposure alone. To remove the manubrium, a finger is inserted underneath the inner surface and all soft tissue structures are bluntly dissected from its undersurface. To remove a portion of the manubrium, as shown in the inset in Figure 13J, we use the B1 cutting bit of the Midas Rex (craniotomy bit). Alternatively, a small portion of the manubrium may be drilled out with a round bur. Brisk bleeding may accompany this maneuver, and all bone edges must be waxed. The most important vascular structure that traverses the superior mediastinum is the innominate vein, which is generally higher in young infants and children. The thymus and surrounding fat may obscure the operative approach and may be resected.

6. The avascular plane between the carotid sheath laterally and the trachea and esophagus medially is identified and developed down to the prevertebral fascia (Fig. 13K). Once the prevertebral fascia and longus coli muscles are identified, handheld Cloward retractors are inserted and the plane expanded in the cephalocaudal direction. In a left-sided exposure, an attempt must be made to identify the recurrent laryngeal nerve, which lies in the tracheoesophageal groove on the left. On the right, it generally crosses the prevertebral area and is more liable to injury. The level of dissection can now be confirmed by intraoperative radiography. The level may be difficult to visualize from lateral views alone, and we generally place a needle at a higher interspace and then count downward to confirm the correct level.

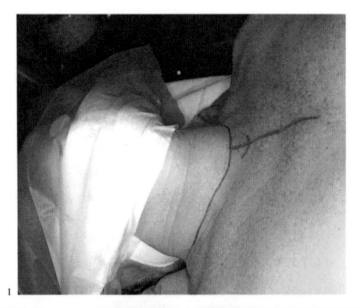

1

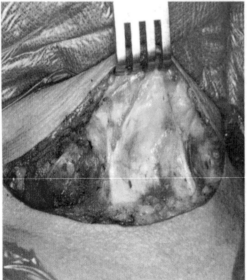
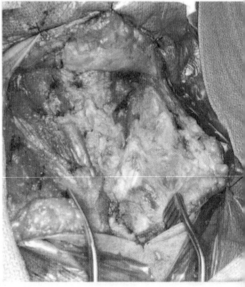

2

FIGURE 13E. (1) The skin incision for the transverse "T" is demonstrated with skin markings. (2) The development of the subplatysmal flaps shows the clavicle visible in the wound. (3) The strap muscles with their insertion into the clavicle and sternum.

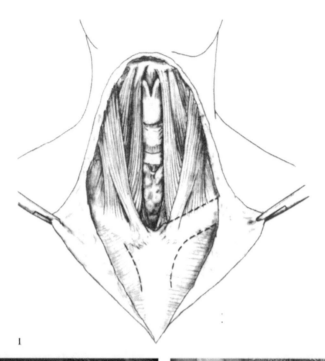

1

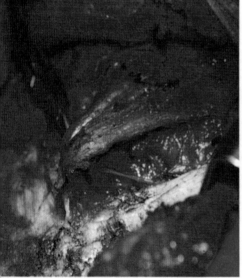

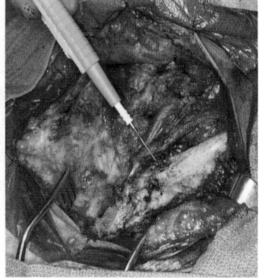

3

FIGURE 13F. (1) The anterior throat with the strap muscles and their incursions onto the clavicle and sternum. The thyroid cartilage and gland are visible in the depth of the wound. (From O'Shea J, Sundaresan N, Stein Berger A, Moore F. In Menezes A, Sonntag VKH (eds): Principles of Spinal Surgery. New York, McGraw-Hill, 1996, p 1257, with permission.) (2) The insertions of the muscular tendon of the clavicle and manubrium are removed, revealing the underlying bony structure. (3) The clavicle is marked for resection.

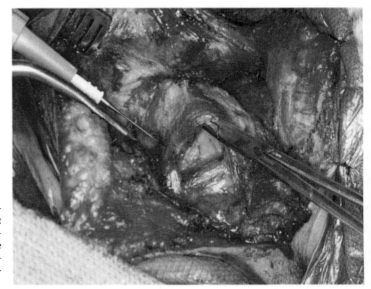

FIGURE 13G. The sternomastoid is resected from the manubrium and left clavicle by cautery, the muscle is retracted superior and laterally, and the strap muscles on the ipsilateral section just above the clavicle are retracted superior and medially.

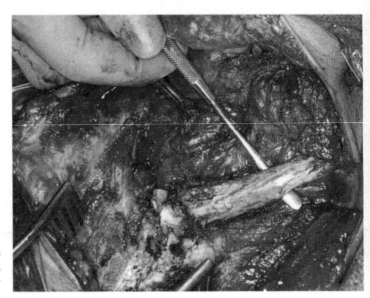

FIGURE 13H. The medial half of the clavicle is removed with the Gigli saw, and the underlying tissue is protected.

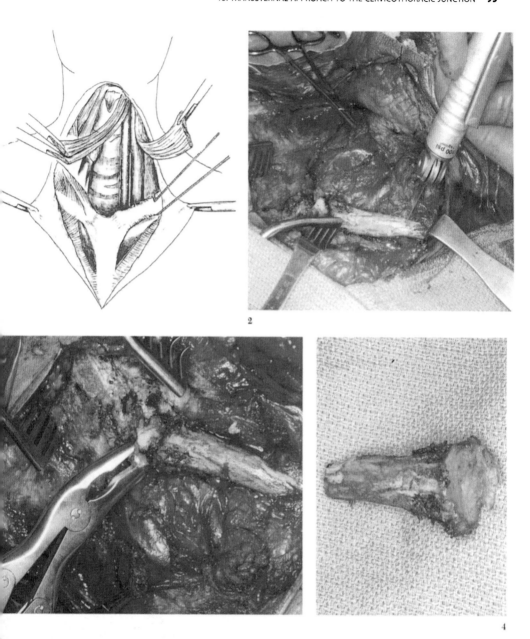

FIGURE 13I. (1) The strap muscles are detached from the clavicle and the Gigli saw is used to section the clavicle. (From O'Shea J, Sundaresan N, Stein Berger A, Moore F. In Menezes A, Sonntag VKH (eds): Principles of Spinal Surgery. New York, McGraw-Hill, 1996, p 1257, with permission.) (2) The clavicle is osteotomized and the cartilage of the sternoclavicular joint exposed. (3) The cartilage of the sternoclavicular joint is removed and the piece of clavicle is freed. (4) The clavicle with its articular cartilage. Removal of this articular cartilage allows use of the clavicle as graft.

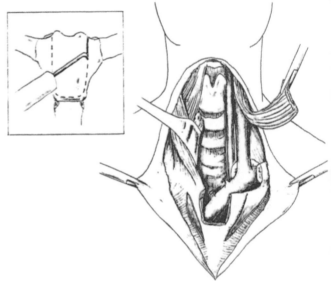

FIGURE 13J. Clavicle, sternohyoid cla-vicular, and manubrium have been sectioned and removed. (From O'Shea J, Sundaresan N, Stein Berger A, Moore F. In Menezes A, Sonntag VKH (eds): Principles of Spinal Surgery. New York, McGraw-Hill, 1996, p 1258, with permission.)

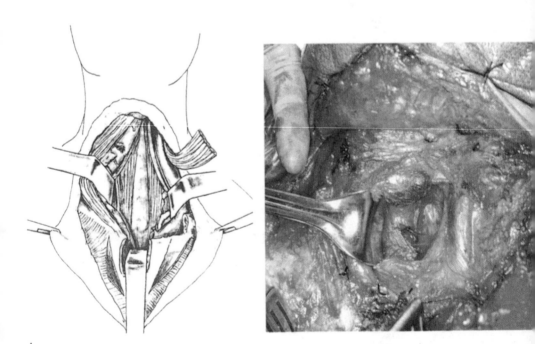

FIGURE 13K. (1) Prevertebral fascia and longus coli exposed. (From O'Shea J, Sundaresan N, Stein Berger A, Moore F. In Menezes A, Sonn-tag VKH (eds): Principles of Spinal Surgery. New York, McGraw-Hill, 1996, p 1258, with permission.) (2) The avascular plane between the carotid sheath laterally and the trachea and esophagus medially is identified and developed down to the prevertebral fascia.

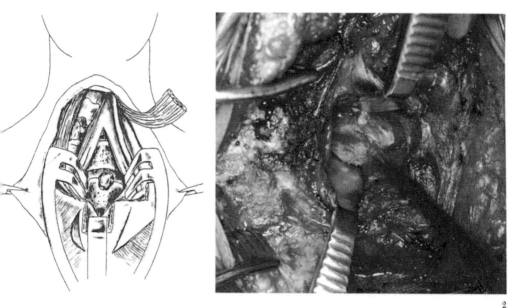

2

FIGURE 13L. (1) Self-retaining retractors are positioned under the longus coli. (From O'Shea J, Sundaresan N, Stein Berger A, Moore F. In Menezes A, Sonntag VKH (eds): Principles of Spinal Surgery. New York, McGraw-Hill, 1996, with permission.) (2) The jugular vein is clearly visible.

7. After identifying the correct spinal levels, the longus coli muscles are stripped from the front of the spine using cautery. In addition, the ligaments and periosteum overlying the vertebral bodies are stripped laterally as far as possible. Self-retaining retractors are then placed with the sharp edges underneath the longus coli muscles (Fig. 13L). The disc spaces above and below the level of involvement are identified and removed with angled curettes and rongeurs. Occasionally, a high-speed drill may be required to drill the bodies if they are sclerotic. All involved bone including the posterior longitudinal ligament should be removed with Kerrison rongeurs. In patients with tumors, the posterior longitudinal ligament is invariably involved by tumor and should be removed. Dissection should be extended laterally to free involved nerve roots that may be compressed by bone fragments. Meticulous hemostasis is obtained using bipolar cautery under constant saline irrigation.

8. Following decompression, stabilization is accomplished in several ways. Following single-level vertebrectomies in cancer patients, immediate stability can be achieved using methyl methacrylate constructs held in place by Steinman pins. In others, bone fusion may be necessary. The resected clavicle is an excellent strut graft; this is cut to an appropriate length with an oscillating saw and positioned in the defect. We currently use titanium plates (Orion or Morscher) in virtually all patients to supplement the bone graft (Fig. 13M). The correct positioning of intraoperative implants is checked by intraoperative X-rays.

9. The wound is closed in anatomical layers. We recommend drainage of the wound with soft suction drains and generally close the skin with staples (Fig. 13N).

10. In patients with three-column involvement, a second-stage or simultaneous posterior fixation is necessary; this can be accomplished by segmental fixation using hook constructs or sublaminar wiring. In some patients, following laminectomy, pedicle, screws (3.5-mm diameter) are used. Pedicle screws in the cervicothoracic region are technically more difficult to place, and we recommend the use of a frameless stereotaxy system such as the Stealth to achieve correct intraoperative placement.

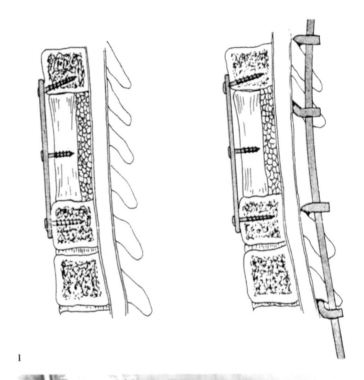

1

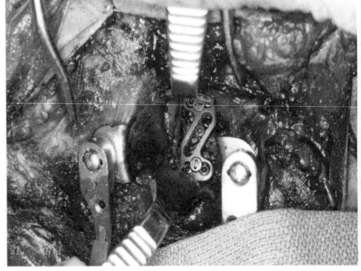

FIGURE 13M. (1) After resection, stabilization is performed with the clavicle as bone graft and anterior plates (Orion or Morscher). If three-column involvement is present, a second-stage or simultaneous posterior instrumentation is performed. (From O'Shea J, Sundaresan N, Stein Berger A, Moore F. In Menezes A, Sonntag VKH (eds): Principles of Spinal Surgery. New York, McGraw-Hill, 1996, with permission.) (2) The spinal plate is inserted through the exposed area, the self-retained retractors demonstrate the spine clearly.

2

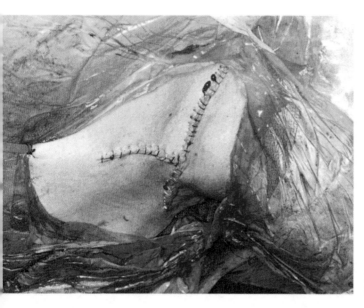

FIGURE 13N. The final closure of the T incision.

Postoperative Management

The length and complexity of the surgery determine the duration of intubation. In long, complicated cases, especially in elderly patients, it may be prudent to leave the endotracheal tube in place for about 12 to 24 hours to allow postoperative laryngeal swelling to subside. Patients undergoing shorter procedures can be extubated early. Many patients may have temporary hoarseness from traction of the recurrent laryngeal nerve. Older patients with prolonged surgery may have superior laryngeal nerve weakness (with inability to clear their secretions and the danger of possible aspiration). Postoperative mobilization is usually begun with patients in a Philadelphia collar, which is kept on for 8 to 12 weeks.

Remember:

1. Always try to perform this exposure from the left side to minimize the possibility of injury to the recurrent laryngeal nerve.
2. Remember that the innominate vein lies underneath the clavicle and is potentially vulnerable to injury.
3. This operative exposure provides as much access as the complete median sternotomy. Several modifications of this procedure have been proposed, the major feature of which is sparing of the clavicle; the alternative is performing a complete sternotomy. Kurtz et al. have proposed several modifications of our approach, which are reasonable.[10] Instead of a T-shaped incision, the horizontal limb is made only on the side of the approach. They leave the manubrium intact and use a combination of methyl methacrylate and bone graft. Nazzaro et al. have described an extension of this procedure that combines a partial medial sternotomy with an anterolateral thoracotomy but requires the services of a thoracic surgeon.[11] Their approach may be appropriate for tumors with extensive anterolateral soft tissue involvement.
4. If there is significant kyphosis with collapse of the vertebra, it may be necessary to remove the normal vertebra above the collapse to reverse the kyphosis and decompress the cord.

References

1. Cauchoix J, Binet J: Anterior surgical approaches to the spine. Ann R Coll Surg Engl 27:237–243, 1957.
2. Micheli LJ, Hood RW: Anterior exposure of the cervicothoracic spine using a combined cervical and thoracic approach. J Bone Joint Surg 65A:992–997, 1983.
3. Sundaresan N, Shah J, Foley KM, Rosen G: An anterior surgical approach to the upper thoracic vertebra. J Neurosurg 61:686–690, 1984.
4. Sundaresan N, Shah J, Feghali JG: Transsternal approach to the upper thoracic vertebra. Am J Surg 198:473–477, 1984.
5. Charles R, Grovender S: Anterior approach to the upper thoracic vertebra. J Bone Joint Surg 71B:81–84, 1989.
6. Krespi YP, Har-El G, Nash M: The transcervical approach to the superior mediastinum. Otolaryngol Head Neck Surg 107(1):7–13, 1992.
7. Johnson RH Jr, Wall MJ Jr, Matto KL: Innominate artery trauma: a thirty-year experience. J Vasc Surg 17(1):134–140, 1993.
8. Clark GC, Lim RC, Rosenberg JM: Cervico-thoracic vascular injuries: presentation, management and outcome. Am Surg 57(9):582–586, 1991.
9. Sundaresan N, Schmidek H, Schiller A, Rosenthal D: Tumors of the Spine: Diagnosis and Management. Philadelphia, Saunders, 1993.
10. Kurtz LT, Pursel SE, Herkowitz HN: Modified anterior approach to the cervicothoracic junction. Spine 16:542–547, 1991.
11. Nazzaro JM, Arbit E, Burt M: Trapdoor exposure of the cervicothoracic junction. J Neurosurg 80:338–341, 1994.

Transaxillary Approach to the Upper Dorsal Spine

Roger C. Breslau

For female patients, and for males of slender build, the transaxillary transthoracic approach is an alternative to the posterior parascapular approach to the upper dorsal spine. The highest dorsal vertebra reached through this approach is the body of T1, although the C7–T1 interspace is often accessible at the extreme apex of the thoracic inlet. The most significant advantage of this approach is that no major muscle groups are sectioned during the procedure, and there is rapid functional recovery of shoulder girdle mobility. The principal disadvantage of the approach is its limited exposure compared with that obtained by complete mobilization of the scapula. The approach is not indicated in obese individuals or in males of substantial muscular build with hypertrophic pectoralis major and latissimus dorsi muscles. The approach described here is from the right side, although the left-side approach is commonly used.

1. Position the patient with the right side of the torso elevated 60 degrees or more. The complete left lateral decubitus position can be used. Carefully protect the wrist and forearm to the elbow with padded circular dressings. Abduct the upper extremity and flex the elbow. Affix the padded forearm to an "L" bar at the anesthesiologist's end of the table. Do not cover the arm with a sterile stockinette, as the operative field can be satisfactorily prepped and draped using standard orthopedic technique, excluding the portion of the upper extremity distal to the midbiceps (Fig. 14A).

2. Place the incision transversely at the base of the natural axillary hairline, and deepen it by electrocautery in the most direct manner to the chest wall. Divide the pectoralis musculature (Fig. 14B).

Caution: It is important to avoid undermining the succulent axillary soft tissues by oblique dissection.

3. Once the chest wall is reached, dissect upward to the apex of the thorax in an avascular plane. By palpation, identify the tight circle of the 1st rib within the circle of

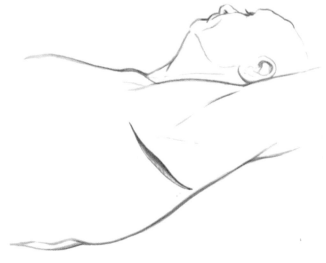

FIGURE 14A. The transaxillary approach to the upper dorsal spine. Position the patient with the left side of the torso elevated 60 degrees or more after protecting the wrist and forearms to the elbow with padded circular dressings. Abduct the upper extremity and flex the elbow. Drape the portion of the upper extremity distal to the midbiceps. The incision is transverse at the base of the natural axillary hairline.

the 2nd rib. The 3rd rib is of principal surgical interest for gaining access to the upper dorsal spine.

4. The relatively large sensory intercostobrachial nerve emerges from the second intercostal space and contributes innervation to the inner aspect of the entire upper arm, as well as a minor sensory "twig" that penetrates he pectoralis major muscle and innervates a patch of prepectoral skin (Figs. 14C, 14D). Avulse this sensory nerve at its point of emergence from the intercostal space and excise a 4- to 5-cm peripheral segment of the nerve. Of course, you should inform the patient preoperatively that this procedure will be done and that there will be postoperative numbness of the denervated area. The altered sensation that follows surgery is not bothersome to most pa-

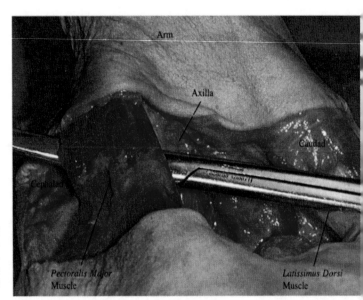

FIGURE 14B. Division of the pectoral muscles is not debilitating and responds to postoperative rehabilitation. Avoid tangential dissection into the succulent axillary tissue and cut directly to the chest wall.

tients and is gradually overcome within several months by sensory ingrowth from adjacent neural segments.

Avulsion of this sensory nerve on a regular basis is preferable to attempting its preservation, because approximately 2%–3% of patients undergoing transaxillary surgery without taking the nerve suffer the late complication of intercostobrachial neuralgia, which is an extremely incapacitating condition requiring frequent axillary blocks and often late neurectomy.

5. After positively identifying the 3rd rib, score the overlying lateral periosteum with electrocautery as far in each direction as possible. Standard periosteal elevators, such as Alexander, Matson, and Doyen instruments, are used to facilitate subperiosteal resection of so long a segment of rib as can be visualized. Use handheld Deaver retractors to maximize exposure between the two major muscles (see Chapter 16).

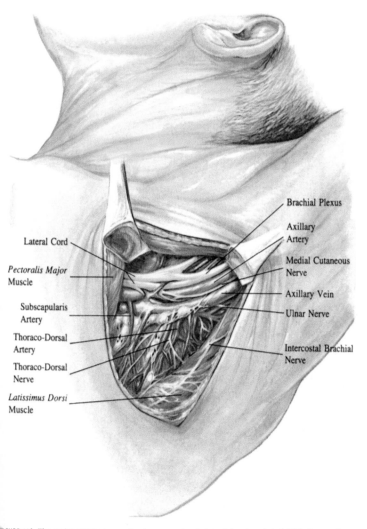

FIGURE 14C. The major arteriovenous structures are retracted medial and cephalad. With direct palpation, feel the ribs and enter the plane just superficial to the chest wall.

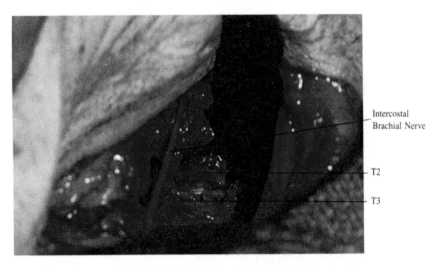

FIGURE 14D. The relatively large sensory intercostal brachial nerve emerges from the second intercostal space and contributes innervation to the inner aspect of the entire upper arm, as well as a minor sensory twig that penetrates the pectoralis major muscle and innervates a patch of prepectoral skin. Avulse this nerve at its point of emergence from the intercostal space and excise a 4- to 5-cm pe-

ripheral segment of the nerve. Removal of the nerve avoids the late complication of intercostal brachial neuralgia, which is an extremely incapacitating condition. The vertebral bodies are visualized in the depth of the wound after removal of parietal pleura and intercostal vessels over the vertebral bodies.

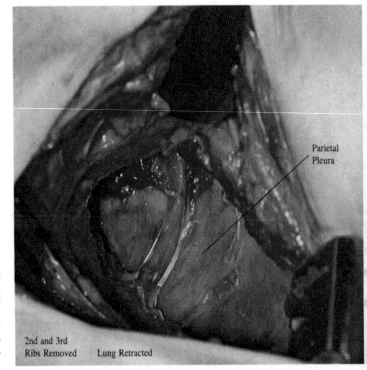

FIGURE 14E. Once the chest wall is reached, identify the 2nd and 3rd ribs, and remove the midportion of the 3rd rib using standard thoracotomy technique (Chapters 15 and 16). After removal of the rib, the rid bed consists of periosteum, fascia, parietal pleura, and sometimes adherent lung.

6. Excise the segment of mobilized rib with Bethune rib shears and smooth the rib ends with box-end Sauerbruch rongeurs. Enter the thorax through the bed of the resected 3rd rib, taking care to avoid injury to the underlying lung. As soon as the parietal pleura is breached (Fig. 14E), the upper lobe of the lung will drop away (Fig. 14F), complete the pleuroperiosteal incision with scissors.

7. Widen the aperture between the 2nd and 4th ribs with a pediatric rib spreader, or even a sternal spreader. Have the anesthesiologist temporarily interrupt positive pressure insufflation of the lung to permit packing of the upper lobe downward with moist laparotomy pads.

8. Carefully incise the pleura overlying the lateral vertebral bodies of T1–T5. Retract the open parietal pleura and dissect bluntly with a Kitner the raised, softer, white intervertebral disc. The intercostal arteries and veins cross the middle of the vertebral body. Dissect out and ligate the intercostal arteries and veins at each level required. Mobilize and retract or divide and oversew the azygous vein (Fig. 14D; also see Chapter 16).

9. Closure: Attempt to close the parietal pleura over the spine. Fully expand the right lung by positive pressure inhalation via the endotracheal tube. Gentle digital massage of the subpleural tissues helps eliminate remaining "islands" of patchy atelectasis. Insert a pleural drainage tube through the 9th intercostal spine to the apex.

To avoid the rare occurrence of postoperative pleural "hernia" through the bed of the missing 3rd rib, resulting in a tender "bursa-like" structure within the axilla, one can loosely tack a patch of Marlex or Mersilene mesh over the rectangular defect between the cut ends of the 3rd rib and the 2nd and 4th ribs. Close the rib bed with interrupted permanent-type sutures of braided Dacron. Monofilament sutures are not

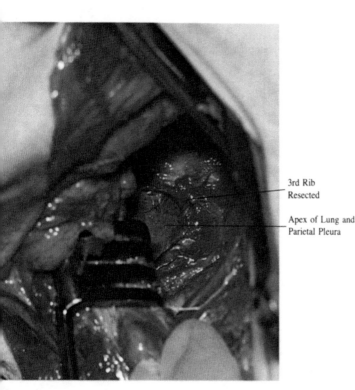

3rd Rib
Resected

Apex of Lung and
Parietal Pleura

FIGURE 14F. Enter the thorax through the bed of the resected 3rd rib. In opening the parietal pleura, take care to avoid injuring the underlying lung. Identify the lung. Bluntly dissect the apex of the lung and extend the opening of the parietal pleura to the full extent of the wound. Pack the upper lobe of the lung downward with moist laparotomy pads. Visualization of the parietal pleura covering and the exposure of the spine is the same as described in Chapters 15 and 16.

recommended. No routine muscular closure is required in the axilla, as no muscles are cut in this approach except for the infrequent need to section partially the pectoralis major muscle for improved anterior exposure. Approximate loosely the axillary soft tissues with interrupted or continuous sutures of the polyglycolic acid type. It is important to leave a suction drain in the depths of the axillary space because of pronounced drainage from transected lymphatic channels during the first 48 to 72 hours following operation. Bring the drain out through a small stab wound inferior to the principal incision. Connect the suction drains to a renewable evacuator of the Jackson–Pratt type. Close the skin with subcuticular 3–0 Prolene.

Additional Anatomy

Important anatomical features that will be noted in the region of primary orthopedic interest are the right innominate vein superiorly; the esophagus, trachea, and superior vena cava medially; and the large azygous vein joining the superior vena cava just above the takeoff of the right mainstem bronchus. The supreme intercostal vein lies just lateral to the insertion of the longus coli muscle, which covers the upper dorsal bodies; sacrifice this vein as the longus coli is reflected (see Fig. 15E). Identify the prominent dorsal sympathetic chain, seen easily through the translucent posterior pleura as it courses over the necks of the upper ribs. The ganglia are easily palpated, and injury to them may be avoided without difficulty; however, the medial rami may have to be sectioned to approach the spinal column.

Remember:

1. Avoid oblique dissection in the axilla.
2. Cut the pectoralis muscles as needed.
3. Identify the 3rd rib in the plane of the chest wall.
4. Identify and avulse the intercostobrachial nerve.
5. Remove the 3rd rib.
6. Incise the parietal pleura over the spine and ligate vascular structures over the vertebral bodies.

Reference

1. Hodgson AR, Yau ACMC: Anterior surgical approaches to the spine. In Apley AG (ed): Recent Advances in Orthopaedics. Baltimore, Williams & Wilkins, 1964, pp 289–323.

Third Rib Resection in the Transthoracic Approach

The 3rd rib resection is used for the transthoracic approach to the T1–T4 area. Resection of the 3rd rib allows greater spreading of the intercostal area than does 2nd rib resection.[1] The cephalad extension of the exposure is enhanced with kyphosis deformity of the cervicothoracic junction area. Exposure of the 3rd rib allows additional removal of the 2nd rib if the operative exposure is inadequate.

1. Place the patient in the lateral decubitus position with the left side up. Prep and drape the entire left upper extremity, draping it sterilely out of the operative field.

2. Incise the skin and subcutaneous tissue from the lateral paraspinous area at T1, along the medial caudal border of the scapula, under the axilla to the costal cartilage of the 3rd rib (Fig. 15A).

3. Carefully divide each subsequent muscle layer down to the level of the rib, sectioning portions of the trapezius, latissimus dorsi, rhomboid major, and serratus posterior (Fig. 15B, 15C), as needed. Careful dissection with electrocautery and meticulous cauterization of each muscle bleeding point allows exposure to the outer periosteum of the 3rd rib with a minimal amount of bleeding. As the muscle layers are divided, retract the scapula cephalad and medially to tense the muscle tissue for easier cutting. Palpate cephalad for identification of the 3rd rib (Fig. 15C). Remember that the 1st rib is situated inside the 2nd; this is important for reaching the correct rib level.

4. For pathology such as large tumors of the cervicothoracic junction, several ribs, including the 1st can be resected, allowing for a large working area to C6. The limiting factor is that a stable rib must be left for support of the scapula.[2]

5. Dissect the external periosteum off the 3rd rib with the rib periosteal elevators (see Chapter 16). Excise the 3rd rib from the angle of the rib to the costal cartilage (Fig. 15D).

6. Open the rib bed as in the standard thoracotomy approach, having provided protection for the lung.

7. Open the intercostal area with the Feochetti rib spreader and retract the lung with the spatula-type lung retractor.

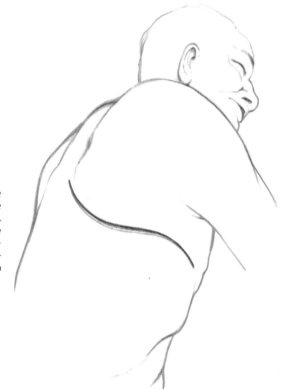

FIGURE 15A. Place the patient in the lateral decubitus position with the left side up. Prep the entire extremity. Drape it out of the sterile operative field. Incise the skin and subcutaneous tissue from the lateral paraspinous area of T2 under the scapula to the costal margin of the 3rd rib.

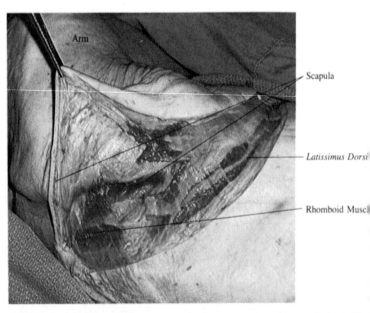

FIGURE 15B. Carefully divide with electrocautery each subsequent muscle area down to the level of the 3rd rib. Section portions of the trapezius, latissimus dorsi, rhomboid major, and posterior serratus as needed. Control the intermuscular bleeding points.

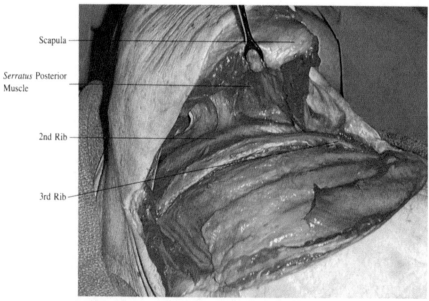

Scapula

Serratus Posterior Muscle

2nd Rib

3rd Rib

FIGURE 15C. Elevation of the scapula aids in the division of the muscles attached to the scapula and allows visualization of the 3rd rib. Palpate cephalad on the chest wall for positive identification of the 3rd rib. Remember, the 1st rib is located inside the 2nd rib and is sometimes missed.

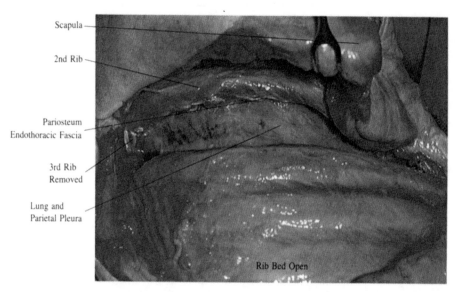

Scapula

2nd Rib

Pariosteum Endothoracic Fascia

3rd Rib Removed

Lung and Parietal Pleura

Rib Bed Open

FIGURE 15D. Excise the 3rd rib from the angle of the rib to the costal cartilage, using the technique described in Chapter 16. The rib bed consists of periosteum, endothoracic fascia, and parietal pleura. Incise this parietal pleura, carefully avoiding damage to the underlying lung. Use small forceps to pick up the rib bed and carefully open it with a knife. If necessary, dissect the lung from the undersurface of the pleura and extend the incision with scissors. Insert the rib spreader and retract the lung with the spatula-type lung retractor.

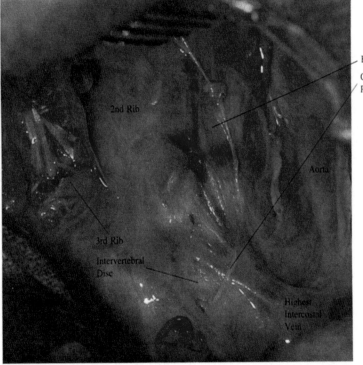

Body of C2

Cut Edge of
Parietal Pleura

2nd Rib

Aorta

3rd Rib

Intervertebral
Disc

Highest
Intercostal
Vein

FIGURE 15E. After insertion of the spreader and retraction of the lung, identify the parietal pleura. Palpate the larger, more prominent white surface of the intervertebral disc, remembering that the major intercostal vessels course over the vertebral bodies, which are the valleys between the discs. As the venous drainage is different on the right side than on the left side of the body, these veins should be identified and not damaged. Elevate the parietal pleura with small forceps and incise with a knife. Extend the incision longitudinally over the vertebral bodies the length of the necessary operative field. Carefully dissect under the pleura as it is opened. By opening only the parietal pleura, the underlying venous and arterial structures can be preserved.

8. Identify in the wound the aorta, the spine, ribs, parietal pleura, and veins under the parietal pleura. The highest intercostal vein is usually well visualized in this area (Fig. 15E).

9. Open the parietal pleura delicately with Adson's pick-ups and Metzenbaum scissors over the costovertebral articulations (Fig. 15F).

10. Identify the prominent soft or white tissue of the intervertebral disc; this is a relatively avascular, safer plane for dissection than the surface of the vertebral body.

11. Dissect, tie, and ligate each intercostal vessel over the vertebral body.

12. Bluntly elevate the soft tissue from the vertebral body.

13. Closure: Visualize the lung fully expanded in all areas. Close the parietal pleura over the spine whenever possible. Place the chest tube through a separate aperture, preferably in the 9th intercostal spine. Protect the lung during closure. Close the chest with the rib approximator. Close the rib bed with interrupted permanent braided Dacron sutures. The chest tube connects to the water seal. With the lung reexpanded the chest tube can usually be removed within 48 to 72 hours, depending on drainage and expansion of the lung.

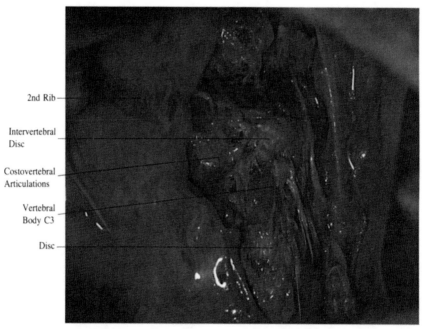

2nd Rib

Intervertebral
Disc

Costovertebral
Articulations

Vertebral
Body C3

Disc

FIGURE 15F. Begin dissection on the intervertebral disc, the safer, more avascular plane. After exposing the necessary intervertebral disc, dissect out and divide the intercostal arterial structures over the surface of each vertebral body. A large vein such as the highest intercostal vein may be ligated and divided as needed. Continue until the necessary vertebral bodies are exposed. With closure the parietal pleura should be resutured.

Additional Anatomy[3]

The venous drainage of the upper thorax is predominantly supplied by the highest intercostal vein. On the left side, this vein drains from the Ist to the 5th or 6th intercostal space. It varies in size inversely to the accessory hemiazygos vein, which is just caudal to this area. The highest intercostal vein passes across the arch of the aorta and left subclavian vein to drain into the left brachiocephalic vein. Variations of venous structures may produce a large, very prominent highest intercostal vein that will need careful ligation. Arterial supply consists of intercostal branches off the aorta posteriorly and anterior intercostal arteries from the internal thoracic artery. The highest intercostal artery ascends under the pleura across the 1st and 2nd ribs in the area of their base to anastomose with the first aortic intercostal. The thoracic sympathetic chain and its ganglia include the first thoracic ganglion, which usually combines the inferior cervical ganglion into a satellite ganglion that lies over the neck of the 1st rib, and the 2nd through 12th cervical ganglia, which lie closer to the intervertebral disc area over the spine.

Remember:

1. Cut the muscles binding the scapula to the chest wall and retract the scapula cephalad.
2. Identify and remove the 3rd rib carefully.
3. Incise the pleura and ligate veins over the vertebral bodies.

References

1. Hodgson AR, Yau ACMC: Anterior surgical approaches to the spinal column. In Apley AG (ed): Recent Advances in Orthopaedics. Baltimore, Williams & Wilkins, 1964, pp 289–323.
2. Dawson E: Personal communication.
3. Goss CM (ed): Gray's Anatomy of the Human Body, 29th edn. Philadelphia, Lea & Febiger, 1973.

Thoracotomy Approach

Use the standard thoracotomy approach for safe exposure of vertebral levels T2–L2. Proper rib selection depends on the pathology for most cases, especially those involving a strut graft. The rib to resect for a certain vertebral level is chosen by one of two methods:

1. When the pathology dictates a direct anterior approach to the vertebral column, that is, kyphotic TB abscess, choose the rib directly horizontal to the vertebral level at the midaxillary line in an anteroposterior (AP) chest X-ray. The rib removed must be cephalad to the lesion to give adequate proximal exposure while working down the lesion.[1]
2. When direct access to the spinal canal is needed at one disc, that is, a thoracic disc excision, resect the rib that leads to that disc, that is, 9th rib to the T8–T9 disc.

There are anatomical variations at the cervicothoracic and thoracolumbar junctions that dictate the rib to be taken. For patients with a large abscess in the right chest or in other circumstances that dictate a right thoracic approach, be prepared to mobilize the vena cava and associated veins from that side.

1. Place the patient in the lateral decubitus position. Approach from the left side, as it is much easier to handle, the aorta and the segmental vessels from the left side.

With the patient in a supine position, insert a double-branched endotracheal tube into the right and left mainstem bronchi to allow selective collapse of the left lung. A standard endotracheal tube may also be used. When the left chest is chosen for the approach, place the patient in the right lateral decubitus position. Center the midthorax of the patient over the break in the table. Pad well under the dependent axilla; pad and protect the left arm. Stabilize the pelvis with a strap to the table, place a pillow between the legs, and pad all bony prominences.

2. Open the skin and subcutaneous tissue from the lateral border of the paraspinous musculature to the sternocostal junction over the rib to be resected. Placing the thoracotomy incision slightly tangential to the rib to be resected allows easier resection of more than one rib if necessary (Fig. 16A).

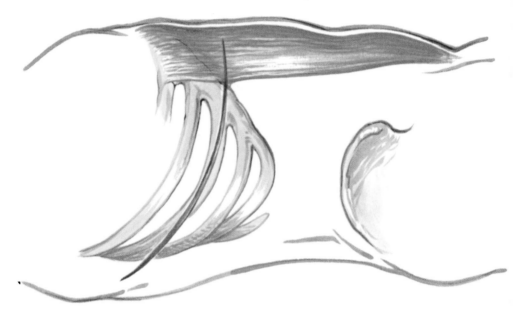

FIGURE 16A. Using the lateral decubitus position, make the standard thoracotomy skin incision over the rib to be resected. The rib to resect for a vertebral level is usually the rib directly horizontal to the vertebral level at the midaxillary line in an anteroposterior (AP) chest X-ray. The approach is cephalad to the lesion, as it is better to resect a rib that allows one to work down on the lesion rather than a more distal rib, which would necessitate working up to the lesion. For sco-liosis, the approach is from the convexity of the lesion, and for non-scoliotic conditions the approach from the left side is preferred. Open the skin of subcutaneous tissue from the lateral border of the paraspinous musculature to the sternocostal junction over the rib to be resected. Placing the thoracotomy incision slightly tangential to the rib to be resected allows easier resection of more than one rib if necessary.

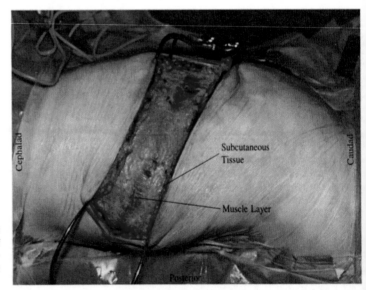

FIGURE 16B. Using electrocautery, cut directly to the outer periosteum of the rib through any intervening muscle or subcutaneous tissue. Obtain adequate hemostasis.

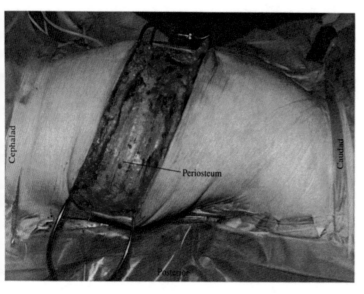

Cephalad

Caudad

Periosteum

Posterior

FIGURE 16C. Cut directly to bone through the outer periosteum of the rib with electrocautery.

Insert self-retaining retractors and extend the wound with electrocautery down through the muscle layers of the thorax. When needed for full exposure, section the latissimus dorsi, trapezius, and rhomboid major and minor muscles.

3. After exposure of the chest wall (Fig. 16B), count the ribs from the 12th up to the appropriate rib or from the 1st rib downward. The 1st rib appears to be inside the 2nd when one is palpating from this angle and it is often difficult to find. Each rib articulates with the superior portion of the body in the area of the disc space of the level above. Therefore, the 12th rib inserts closer to the T11–T12 intervertebral disc space. X-ray confirmation can be obtained if necessary.

4. Expose the outer periosteum of the rib with the electrocautery and cut directly to bone through the periosteum from the angle of the rib to the costal cartilage (Fig. 16C). Elevate the periosteum off the outer rib surface (Fig. 16D). Use the curved-tip rib elevator to strip the superior and inferior borders of the rib, maintaining an intact elevated periosteum, and use the Doyen to elevate the inner periosteum of the under-surface of the rib (Fig. 16E).

Caution: Avoid damaging the intercostal vessels that course on the inferior surface of the rib. Elevate the periosteum of the rib by cutting with the elevator directly on bone. Avoid plunges that might inadvertently enter the pleura.

5. With the intact periosteum freed from the rib, cut the rib with the rib cutter as far posteriorly as necessary between the costotransverse joint and the angle of the rib, and anteriorly at the costal junction (Fig. 16F). Remove the rib and save it for bone graft. Bone wax the end of the rib lightly after rasping to make sure there are no ragged edges. Tie a sponge on the tip of the stump for protection to the surgeon during the procedure.

6. Pick up the inner periosteum of the rib bed with Adson forceps and open the rib bed with scissor tips (Fig. 16G). To avoid lung and pleural adhesions just under the rib, complete the opening of the rib bed with a semiclosed scissor after using a finger to clear lung from the undersurface. When pleural adhesions exist, first attempt to dis-

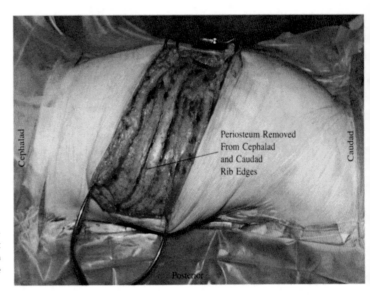

Cephalad

Periosteum Removed
From Cephalad
and Caudad
Rib Edges

Caudad

Posterior

FIGURE 16D. Using the periosteal elevator, elevate the periosteum first from the outer surface of the rib, then the superior surface, followed by the inferior surface of the rib.

sect bluntly with the finger or a sponge stick. If necessary, sharply dissect dense adhesions and ligate vascular structures.

7. Retract the lung medially with the spatula lung retractor. Remove retraction of the lung at least every 20 min to allow adequate expansion of the lung and to prevent postoperative atelectasis. Insert the Feochetti separator in the rib resection defect with moist lap sponges over the edges. Expand the Feochetti to allow adequate visualization inside the thoracic cavity. Flexion of the table may be of benefit.

8. The anatomy of the spine at this point is obscured by the reflection of the parietal pleura as it covers the soft tissue structures over the spinal column

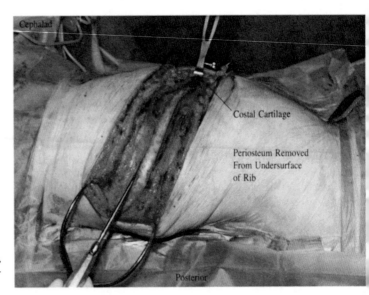

Cephalad

Costal Cartilage

Periosteum Removed
From Undersurface
of Rib

Posterior

FIGURE 16E. Using the Doyen elevator, remove the periosteum from the undersurface of the rib.

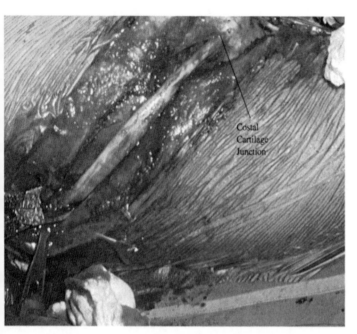

Costal
Cartilage
Junction

FIGURE 16F. Cut the rib as far posteriorly as necessary between the costotransverse joint and the angle of the rib and anteriorly at the costal cartilage junction. Remove the rib. Bone wax lightly the end of the rib after rasping to make sure there are no ragged edges. If necessary, tie a sponge on the tip of the stump for protection to the surgeon during the procedure.

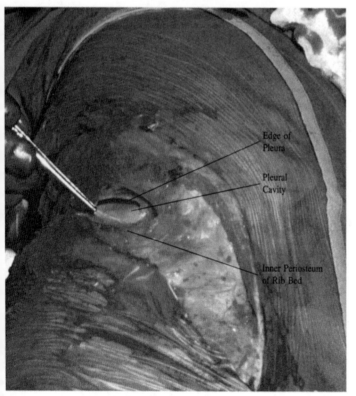

Edge of
Pleura

Pleural
Cavity

Inner Periosteum
of Rib Bed

FIGURE 16G. Pick up the inner periosteum of the rib bed with Adson forceps and open the rib bed with scissor tips or fine dissection with a knife blade. To avoid lung and pleural adhesions just under the rib, complete the opening of the rib bed with a semiclosed scissor, using a finger to clear lung from the undersurface. With the rib bed open, place the Feochetti rib-separating retractor and retract the lung with a spatula lung retractor.

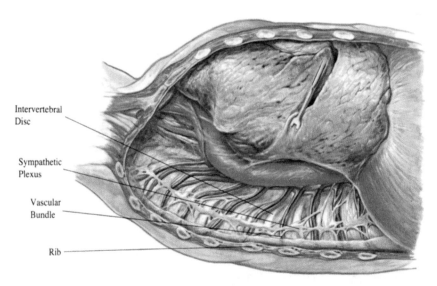

Intervertebral
Disc

Sympathetic
Plexus

Vascular
Bundle

Rib

FIGURE 16H. The spine, aorta, intercostal vessels, and parietal pleura. Under the parietal pleura, the intercostal artery and vein cross the vertebral body at each level. The prominent disc space is the raised, white, firm, and avascular landmark that will allow delineation of the intercostal vessel at each level as it passes over the midvertebral body. The thoracic duct may pass from right to left in the T4–T5 area. The sympathetic plexus ideally should be preserved, but interruption at this level is not of major consequence.

(Figs. 16H, 16I, 16J). Elevate the parietal pleura with Adsons and open it with Metzenbaum scissors. Extend the opening of the parietal pleura in a cephalad and caudad direction on the spine by cutting over a peon dissected under the pleura. The presence of a large para-vertebral abscess at this point means only that the abscess should be exposed just as the spine would be. When present, cut the outer wall of the abscess longitudinally and approach the spine through the abscess.

9. Identify the disc, which is the more prominent, softer, white structure of the spine (Fig. 16K). The discs are relatively avascular and a much safer area for dissection. An intercostal vein and artery cross the midportion of each vertebral body.

10. Bluntly dissect the cut edges of the parietal pleura off the spine with a "Kitner" or sponge (Fig. 16L). Elevate it on the discs and lift it off the vessels on the vertebral body. Dissection begun over the disc is less likely to cause bleeding. After the parietal pleura is opened, it may be sutured back on itself laterally with two stay sutures.

11. Separate, sever, and ligate each of the intercostal vessels over the vertebral body. If there is a large paravertebral abscess, the arteries enter the abscess. Care should be taken to avoid clamping segmental arteries too close to the aorta, so as to lose the tie, or too close to the intervertebral foramen. Tie arteries and veins separately or together depending on their size. Pass the right-angle clamp under the vessels and use a woven 2–0 suture in a free tie to tie off first the medial and then the lateral exposed vessels, or use vascular clips in a similar fashion.

Caution: Take care to dissect adequately under the vessels, as a common mistake is to have both ligature sutures in the same place under the vessel and not have adequate room for cutting between them. Handle every segmental vessel in the area of the bony work in this manner. A vascular etiology for paralysis due to ligation of a segmental artery on the vertebral body has not been a problem.[1]

Caution: Do not dissect into the intervertebral foramen.

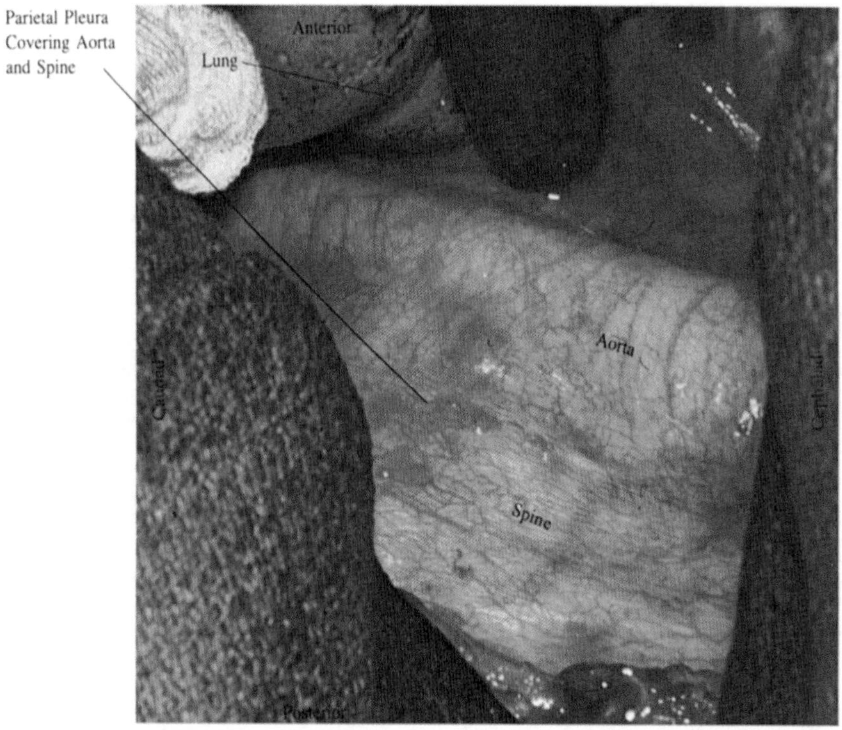

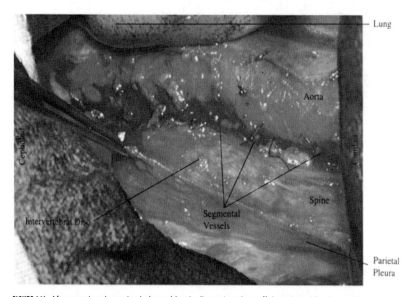

Parietal Pleura Covering Aorta and Spine

Anterior

Lung

Caudad

Aorta

Cephalad

Spine

Posterior

FIGURE 16I. The parietal pleural covering of the aorta and spine. Elevate the parietal pleura with Adson forceps and open it carefully with Metzenbaum scissors. Extend the opening of the parietal pleura in a cephalad and caudad direction by gently dissecting the soft tissues from the undersurface of the pleura, passing a peon under the parietal pleura and opening it safely with scissors. A large paravertebral abscess encountered at this time should be opened, exposing the spine just as one would in a nonabscessed case. It is sometimes difficult to remove the parietal pleura from the abscessed cavity itself, and it can be opened simultaneously.

Lung

Aorta

Cephalad

Caudad

Spine

Intervertebral Disc

Segmental Vessels

Parietal Pleura

FIGURE 16J. After opening the parietal pleura, bluntly dissect its edges off the spine with a "peanut" or sponge. The parietal pleura may be sutured back laterally with stay sutures when necessary for continued retraction.

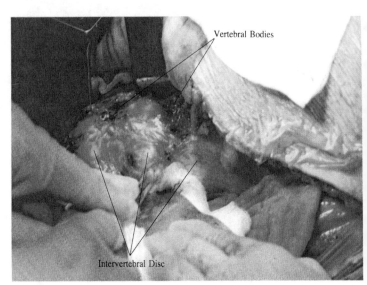

FIGURE 16K. Begin this dissection by first identifying the intervertebral disc—the prominent, softer, whiter structure of the spine.

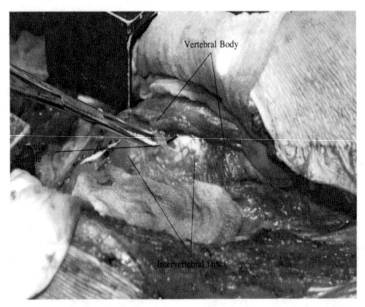

FIGURE 16L. Separate, cut, and ligate each of the intercostal vessels over the vertebral body. Care should be taken to avoid tying segmental arteries too close to the aorta, as the tie might loosen. Tie arteries and veins either separately or together depending on their size. Pass the right-angle clamp under the vessels and use a woven 2-0 suture as a free tie to tie off the exposed vessels first medially and then laterally. Avoid dissection of vessels into the intervertebral foramen. When a paravertebral abscess is present, cut directly through the abscessed wall and clamp and ligate intercostal vessels as they are encountered in the abscessed wall. According to need, all the soft tissue can be dissected bluntly from the midline outward to expose the spine and remove all soft tissue from the surface of disc and vertebral bodies.

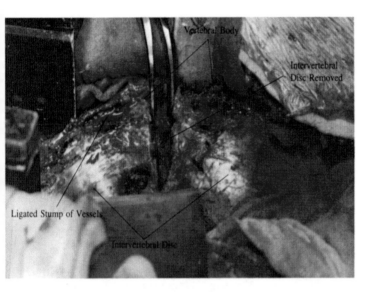

Vertebral Body

Intervertebral
Disc Removed

Ligated Stump of Vessels

Intervertebral Disc

12. After division of the segmental vessels, bluntly expose the outer surface of the spine (Fig. 16M). When bone and disc exposure is needed, cut with the cautery directly to bone. Use the periosteal elevator to dissect the annulus of the disc and the periosteum of the bone medially and laterally to expose the entire disc and vertebral column. The tendency is to not dissect the soft tissue laterally enough off the spine (Figs. 16N, 16O, 16P). The rib head articulates with the cephalad half of its appropriate vertebral

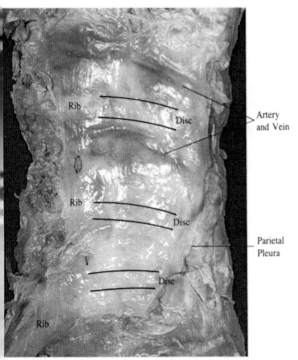

Rib

Disc

Rib

Disc

Disc

Rib

Artery
and Vein

Parietal
Pleura

FIGURE 16N. The parietal pleural covering of the spine, intervertebral disc, vertebral bodies, intercostal vessels, and rib articulations.

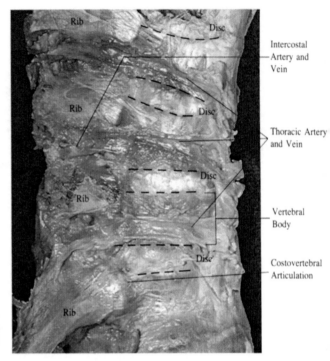

FIGURE 160. After removal of the parietal pleura, the disc spaces are easily visualized along with the intercostal vessels.

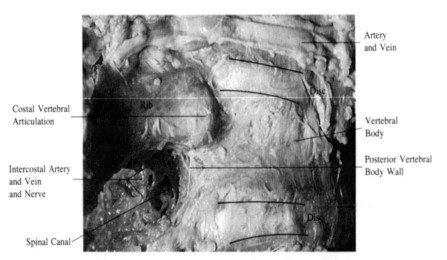

FIGURE 16P. The rib articulates with the cephalad half of its appropriately numbered vertebral body and with the disc space above. Therefore, the 10th rib articulates at T9–T10. Removal of the head of the rib and its articulation allows excellent exposure of the posterior lateral aspect of the intervertebral disc. After removal of rib head and disc, identify the intercostal nerve, dural sac, posterior vertebral body wall, and spinal canal. The costal vertebral articulation is a major stabilizing structure in the thoracic spine.

For exposure of the spinal canal from the anterior approach, one may dissect in the midline or anterolaterally directly through the intervertebral disc, removing intervertebral disc above and below the vertebral body to be resected. This method maintains an avascular field while identifying the posterior annulus of the disc and the posterior body wall. Using the electric bur, dissect directly through the vertebral body after having previously identified its posterior wall at the disc space above and below.

body and the disc space above (Fig. 16M). Resection of the rib head can be used to gain access to the posterior disc and the spinal canal. Identification of the left pedicle in a left-sided approach helps locate the spinal canal for orientation. For complete exposure of the vertebral body, resect the disc above and below to identify the posterior body wall and spinal canal and dissect laterally to identify the pedicle and spinal canal.

13. Closure: Visualize the lung fully expanded in all areas. Close the parietal pleura over the spine whenever possible. Place the chest tube through a separate aperture, preferably in the 9th intercostal space. Protect the lung during closure. Close the chest with the rib approximator. Close the rib bed with interrupted permanent braided Dacron sutures. The chest tube connects to the water seal. With the lung reexpanded, the chest tube can usually be removed within 48 to 72 hours, depending on drainage and expansion of the lung.

Remember:

1. Beware of the intercostal artery and vein on the inferior surface of the rib when removing the periosteum of the rib.
2. Beware of the lung when opening the floor of the rib bed.
3. Open the parietal pleura over the spine approximately $1^1/_2$ inches from the head of the rib.
4. Identify the disc as an avascular area.
5. Tie segmental vessels, leaving an adequate proximal stump.
6. Identify the costovertebral articulation, head of the rib, and pedicle.
7. Close the parietal pleura over the spine.
8. Reapproximate the ribs with woven Dacron suture.

Reference

1. Hodgson AR, Yau ACMC: Anterior surgical approaches to the spinal column. In Apley AG (ed): Recent Advances in Orthopaedics. Baltimore, Williams & Wilkins, 1964, pp 289–323.

17 | The Thoracolumbar Junction

For approaches to the thoracolumbar junction (T10–L1), Hodgson recommends a 9th rib resection.[1] Dwyer recommends a 10th rib resection with the standard thoracolumbar approach.[2] For T12–L1, Perry[3] recommends a 10th rib resection. The rules for resecting the best rib for exposure are much the same in this area as in the rest of the thoracic spine. Ideally, choosing the rib in the midaxillary line opposite the lesion or the apex of a curve allows adequate proximal exposure for working "down" or caudad on the lesion.

For maximum exposure of T11–T12, transthoracic resection of the 9th rib is usually best, and at T12–L1 a 10th rib thoracoabdominal approach is preferred; these involve detaching the diaphragm at its circumference. In patients in whom it is imperative that the diaphragm not be taken down, or when less exposure is needed, that is, resection of one disc with grafting, the 12th rib approach is used. For L1–L2 exposure, a 12th rib extrapleural, retroperitoneal approach is recommended.

Three additional approaches have use in special situations. The 11th rib approach is the highest practical, extrapleural, retroperitoneal, anterior approach for exposure of T10–L2. It is a more demanding approach with less expansive exposure, but avoids opening the pleural cavity and cutting the diaphragm in potentially high-morbidity patients.

The posterior costotransversectomy approach is a viable alternative for limited extrapleural exposure with low morbidity. By following the 12th subcostal nerve to T12–L1, the vertebral body and spinal canal can be exposed. The visualization needed for total discectomy, vertebrectomy, and strut grafting is inferior when compared with the anterior approach, unless at least two levels are costotransversectomized.

Use the 10th rib thoracolumbar approach for long exposures of the thoracic and lumbar spine because this allows proximal and distal extension for multilevel operations and optimum exposure for bony work.

Caution: Make an exposure that is cephalad enough to be above the entire working area.

Additional Anatomy

For thoracolumbar approaches, the anatomy of the diaphragm is most important. The diaphragm itself is markedly dome shaped, arching cephalad to approximately the T7 level. It is attached distally to the sternal part of the xyphoid process, the costal part to the inner surface of the costal cartilages and ribs 6–12, and to the lumbocostal arches, the crus of the diaphragm, and the lumbar vertebrae. There is a medial and lateral lumbocostal arch (Fig. 17A). The medial lumbar costal arch extends from the crus of the diaphragm and vertebral body, arches over the cephalad portion of the psoas major muscle, and inserts on the anterior surface of the transverse process of L1. The lateral lumbocostal arch extends from this transverse process of L1, arching over the quadratus lumborum muscle to the tip of the 12th rib. The crura of the diaphragm consists of

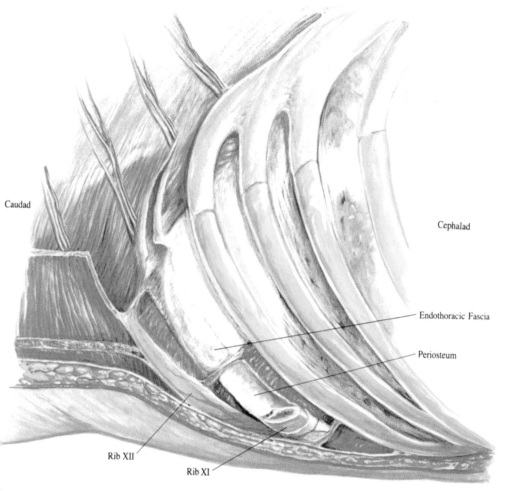

Caudad

Cephalad

Endothoracic Fascia

Periosteum

Rib XII

Rib XI

FIGURE 17A. The extrapleural space may be entered at the tip of the costal cartilage or, sometimes, at the angle of the rib. The extent of the pleura over the 12th rib varies according to its length. In a long 12th rib, there should be a relatively safe area at the tip of the rib to allow entrance into the extrapleural space and identification of the pleura, followed by a blunt dissection of the pleura off the undersurface of the rib bed. The rib bed itself consists of periosteum of the rib, endothoracic fascia, and the parietal pleura.

a large right crus extending down the right side of the L1, L2, and L3 vertebral bodies and a smaller left crus attaching to L1 and L2 (see Fig. 18G). These crura extend cephalad and anterior to approximately the T11–T12 area medially in the midline to form the aortic hiatus. The esophageal hiatus and vena cava foramen lie in the anterior wall of the diaphragm. The aortic hiatus itself also gives passage to the azygos vein and the thoracic duct as well as the aorta. The esophageal hiatus at the approximate level of the 10th thoracic vertebra transmits the vagus nerve and the esophagus. Smaller apertures include those for the splenic nerves and hemiazygos vein. The sympathetic trunk usually enters under the medial lumbocostal arch.

The innervation of the diaphragm is of a central origin and resection should be circumferential approximately 1 inch from the outer perimeter, leaving enough diaphragm to reattach. This procedure should not interfere with innervation of the diaphragm or its function.

The fascial lining of the undersurface of the diaphragm is the transversalis fascia. Its counterpart inside the thorax is the endothoracic fascia, which is the internal investing fascia of the entire inner thoracic cavity. Just as the transversalis fascia covers all muscles, that is, the psoas, quadratus lumborum, and all vascular and bony structures in the abdomen, the endothoracic fascia covers the internal surfaces of the ribs, the superior surface of the cephalad, interthoracic portion of the diaphragm, and includes the paravertebral fascia covering the vertebrae and discs. In a cephalad direction, the endothoracic fascia is continuous with the cervical paravertebral fascia and caudally is continuous with the transversalis fascia, or endoabdominal fascia, as it is sometimes called. The insertion of the diaphragm into the ribs interdigitates with the insertion of the transversus abdominus muscle. These interdigitating slips can be used to reapproximate the slips of diaphragm to their anchoring attachments, especially at the tips of the 11th and 12th ribs (Fig. 17A). Division of the diaphragm should proceed to the crus of the diaphragm. Elevation of the crus of the diaphragm off the involved vertebral bodies to be worked on would usually allow a cephalad retraction of the diaphragm for work on vertebral bodies through L2. By placement of small stay sutures, the location of reattachment areas can be marked as each is taken down. Any costal cartilage that is divided off the tip of the rib on combined thoracoabdominal approaches can, of course, be reapproximated (see Fig. 18D).

The pleural cavity extends over the majority of the 11th rib and the midportion of the 12th rib (see Chapter 20 and Fig. 17A).

References

1. Hodgson AR, Yau ACMC: Anterior approach to the spinal column. In Apley AG (ed): Recent Advances in Orthopaedics. Baltimore, Williams & Wilkins, 1964, pp 289–326.
2. Dwyer AF, Newton NC, Sherwood AA: An anterior approach in scoliosis. Clin Orthop 62:192, 1969.
3. Perry J: Surgical approaches to the spine. In Pierce N, Nichol V (eds): The Total Care of Spinal Cord Injuries. Boston, Little, Brown, 1977, pp 53–79.

Tenth Rib: Thoracoabdominal Approach

1. Place the patient in the lateral decubitus position. Approach from the convexity of the scoliosis or from the left side when possible. A left-sided approach is preferred because of ease of mobilization of the aorta compared with the vena cava. In addition, splenic retraction is easier than hepatic. Incise the skin and subcutaneous tissue from the lateral border of the paraspinous musculature over the 10th rib to the junction of the 10th rib and costal cartilage.[1] Curve the incision anteriorly from the tip of the 10th rib to the lateral rectus sheath and distally down the edge of the sheath as far as necessary for exposure (Fig. 18A). Extend the wound slowly through each muscle layer with the electrocautery. The assistant aggressively picks up bleeders with two Adson forceps.

2. Open the superficial periosteum of the 10th rib to the costal cartilage. A sharp curved periosteal elevator removes the superficial and deep periosteum off the rib. Take care to avoid the neurovascular bundle on the inferior surface of the rib. Cut posteriorly at the angle of the rib and cut at the junction of rib and costal cartilage. Remove the rib. On opening the pleural space, retract the lung and open the rib bed fully with scissors (Fig. 18B). (See Chapter 16.)

3. Split the costal cartilage with a knife along its length (Fig. 18C). Open the undersurface of the costal cartilage and retract the two tags of cartilage[1–3] (Fig. 18D).

4. Bluntly dissect under the retracted split tips of costal cartilage to identify the retroperitoneal space (Fig. 18E). The light areolar tissue of the retroperitoneal fat is the guide to the retroperitoneal space.

5. Bluntly dissect the peritoneum off the inferior surface of the diaphragm. Use a sponge to sweep the peritoneum from the undersurface of first the diaphragm, then the transversalis fascia and abdominal wall.

6. With the peritoneum thus retracted, open the abdominal musculature (the external oblique, the internal oblique, and the transverse abdominis) carefully one layer at a time with complete hemostasis. At this point, the chest and retroperitoneal space are open and the diaphragm is the intervening structure in the wound (Figs. 18E, 18F).

7. Incise the diaphragm from inside the chest with clear visualization under the diaphragm in the retroperitoneal space (Fig. 18G). Extend the incision in the diaphragm circumferentially 1 inch from its peripheral attachment to the chest wall.[4] Use marker clips throughout the takedown of the diaphragm to allow accurate reapproximation.

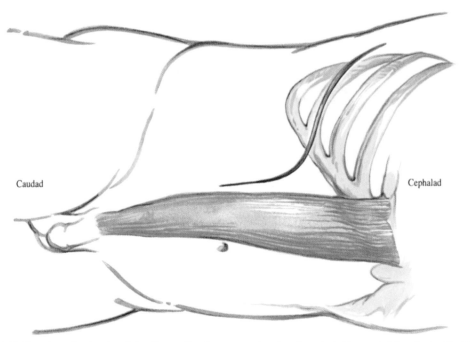

FIGURE 18A. Place the patient in a lateral decubitus position. Approach from the convexity of the scoliosis or from the left side as indicated. A left-sided-approach is preferred because of ease of mobilization of the aorta compared with the vena cava. Incise the skin and subcutaneous tissue from the lateral border of the paraspinous musculature over the 10th rib to the junction of the 10th rib and costal cartilage. Curve the incision anteriorly from the tip of the 10th rib to the lateral rectus sheath and distally down the edge of the sheath as far as necessary for exposure. Extend the wound slowly through each muscle layer to the periosteum of the 10th rib, and remove the 10th rib from the angle of the rib to the costal cartilage as in Chapter 16.

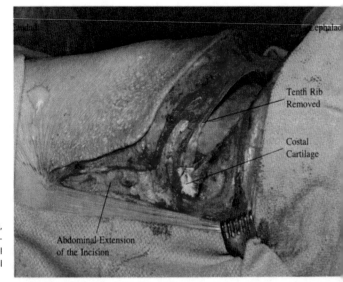

FIGURE 18B. With the rib removed, carefully delineate the costal cartilage. At this point, the intrapleural cavity is opened; the retroperitoneal cavity is still closed.

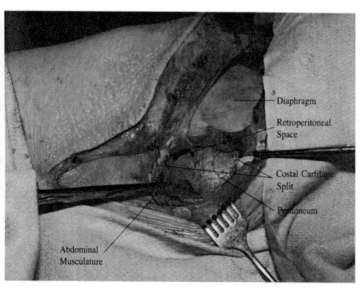

Diaphragm

Retroperitoneal
Space

Costal Cartilage
Split

Peritoneum

Abdominal
Musculature

FIGURE 18C. Split the costal cartilage. Open only the most superficial layer of soft tissue under the costal cartilage enough to allow retraction of the cartilage tips.

8. For work on T12–L1: Resect the diaphragm to the spine. Cut the crus of the diaphragm and elevate it off the spinal column (Fig. 18H). Use protected Deaver retractors to retract the peritoneal sac anteriorly. Use a large rib retractor such as the Feochetti to open the 10th rib incision in the chest. The spine is visualized from approximately T6 as far distally in the lumbar spine as is necessary. In the lumbar spine, remove the attachments of the psoas and the crus of the diaphragm from the spine for proper visualization. In the thoracic spine, open the parietal pleura as in the standard thoracotomy approach. Tie and ligate each intercostal artery and vein to allow mobilization of the major

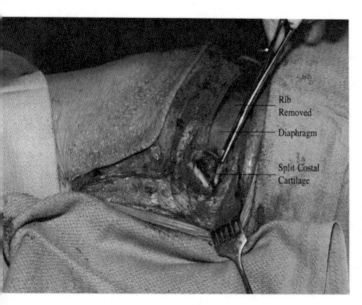

Rib
Removed

Diaphragm

Split Costal
Cartilage

FIGURE 18D. Retract the split tips of costal cartilage. Identify the insertion of the diaphragm into the cephalad cartilage tip and the insertion of the abdominal musculature into the caudad cartilage tip. Bluntly dissect under the retracted tags of cartilage and attached musculature to locate the peritoneum and retroperitoneal space. The light areolar texture of the retroperitoneal fat is the guide to the retroperitoneal space.

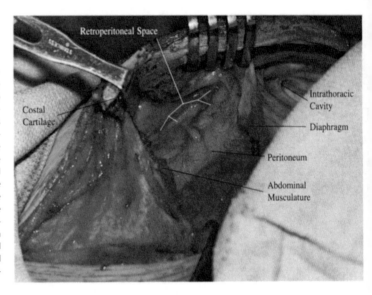

FIGURE 18E. Bluntly dissect the peritoneum off the inferior surface of the diaphragm. Use a sponge to sweep the peritoneum from the undersurface of the diaphragm. The space is expanded under the diaphragm to allow the peripheral detachment of the diaphragm without damaging the peritoneum. Visualize the intrapleural cavity and the retroperitoneal space with the intervening diaphragm. The interpleural cavity and lung and the retroperitoneal space are now well visualized. Sweep the periosteum from the undersurface of the abdominal musculature and open the abdominal wall musculature in the line of incision. (Posterior view.)

vascular trunks. When possible, tie off the thoracic duct, which usually crosses right to left around T4–T5, and avoid the sympathetic plexus. After removal of the intercostal vessels, cut directly to the spine. Dissect on the spine to remove the soft tissue laterally.

9. Closure: The key to closure is the reapproximation of the costal cartilage. After resuturing the diaphragm with multiple interrupted sutures and reapproximating the split cartilage, insert the chest tube in the 8th intercostal space and pass it posterosuperior. Attached to the cephalad half of the costal cartilage is the insertion of the diaphragm and the interthoracic fascia. Inserting into the distal split of costal cartilage is the transverse abdominal fascia and attachment for the abdominal musculature. With

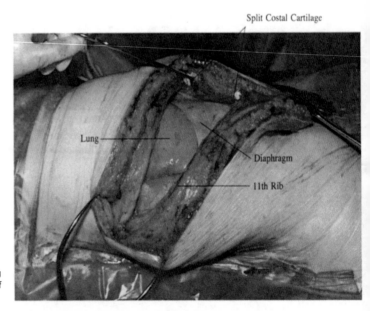

FIGURE 18F. The peritoneum and lung are now protected to allow division of the diaphragm.

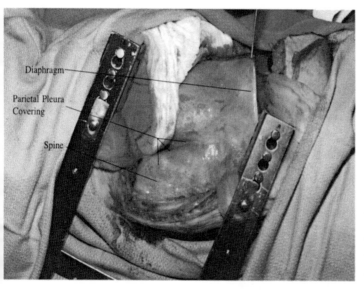

FIGURE 18G. Incise the diaphragm from inside the chest with clear visualization under the diaphragm in the retroperitoneal space. Extend the incision in the diaphragm circumferentially 1 inch from its peripheral attachment to the chest wall. Use marker clips throughout the takedown of the diaphragm to allow accurate reapproximation, The diaphragm is innervated predominantly from a central distribution. The nerve supply should not be damaged with this peripheral detachment. A 1-inch margin allows adequate tissue for suturing and reapproximation. The insertion of the diaphragm on the spine must be removed for bony work on T12–L2.

reapproximation of the costal cartilage, the layers of the abdominal musculature are much better defined. Close each layer of the abdominal wall separately when possible and close the chest as in a standard thoracotomy.

Remember:

1. Split the costal cartilage.
2. Bluntly dissect under the costal cartilage, as the split tags of the cartilage are retracted cephalad and caudad.

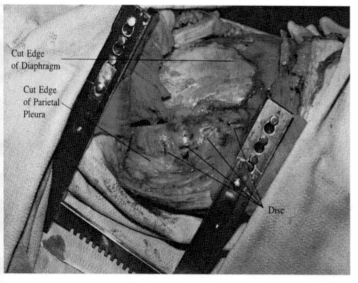

FIGURE 18H. After detachment and retraction of the diaphragm, expose the spine as in Chapter 16. Identify the disc space and clear tissue from it, isolating the intercostal arteries, and severing and ligating each over the vertebral bodies.

3. Identify the soft bubbly character of the retroperitoneal fat.
4. Remove peritoneum from undersurface of the abdominal wall and the diaphragm before incising those areas.
5. Identify the psoas and crus of the diaphragm.
6. Isolate and ligate intercostal vessels over each vertebra. Remember, the 12th and 1st vessels may be covered by the muscular crus of the diaphragm.
7. Reapproximate the split costal cartilage to initiate closure.
8. Close the diaphragm, rib bed, and each muscle layer.

References

1. Riceborough EJ: The anterior approach to the spine for correction of the axial skeleton. Clin Orthop 93:207–214, 1973.
2. Dwyer AF, Newton NC, Sherwood AA: An anterior approach to scoliosis. Clin Orthop 62:192, 1969.
3. Dwyer AF: Experience of anterior correction of scoliosis. Clin Orthop 93:192–201, 1973.
4. Scott R: Innervation of the diaphragm and its practical aspects in surgery. Thorax 20:357, 1965.

Eleventh Rib Approach

1. Make a standard skin incision over the entire length of the left 11th rib. Extend the incision from the rib tip medioinferiorly to the edge of the rectus sheath (Fig. 19A). You can expand the incision by curving the posterior arm cephalad to allow for removal of additional rib and by extending the anterior arm down the abdominal wall vertically for exposure of more of the lumbar spine retroperitoneally.

2. Resect the 11th rib from the angle of the rib to the junction of rib and costal cartilage, leaving the rib bed intact.

3. The most crucial step of the operation is to remain in the extrapleural and retroperitoneal plane at this point.

4. Split the costal cartilage. The insertion of the diaphragm is into the cephalad edge of costal cartilage and adjacent rib bed; likewise, the insertion of the transversus abdominus musculature and transversalis fascia is into the caudad portion. The pleura and the pleural cavity are under the rib bed.

5. The key is to open the split cartilage and dissect carefully under the costal cartilage several inches toward the rib bed to protect the parietal pleura (Figs. 19B, 19C). Do not damage the pleura while the retroperitoneal space is being opened.

6. Bluntly dissect the upper cartilage tag cephalad and the lower tag caudad (Fig. 19C). At this point, identify the retroperitoneal space and the peritoneum. Extend this incision from the level of the costal cartilage medially 3 inches. Divide each muscle layer (external oblique, internal oblique, transversus abdominis) from the tip of the 11th rib.

Caution: The muscle layers thin out dramatically medially and the peritoneum is easily entered. If this happens, repair it immediately with pursestring sutures. After the peritoneum is reached, it is bluntly dissected from the undersurface of the transversalis fascia, the fascia opened, and the peritoneal retracted (Fig. 19D).

7. After exposure of the peritoneum, the parietal pleura must be identified and dissected free intact. Occasionally the pleura extends to the tip of the 11th rib, but usually it passes slightly more proximal to the tip of the 11th rib and across the midportion of the 12th rib (Fig. 19C). The rib bed has three layers: periosteum, endothoracic fascia, and parietal pleura. Open only the periosteum and muscle of the rib bed. Identify

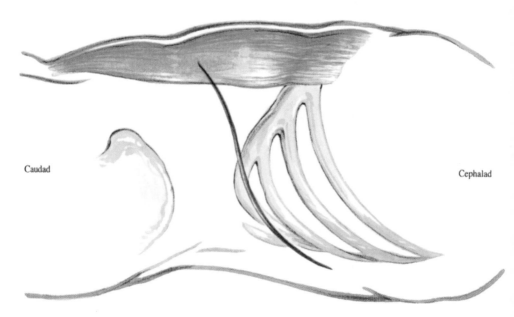

Caudad

Cephalad

FIGURE 19A. Make a standard incision over the left 11th rib extending from the tip of the 11th rib to the edge of the rectus sheath. Remove the 11th rib and split the costal cartilage (as demonstrated in Chapter 18). Separate the split cartilaginous tips and bluntly dissect with utmost care the separating leaves of tissue. Dissect the parietal pleura from the undersurface of the rib bed, starting at the split cartilage.

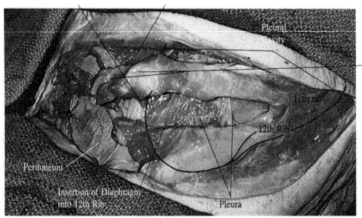

Cartilagenous
Tip of 11th Rib

FIGURE 19B. In a dissected specimen, note the important relationships of the pleura and peritoneum to the cartilage at the tip of the 11th rib. Understanding the anatomy of the undersurface of the 11th rib bed is important in maintaining an extrapleural retroperitoneal approach.

The intimate relationship of the pleural cavity and the peritoneal cavity is seen under the 11th and 12th ribs. The attachment of the abdominal musculature to the cartilage tip of the 11th rib has been removed. The diaphragmatic insertions into ribs 11 and 12 are present. The objective of the dissection is to enter the space between the peritoneal cavity and the pleural cavity.

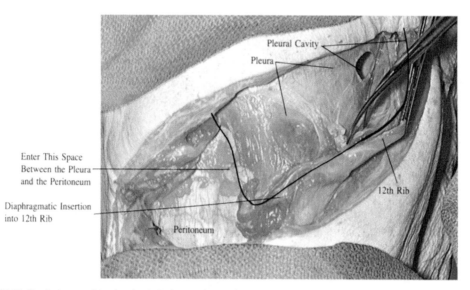

FIGURE 19C. The distal extent of the pleural cavity in close proximity to the peritoneal cavity. Dissection takes place between these two planes in the retroperitoneal, extrapleural space, reflecting cephalad the parietal pleura seen here.

the parietal pleura. Begin the crucial dissection of pleura from the endothoracic fascia of the rib bed. Use cotton gloves or gauze wrapped around the dissecting finger to dissect bluntly toward the spine under the rib bed. Pushing the soft tissue off, dissect very carefully the undersurface of the rib bed. If the pleura is damaged, it should be sutured. After dissection of the pleura, open the rib bed with a scissor. It is the strong fascia of the rib bed that prevents exposure. After the rib bed is opened, insert the Feochetti retractor. If the Feochetti is ineffective because of a small lower rib to retract against, use Deavers. The diaphragm is attached to the tip of the 12th rib. Often this

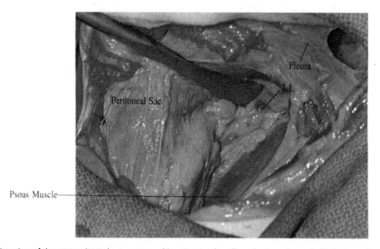

FIGURE 19D. Another view of the retroperitoneal space approaching L1 extrapleurally and retroperitoneally. With the peritoneal sac forward, dissect and retract the pleura cephalad.

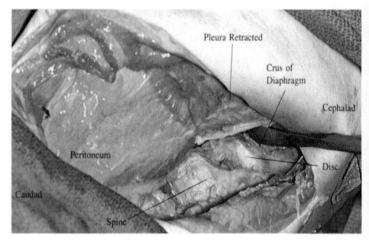

FIGURE 19E. Exposure of the spine consists of identification of disc spaces, blunt dissection on the disc space, isolation of intercostal arteries and veins, and removal of the insertion of the crus of the diaphragm. Beware of the 12th intercostal artery and vein under the crus of the diaphragm.

is a direct tether to adequate expansion of the wound. With the pleura having been reflected off the undersurface of the diaphragm in this area, cut the insertion of the diaphragm off the tip of the 12th rib.

8. Remember: The approach is under the diaphragm, which has been retracted cephalad. The peritoneum is bluntly dissected from the undersurface of the diaphragm. Retract the peritoneum and contents anteriorly. Enter the retroperitoneal space and identify the psoas muscle over the transverse processes.

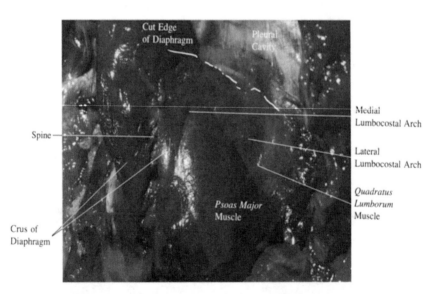

FIGURE 19F. Extending the exposure in Figure 19D cephalad on the psoas major muscle, one encounters the crus of the diaphragm, medial lumbocostal arch, and insertion of the psoas muscle. The spine is obscured by the often bulky muscle mass that in this area hides the intercostal vessels and the peripheral extent of the pleura. Remember, at any time when one dissects cephalad to the L1 transverse process the pleura may be inadvertently entered. To extend the 11th rib approach cephalad, identify the origin of the psoas muscle over the transverse processes and bodies of T12, L1. The transverse process of L1 is the junction of the medial and lateral lumbocostal arches. The left and right crura of the diaphragm are identified as they extend over the spine.

9. Identify the origin of psoas muscle over the transverse processes and bodies of T12 and L1 (Figs. 19D, 19E, 19F). Identify the transverse process of L1, which is the junction of the medial and lateral lumbocostal arches. Identify the crus of the diaphragm over L1.

10. Cut the attachment of the lumbocostal arches from the transverse process of L1.

11. Cut and elevate the left crus of the diaphragm from the vertebral bodies of L1 and L2 (Fig. 19G). Identify and ligate segmental vessels at each vertebral body level.

Caution: Do not neglect the segmental vessels over L1. Blunt dissection can be carried proximally on the spine to the level of T11. The pleura often extends into the costophrenic sulcus medially at the 12th vertebral body. There is the danger of entering the pleura with the proximal blunt dissection, even after the pleura has been identified over the midportion of the 11th rib.

12. Often the psoas muscle bulges medially and obscures the spine and the crus of the diaphragm. Use finger palpation to differentiate the texture of the intervertebral disc from the vertebral bodies. Take down the psoas from its insertion onto the body of T12–L1 and the transverse processes of T12 and L1. Control the bleeding in the attachments of the psoas by electrocautery. The T11–T12–L1 vertebral bodies are exposed in the wound extrapleurally and retroperitoneally (Fig. 19H).

13. Closure: Expand the lung before closure to observe for any air leak. Attach the

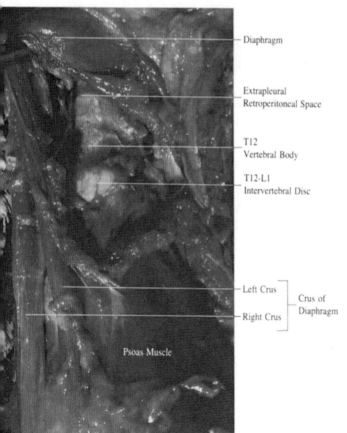

Diaphragm

Extrapleural
Retroperitoneal Space

T12
Vertebral Body

T12-L1
Intervertebral Disc

Left Crus ⎤
　　　　　 ⎬ Crus of
Right Crus ⎦ Diaphragm

Psoas Muscle

FIGURE 19G. Expose the T12–L1 disc space and dissect cephalad on the spine, leaving the diaphragm and pleural cavity cephalad. It is technically possible to extend the approach up to T9.

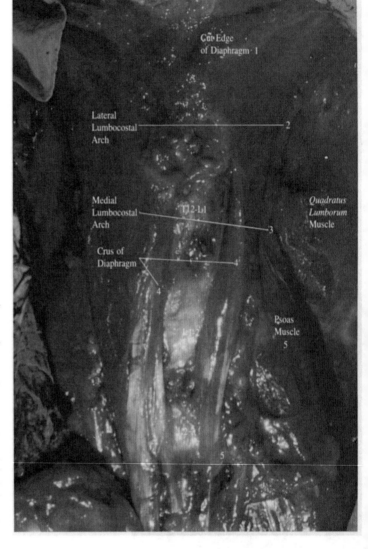

FIGURE 19H. Remove the crus of the diaphragm from the vertebral body. The right crus of the diaphragm is large and extends down the right side of the L1, L2, L3 vertebral bodies. The left crus extends to L2. The crui extend anteriorly into the substance of the diaphragm, forming the aortic hiatus. The insertion of the diaphragm into the transverse process of L1 is in the form of a medial and lateral lumbocostal arch. The medial lumbocostal arch extends from the crus of the diaphragm and vertebral body, arches over the cephalad portion of the psoas major muscle, and inserts into the anterior surface of the transverse process of L1. The lateral lumbocostal arch expands from this transverse process of L1, arching over the quadratus lumborum muscle to the tip of the 12th rib. Beware of the intercostal vessels over T12–L1 and L1–L2 when removing the diaphragmatic crura.

lumbocostal arch to the transverse process of L1, the crus of the diaphragm to the vertebral body, and the insertion of the diaphragm into the tip of the 11th and 12th ribs.

Again, the key to closure is in reapproximating the costal cartilage on the tip of the 11th rib. Close the rib bed with interrupted suture. Then each layer closure follows with running absorbable suture.

Additional Anatomy

Beware of the muscle-covered intercostal vessels crossing the midbody of T12, and do not damage the pleura over the vertebral body when dissecting proximally toward the T11–T12. The crus of the diaphragm forms a sling, anteriorly at which is the aortic hiatus. The thoracic duct enters through the aortic hiatus anterior to the aorta. The renal artery and kidney have been reflected anteriorly and to the right from this left lateral approach.

The sympathetic chain is in its paraspinous location entering the diaphragm. Although often sectioned in the approach, it sometimes can be identified and preserved. There should be no permanent sequelae from unilateral transection of the sympathetic chain.

Remember:

1. Identify the costal cartilage at the tip of the 11th rib.
2. Identify attachment of diaphragm, endothoracic fascia, and transversalis fascia to the tip of the 11th rib.
3. Split the cartilage of the 11th rib and enter the area beneath the rib bed only at the extreme tip in the area of the costal cartilage.
4. Dissect the pleura bluntly off the undersurface of the 11th rib bed.
5. Detach the insertion of the diaphragm from the tip of the 12th rib.
6. Elevate the lumbocostal arches from the psoas muscle and the crus of the diaphragm from the vertebral body. Beware of damage to the 12th intercostal artery and vein.
7. Beware of damage to the pleura in the area of the paravertebral sulcus.
8. The costal cartilage is the key to closure.

References

1. Hodgson AR, Yau ACMC: Anterior surgical approaches to the spinal column. In Apley AG (ed): Recent Advances in Orthopaedics. Baltimore, Williams & Wilkins, 1964, pp 289–323.
2. Mouat TB: The operative approach to the kidney of Bernard Fey. Br J Urol 2, 1939.

19B

Trans-Eleventh Rib Extrapleural Approach

Yutaka Hiraizumi

The trans-11th rib extrapleural approach is less traumatic to the respiratory system[1] and has the advantage that a patient does not necessarily need either thoracic drainage or a postoperative intensive care unit (ICU) stay. The incidence of postoperative atelectasis is very rare, because ventilation is maintained and no direct mechanical pressure is applied to the lung tissue during the spinal procedure; this is beneficial for geriatric or ventilatory poor-risk patients. Even if the parietal pleura is accidentally perforated, suturing the injured pleura requires less intensive postoperative management compared to the ordinary thoracotomy procedure.

1. The exposable cephalad operative field for 11th rib resection is the T11 vertebral body and the intervertebral disc of T11–T12. Likewise, caudad exposure is the L2 vertebral body. Pathology that has occurred around T12 or L1 is the most convenient target. If the skin incision is extended toward the symphysis pubica caudally, the L5–S1 disc space can be reached with this approach.

2. Indications for this approach are determined by pathology that exists anterolateral to the following spinal levels:

- Disc herniation at T11–T12, T12–L1, L1–L2
- Burst fracture, tumor, spondylitis, or ossification of the posterior longitudinal ligament (OPLL) at T12, L1, L2
- Scoliosis or kyphotic deformity at the thoracolumbar junction

3. Contraindications for this approach include previous thoracotomy. Spinal infection, either pyogenic or tuberculous, or metastatic spinal tumor is not necessarily a contraindication unless severe adhesive pleuritis is expected. Rather, these diseases can be good indications because the parietal pleura plays a role in barricading disease dissemination.

The patient is placed in either right or left lateral decubitus position depending on convenience in approaching the spinal pathology. As in ordinary thoracotomy, the upper extremity of the open side is lifted forward and an axillar pad is placed under the dependent axilla. The operating table should be slightly bent to maintain the coronal spinal physiologic alignment.

1. In the same fashion as in ordinary trans-11th rib thoracotomy, a curved oblique incision is made over the 11th rib. The posterior border of this incision is placed just lateral to the margin of the paravertebral muscles, and the anterior border is 3 to 5 cm beyond the tip of the 11th rib (Fig. 19I). The incision can be extended toward the symphysis pubica depending upon how far down the exposure to the lumbar spine is needed.

2. Along this incision line, m. latissimus dorsi is undermined and the muscle belly is clamped with two Pean's or Kelly's forceps in parallel. Between those two clamps, the muscle belly is incised using electric cautery. In the same manner, the underlying m. serratus anterior is incised (Fig. 19J).

3. Underneath those separated muscle layers, the 11th rib appears and the superficial periosteum is opened. The superior surface, then the inferior surface, followed by the undersurface of the 11th rib are carefully released subperiosteally using periosteal elevators such as Cobb and Dwyer instruments. Then, the 11th rib is harvested from the angle of the rib to the costal cartilage junction for bone grafting,

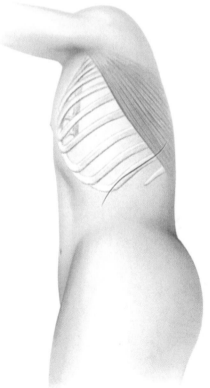

FIGURE 19I. A curved oblique incision is made along the 11th rib.

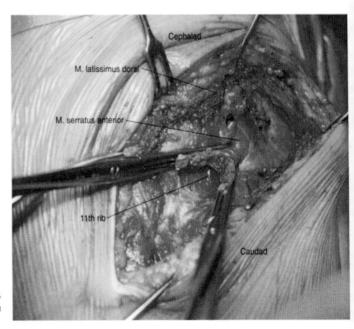

FIGURE 19J. Excision of m. latissimus dorsi and m. serratus anterior along the 11th rib.

leaving the 11th costal cartilage as the entrance to both the retroperitoneal and the extrapleural spaces. This cartilage, which forms a part of the arcus costalis, is then split with a sharp knife. The proximal stump of the 11th rib is packed with bone wax for hemostasis (Fig. 19K).

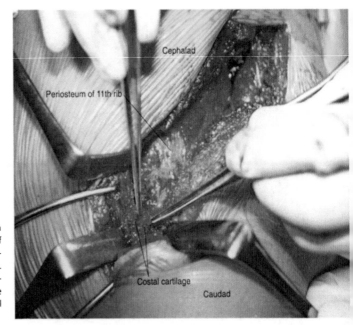

FIGURE 19K. After removal of the 11th rib. The bed of the 11th rib is made of the inner periosteum, the endothoracic fascia, and the parietal pleura. The interspace of the split costal cartilage, which is the entry zone to the retroperitoneal and the extrapleural spaces, is shown.

Caution: The rib bed of the 11th rib is composed of three layers; the inner periosteum of the 11th rib, endothoracic fascia, and the parietal pleural. The rib bed should be maintained intact so as not to converge to thoracotomy.

4. Because the diaphragm inserts to the 11th and the 12th costal cartilage in the lateral aspect of the thoracic cage, immediately after splitting the 11th costal cartilage, muscle fibers of the diaphragm spontaneously separate about 2 cm along its fibrous orientation. When both sides of the split cartilage are retracted, the m. obliquus externus abdominis is easily separated along its fibrous orientation, and the underlying m. obliquus internus abdominis and m. transversus abdominis appear. Both the m. obliquus internus abdominis and the m. transversus abdominis are carefully undermined and detached from the underlying peritoneum and then clamped with two Pean's or Kelly's forceps in parallel. Between those two forceps, muscle bellies are incised with electric cautery 3 to 5 cm along the incision line, until the underlying thin peritoneum becomes visible. M. transversus abdominis inserts to the arcus costalis and is interdigitated with insertion of the diaphragm (Fig. 19L).

Caution: Care must be taken not to spread this entry zone too wide, to avoid injuring the underlying peritoneum and parietal pleura.

5. The interspace between the deep fascia of m. transversus abdominis and the peritoneum is bluntly dissected toward the retroperitoneal space using the fingertips until the fingertips feel the vertebral body surface and the overriding aorta. The fingertips are first oriented posteriorly toward the m. quadratus lumborum and m. psoas major and then medially toward the vertebral body surface (Fig. 19M).

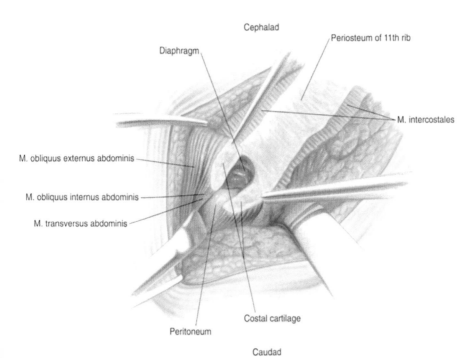

Cephalad

Diaphragm

Periosteum of 11th rib

M. intercostales

M. obliquus externus abdominis

M. obliquus internus abdominis

M. transversus abdominis

Costal cartilage

Peritoneum

Caudad

FIGURE 19L. By splitting the 11th costal cartilage, the underlying diaphragm spontaneously separates for a few centimeters along its fibrous orientation. This space becomes the entry zone into the retroperitoneal and the extrapleural spaces.

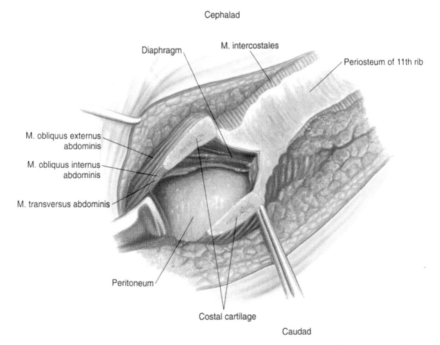

Cephalad

Diaphragm

M. intercostales

Periosteum of 11th rib

M. obliquus externus abdominis

M. obliquus internus abdominis

M. transversus abdominis

Peritoneum

Costal cartilage

Caudad

FIGURE 19M. The retroperitoneal space is bluntly dissected between the peritoneum and the deep fascia of m. transversus abdominis until the surgeon's fingertips feel the vertebral body surface and the overriding aorta.

Caution: Blunt dissection of the peritoneum should include the inferior surface of the diaphragm until its insertion to the L1 vertebral body; otherwise, incision of the diaphragm may cause peritoneal injury. During blunt separation, to avoid perforation the fingertips should never be directed toward the thin peritoneum. As the peritoneum is reversed until the L1 vertebral body is exposed, there is adipose tissue, which includes the sympathetic trunk at the medial border of m. psoas major. This sympathetic trunk should be preserved if possible. The ureter, which attaches to the peritoneum, is usually retracted with the peritoneum.

6. The entry zone to the extrapleural space, which exists between the rib bed and the insertion of the diaphragm under the split 11th costal cartilage, is carefully dissected along the diaphragmatic insertion, orienting toward the 12th costal cartilage, using a curved mosquito or Kelly's forceps. One suture is placed on each side of the split cartilage as landmarks; these are used when repairing the arcus costalis. Once diaphragmatic dissection is started, the marginal line of the transparent parietal pleura becomes distinguishable by the ebb-and-flow motion of the lung surface. Then, the insertion of the diaphragm is clamped by a couple of curved Pean's or Kelly's forceps in parallel and is incised with careful attention to the lung motion. Sutures should be placed every inch in pairs to ensure against perforation of the parietal pleura. They also serve as landmarks and anchoring sutures when repairing the diaphragm. The parietal pleura attaching to the endothoracic fascia is bluntly dissected with most careful attention to avoid perforation; then, the remaining 11th rib bed can be incised to establish a wide operative (Fig. 19N).

Caution: Three-dimensional anatomical knowledge of the diaphragm is mandatory to avoid incisional disorientation. The insertion of the diaphragm orients laterally to the

Cephalad

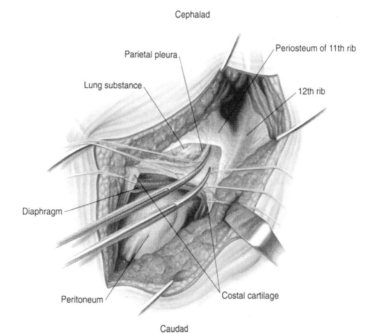

Parietal pleura

Periosteum of 11th rib

Lung substance

12th rib

Diaphragm

Peritoneum

Costal cartilage

Caudad

FIGURE 19N. The entrance to the extrapleural space is between the rib bed of the 11th rib and the diaphragmatic insertion under the split 11th costal cartilage. The parietal pleura usually does not reach this aspect. Incision of the diaphragm starts from its insertion to the 11th costal cartilage, orienting to the insertion to the 12th costal cartilage along the diaphragmatic peripheral margin. Sutures are placed on each side of the spit cartilage and also on each side of the incised diaphragmatic margin for landmarks and anchors for repairing the diaphragm and the arcus costalis. These stitches are also important to avoid iatrogenic pneumothorax. The parietal pleura is transparent, and one can distinguish its presence by the rise and fall of the lung.

11th and the 12th costal cartilage, posteriorly to the L1 transverse process and the L1 vertebral body, so that one should never make a diaphragmatic incision along the 11th or 12th rib curvature. Once the incision reaches the tip of the 12th costal cartilage, then orient toward the L1 transverse process and L1 vertebral body; otherwise, thoracotomy will occur. This is the point most different from the conventional thoracotomy. Dissection of the diaphragm is started blind, close to its insertion to the 11th costal cartilage. The parietal pleura does not usually reach this aspect and remains slightly more proximal; however, this is the most technically demanding point for this approach. The parietal pleura is very thin and transparent. Usually, it is difficult to discriminate its marginal line if ventilation has ceased. Ventilation should be maintained during this procedure so that one can clearly observe the rise and fall of the lung surface. Placing sutured in pairs when incising the diaphragm is important to avoid accidental pleural perforation during this dissecting procedure. When repairing the diaphragm, tying each pair of sutures enables accurate reapproximation of the detached diaphragm; these then also work as anchoring sutures. The diaphragm in geriatric patients is usually very thin so that those stitches reinforce closure of the thoracic cage and ensure postoperative respiratory function. Keep in mind that in the case of a short 12th rib the parietal pleura often covers the entire length of the 12th rib.

7. The incision of the diaphragm is continued circumferentially along the insertion of the diaphragm at the 12th costal cartilage and the L1 transverse process and terminates at the L1 vertebral body. The incision line is placed 2 cm medial from its peripheral attachment to the chest wall. During this procedure, the parietal pleura that attaches to the endothoracic fascia and vertebral bodies is bluntly dissected by sponge or fingertips, and the T11 and T12 vertebral bodies are exposed. The T11–T12, T12–L1, and L1–L2 disc levels can be determined by probing elastic prominences between concave vertebral bodies. In the thoracic spine, costovertebral articulation occupies the posterior third and the anterior longitudinal ligament covers the anterior third of the lateral surface of the vertebral body. Likewise, in the lumbar spine, the m. psoas major covers the lateral surface of the vertebral body, and the crus and the anterior longitudinal ligament cover the anterior third of the vertebral body (Fig. 19O).

Caution: The incision line of the diaphragm should be placed 2 cm medial from the peripheral attachment to preserve a margin for reattachment and central innervation by the phrenic nerve. Dissection of the parietal pleura is easier at the undersurface of the rib bed and the oversurface of the diaphragm; however, the pleura should be carefully dissected around the costovertebral articulation in which it forms a paravertebral sulcus. The diaphragmatic attachment to the L1 vertebral body also requires attention because a deep and blind maneuver is needed. To avoid perforation, the fingertips should never be directed toward the parietal pleura. Once perforation occurs, closure is difficult.

8. To expose the L1 vertebral body, the origin of the m. psoas major to the T12 and L1 vertebral bodies and the L1 transverse process must be detached by electric cautery, leaving stay sutures for reapproximation; then, the muscle belly is retracted inferiorly (Fig. 19P). If the head of the ribs obstructs operative procedures, they can be resected with an osteotome. The insertion of the diaphragm to the L1 vertebral body

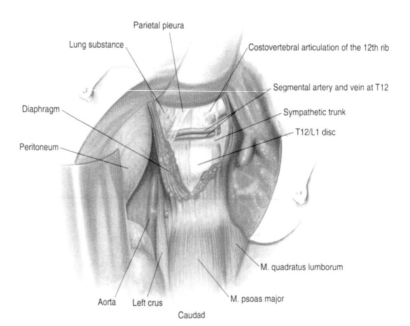

Cephalad

Parietal pleura

Lung substance

Costovertebral articulation of the 12th rib

Segmental artery and vein at T12

Diaphragm

Sympathetic trunk

T12/L1 disc

Peritoneum

M. quadratus lumborum

Aorta   Left crus   M. psoas major

Caudad

FIGURE 19O. The insertion of the diaphragm attaches to the 12th costal cartilage laterally and to the L1 transverse process and the L1 vertebral body posteriorly. The incision will extend to its insertion to the L1 vertebral body.

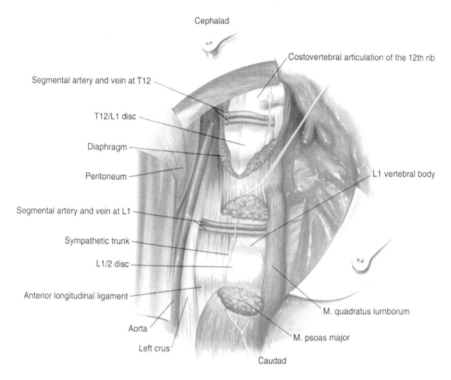

Cephalad

Costovertebral articulation of the 12th rib

Segmental artery and vein at T12

T12/L1 disc

Diaphragm

Peritoneum

L1 vertebral body

Segmental artery and vein at L1

Sympathetic trunk

L1/2 disc

Anterior longitudinal ligament

M. quadratus lumborum

Aorta

M. psoas major

Left crus

Caudad

FIGURE 19P. The m. psoas major obstructs exposure of the L1 vertebral body, so its origin is separated and reversed.

obstructs operative procedures at this aspect; often, it must be detached from the L1 vertebral body. The crus of the diaphragm can be incised if it is obstructing spinal procedures.

Caution: The aorta descends on the left side of the thoracic spine and descends anteriorly at the lumbar spine. The head of the 12th rib and the insertion of the diaphragm to the L1 vertebral body are good landmarks to identify the disc level or vertebra. However, intraoperative radiographic identification of disc and vertebral levels is required. Do not coagulate segmental vessels, but ligate or staple them carefully first medially then laterally. As far as the subperiosteal approach is applied, injury to the parietal pleura, peritoneum, major vessels, and the thoracic duct can be avoided.

9. Because ventilation is maintained and no direct mechanical pressure to the lung is applied during spinal procedures, postoperative atelectasis is rare. Once the spinal procedure is completed, any trauma to the parietal pleura is investigated with saline filled into the thoracic cage before closing the wound. If a major pleural tear is detected, thoracic damage with negative pressure is required; however, a pinhole injury can be ignored. The diaphragm is resutured, reinforced by anchoring stitches that were previously prepared. The split costal cartilage is then reapproximated, tying up the previous stitches. Each layer of the separated muscles is closed in layer-to-layer fashion.

Caution: Equal tension on the repaired diaphragm through accurate reapproximation is essential. Suturing of the diaphragm must be reinforced by anchoring stitches.

Acknowledgment

The author thanks Mr. Hitoshi Asano, medical illustrator, for his contribution.

Reference

1. McMinn RMH, Hutchings RT: A Color Atlas of Human Anatomy. London, Wolfe, 1977.

Twelfth Rib Approach

The 12th rib resection with flank incision was developed to allow better exposure of the kidney (Fig. 20A).[1-3] The 12th rib and its periosteal bed are joined at the rib's tip by the insertion of the diaphragm and of the transversus abdominis fascia and muscle. They form an anchoring point to resist cephalad retraction. By removing the 12th rib, opening the 12th rib bed, and freeing the muscle insertions of the tip of the 12th rib, one has greater exposure for cephalad retraction when exposing the kidney, retroperitoneal space, or spine. Resection of the rib and the periosteum of the rib bed allows release of the posterior lumbocostal ligament, which is a strong tether against cephalad retraction, and frees the fibers of the internal/external oblique muscles. With the added exposure, the L1 vertebral body and distal segments can be adequately visualized.

One of the major complications of the thoracolumbar approach is damage to the pleura in the region of the 12th rib. The relationship of the pleura to the 12th rib, as presented by Myney and Hughes,[1] begins with a classification of 12th ribs into a long type of 11–14 cm and a short type of 1.5–6 cm. In the more common long rib the pleura are usually on the undersurface of the posterior 6 cm of the rib. The pleura may extend over the T11–T12 interspace anteriorly as far as 10–11 cm from the midline. With short 12th ribs, the entire length of the rib should be considered to be covered with pleura (see Figs. 17A, 19C, 20B). With this location of the pleura in mind, one may follow the four steps outlined by Digby for avoiding the pleura:

1. Study the maximum inspiration chest X-ray taken before the operation to show the lower extent of the pleura.
2. Expose the periosteum on the outer side of the rib before incising it to avoid deep plunges that can section the pleura off the rib surface.
3. Avoid sharp projecting fragments on the stump of the last rib and cover the stump with a tethered gauze roll.
4. Make the longitudinal incision in the periosteum and inner aspects of the last rib sufficiently far out to be below and beyond the pleura reflection.[3]

1. Place the patient in the right lateral decubitus position over the break in the table; this increases the distance between the iliac crest and costal margin and aids in the exposure (see Fig. 20A).

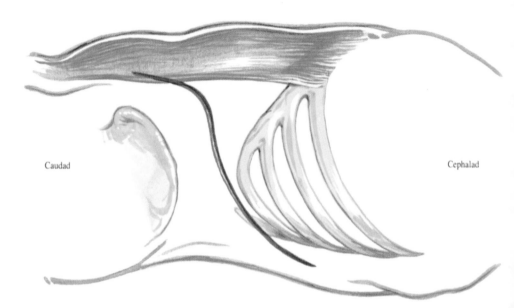

Caudad   Cephalad

FIGURE 20A. Incise the skin and subcutaneous tissue from the costo-transverse junction to 6 inches anterior to the tip of the 12th rib. Resect the 12th rib with a standard thoracotomy technique. and extend the anterior incision to open the abdominal musculature as described in Chapter 18. The chief advantage of the 12th rib excision is that it allows easier retraction and exposure of the upper lumbar spine. Removal of the rib and preservation of the rib bed does not add greatly to ease of retraction; therefore, the rib bed should be opened as in a standard thoracotomy technique except extrapleurally, as described in Chapter 19. The approach is an extrapleural approach; therefore, identification of the peripheral extent of the pleura should follow Digby's rules. 1. Study the maximum inspiration chest X-ray taken before the operation to show the lower extent of the pleura. 2. Exposing the periosteum on the outer side of the rib before incising it avoids deep plunges that can section the pleura off the rib surface. 3. Avoid sharp projecting fragments on the stump of the last rib and cover the stump with a tethered gauze roll. 4. Make the longitudinal incision in the periosteum and inner aspects of the last rib sufficiently far out to be below and beyond the pleura reflection.

2. Incise the skin and subcutaneous tissue from the costotransverse junction to 6 inches anterior to the tip of the 12th rib. Divide muscle layers with the electrocautery to the surface of the 12th rib. Take care to cut the latissimus dorsi and serratus posterior musculature directly in line with the incision to the rib. Do not slide off the rib inferiorly and damage the subcostal nerve and vessels.

3. Open the periosteum of the rib and elevate the superficial and deep surfaces of the periosteum off the rib (see Chapter 16).

4. Cut the rib at the costotransverse junction and elevate with a bone clamp the cut rib from the rib bed, leaving it attached anteriorly. Attached to the tip of the 12th rib is the diaphragm superiorly and the transverse abdominis musculature and fascia inferiorly. The pleura is safely protected under the rib bed (see Fig. 20B). The safest area to enter the rib bed of the 12th rib is at the tip.

Caution: If it is a short rib, the pleura will be at the tip of the 12th rib.

5. While elevating the rib, split the tissue on the tip of the 12th rib and remove the rib. Retract slightly the diaphragmatic insertion cephalad, the abdominal musculature caudad.

6. Identify the foamy fat of the retroperitoneal space. Open this carefully and identify the peritoneum. Bluntly dissect the peritoneum from the undersurface of the abdominal wall for further opening of muscle layers.

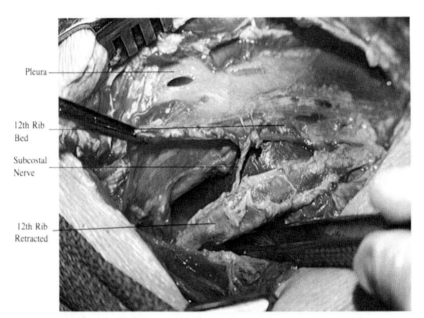

Pleura

12th Rib
Bed

Subcostal
Nerve

12th Rib
Retracted

FIGURE 20B. The rib bed of the 12th rib and its relationship to the pleura. This rib bed must be opened while maintaining an extrapleural position. With a long 12th rib the pleura usually only extends medially as far as the lateral three-fourths of the rib bed. Therefore, it is easier to begin the plane of dissection at the medial tip of the rib bed, progress laterally, find the pleura, and dissect it off. With a short (6-inch or smaller) 12th rib, dissection at the tip of the rib must be done as carefully as described in Chapter 19 because pleura covers the entire rib.

7. Extend the incision through the external oblique and internal oblique musculature with the electrocautery. Identify the transversus abdominis musculature and carefully spread this muscle to expose the transversalis fascia.

8. Retract the peritoneum anteriorly and expose the retroperitoneal space (see Fig. 20C).

9. The endothoracic fascia lines the undersurface of the rib bed. Dissect bluntly the pleura from the endothoracic fascia. Sweep the pleura off from the tip proximally. With the pleura removed from the undersurface, open the rib bed.

10. The 12th intercostal nerve runs under and through the internal oblique. In opening the abdominal musculature, identify and protect the 12th intercostal nerve. Now identify the retroperitoneal space, the opened rib bed, the cephalad retracted diaphragm and pleura, each layer of the abdominal musculature, the peritoneum, and the psoas.

11. Locating the psoas muscle is the critical factor at this point.[3] Use Deaver retractors to hold the peritoneal sac and its contents anteriorly (Figs. 20C, 20D). Take care not to enter the retropsoas space, which is a blind pouch.

12. With the kidney retracted forward, identify the ureter on the undersurface of the peritoneum. It need not be dissected free and is retracted with the peritoneum.

13. Palpate the spine to find the soft prominent disc spaces.

14. Bluntly spread the retroperitoneal soft tissue on the first identifiable disc. Stay on the surface of the disc and not on the vertebral body, where the intercostal vessels are.

15. With the clearing of one disc, insert a needle for X-ray confirmation of the level.

16. The psoas frequently bulges over the midline and obscures the spine as it inserts on the 12th and 1st bodies and on the lumbocostal arches. Remove the psoas muscle initially from the disc area, then from the vertebral bodies.

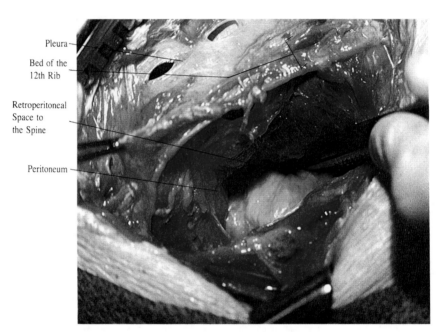

Pleura

Bed of the
12th Rib

Retroperitoneal
Space to
the Spine

Peritoneum

FIGURE 20C. Exposure of the spine through the retroperitoneal space with protection of the pleura.

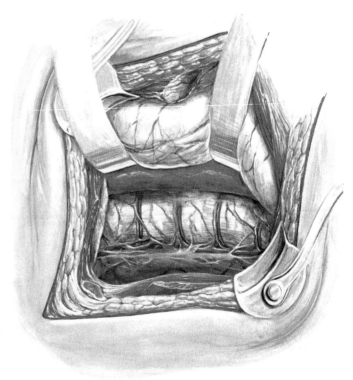

FIGURE 20D. With retraction of the pleural sac, the abdominal aorta is located by palpation and the spine exposed.

Caution: Cauterize or tie vascular structures in the midportion of the vertebral body and control bleeding from the origin of the psoas.

17. Cut the crus of the diaphragm from the spine and elevate in a cephalad direction with the periosteal elevator. With the crus of the diaphragm elevated cephalad and with the psoas muscle retracted laterally and inferiorly, the T12–S1 discs should be well visualized. Remove the insertion of the lumbocostal arch on the transverse process of L1 for additional visualization cephalad. Theoretically this area can be expanded to the 10th thoracic vertebra, but the exposure will be confining in any level above T12.

Caution: The pleura in the sulcus is immediately over the spine and the rib heads. Continue blunt dissection of the pleura toward the spine until this is sufficiently elevated.[4]

18. Closure: Close the rib bed, approximate the cartilaginous tip of the rib, and close each abdominal muscle layer.

Remember:

1. Do not plunge off the tip of the 12th rib.
2. Use the split costal cartilage tips to separate the diaphragmatic insertion from the transversus abdominis insertion.
3. Follow the Digby rules to avoid pleural damage.
4. Use blunt dissection on peritoneum and pleura.
5. Identify and ligate each intercostal artery and vein over *each vertebral body.*
6. Find the psoas muscle, transversus process of L1, and the crus of the diaphragm.

References

1. Hughes J: Urology 61(2):159–162, 1949.
2. Hodgson AR, Yau ACMC: Anterior surgical approaches to the spinal column. In Apley AG (ed): Recent Advances in Orthopaedics. Baltimore, Williams & Wilkins, 1964, pp 289–323.
3. Digby KH: 12th rib incision as an approach to the kidney. Surg Gynecol Obstet 73:84–85, 1941.
4. Rothman R: Anterior Sequential Approach to the Spine, Vol. I. Philadelphia, Saunders, 1975, pp 124–125.

21

Anterior Retroperitoneal Flank Approach to L2–L5 of the Lumbar Spine

1. Place the patient in the left lateral decubitus position. The radiopaque "bean-bag" for positioning allows adequate intraoperative X-ray visualization. Slightly flex the knees, place the axillary pad, and support the head sufficiently. Too much hip flexion at this point will limit the operative exposure anteriorly. Position the left hip flexed less than the right.

2. The surgeon stands anterior to the patient. The assistant stands posterior to the patient. Begin the incision equidistant between the lowest rib and the superior iliac crest in the midaxillary line and extend it approximately to the edge of the rectus sheath. The level of the incision varies according to the level of the spine approached. L5–S1 is in the lower half of the distance between umbilicus and symphysis, L4–L5 is in the upper half, L3–L4 at the umbilicus, and L2–L3 above it (Fig. 21A). With self-retaining retractors, the assistant spreads the skin and subcutaneous tissue, using two Adson pick-ups for rapid cauterization of bleeders in the subcutaneous tissue.

3. Muscle relaxation allows greater mobility to the abdominal wall and decreases the contractility of the muscle as it is incised. Expose the fascia of the external oblique muscle. The surgeon cauterizes through the muscle, and the assistant picks up bleeding points before and after they are cut. Dissect through the external oblique to the internal oblique muscle (Fig. 21B); use the same procedure through the internal oblique. Inferior to the internal oblique is the transversus abdominis. Care must be used in inserting the self-retaining retractors into the muscle layers so as not to damage the peritoneum. If the transversus abdominis muscle is well developed, cauterize it down to its lower layers (Fig. 21C). Often, this is a very thin or absent muscle layer. Bluntly spread the thin muscle in line with its fibers to expose the transversalis fascia (Fig. 21D).

4. Open the transversalis fascia in the posterior portion of the wound. Lift the transversalis fascia with the Adson and carefully open it with blunt scissors. The retroperitoneal fat allows room to enter the extraperitoneal space. Dissection of the muscle layers becomes more difficult medially. The muscle layers thin out and the layers of fascia become almost joined medially. The peritoneum is very superficial (Fig. 21E). Inadvertent penetration of the peritoneum is most likely just lateral to the rectus sheath.

5. Enter the retroperitoneal space laterally (Fig. 21F). Identify the peritoneum and the fat of the retroperitoneal space. Remove the peritoneum from the remaining trans-

154

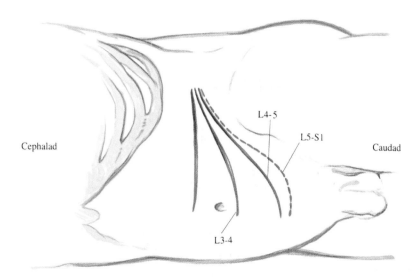

FIGURE 21A. Patient in left lateral decubitus position. Using the radiopaque beanbag for positioning allows adequate intraoperative X-ray visualization. Slightly flex the knees, place the axillary pad, and support the head sufficiently. Too much hip flexion at this point will limit the exposure anteriorly. Have the left hip only slightly flexed. Begin the incision equidistant between the lowest rib and superior iliac crest in the midaxillary line (it may be closer to the crest for lower levels) and extend it proximally to the edge of the rectus sheath. The level of incision varies according to the level of the spine approached. L5–S1 is in the lower half of the distance between the umbilicus and the symphysis pubis. L4–L5 lies in the upper half of this distance, L3–L4 at the umbilicus, and L2–L3 above. Incise through the skin and subcutaneous tissue, retracting with self-retaining retractors.

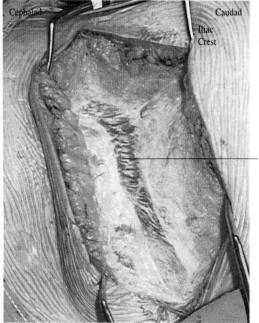

FIGURE 21B. With the surgeon standing anterior to the patient and the assistant posterior, incise through each muscle layer of the abdominal wall with electrocautery.

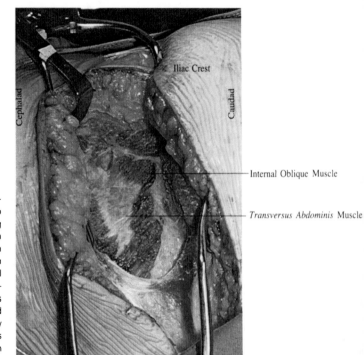

Iliac Crest

Cephalad

Caudad

Internal Oblique Muscle

Transversus Abdominis Muscle

FIGURE 21C. The assistant standing behind the patient should use forceps to pick up each intramuscular bleeding point for cauterization as the surgeon cuts through the muscle layers with the electrocautery. Muscle layers thin out anteriorly into a more superficial fascial layer. Penetration of the peritoneum is common near the rectus sheath, and caution should be used as the incision is taken more medially as one leaves the muscle layers. It is safer in the lateral, muscular portion of the wound.

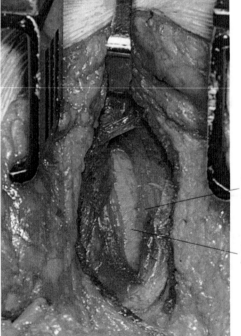

Transversus Abdominis Muscle

Transversalis Fascia and Peritoneum

FIGURE 21D. The transversus abdominis muscle layer, often the thinnest of the three muscle layers of the abdominal wall, must be opened very carefully. The transversalis fascia underneath the transversus abdominis muscle should also be opened very carefully, as the peritoneum is the next most immediate layer under the transversalis fascia. Spread through the transversalis muscle, identify the transversalis fascia, penetrate the transversalis fascia in the more lateral aspect of the wound, and identify the peritoneum.

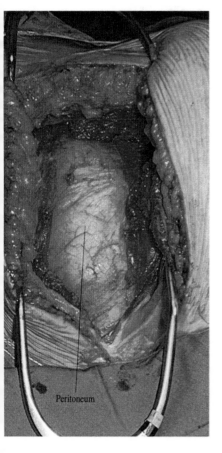

Peritoneum

FIGURE 21E. The peritoneal layer under and adjacent to the transversalis fascia layer should be bluntly swept forward.

versalis fascia medially, with the surgeon in the anterior position lifting the abdominal wall and the assistant in the posterior position peeling the peritoneum off the undersurface of the fascia with a 4 × 4 sponge. Extend the incision medially, after the peritoneum has been safely removed. Take the dissection to the edge of the rectus sheath. The sheath may be incised for added exposure. Torn peritoneum should be repaired promptly.[1]

6. Identification of the psoas muscle is the key to the retroperitoneal space. Pass your hand directly to the psoas (Fig. 21G). One must avoid opening the retropsoas space, which is a blind pouch. Feel through the retroperitoneal tissue for the psoas muscle. The genitofemoral nerve can be identified on this structure. The spine is immediately medial to the psoas and can be partially obscured by it. Now palpate four structures: the psoas muscle, the intervertebral disc, the aorta, and the vertebral, body. Palpate for texture and consistency to determine the appropriate structures.[1] Make any deep retraction with a padded malleable retractor or Deaver. The paravertebral sympathetic chain lies medial to the psoas muscle. The ureter will be reflected medially with the undersurface of the peritoneum (Fig. 21H). If a retroperitoneal abscess is well developed, open it and dissect inside the abscess to the spine (Fig. 21I).

7. The key at this point is to identify the raised, white, softer disc by direct palpation with the finger, as opposed to the lower, concave vertebral body where the lumbar vessels are found. The discs are the hills and the vertebral bodies are the valleys. The vessels are in the valleys.

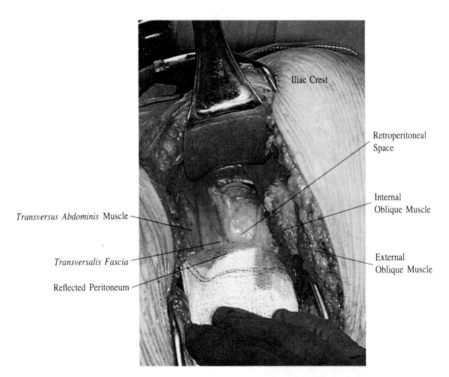

Iliac Crest

Retroperitoneal Space

Internal Oblique Muscle

External Oblique Muscle

Transversus Abdominis Muscle

Transversalis Fascia

Reflected Peritoneum

FIGURE 21F. Identify the fatty layer of the retroperitoneal space as the peritoneal sac and cavity is brought medially. Bluntly penetrate the retroperitoneal space with the hand. In addition, remove the peritoneum from the remaining transversalis fascia medially by having the surgeon in the anterior position lift the abdominal wall and the assistant in the posterior position peel the peritoneum off the undersurface of the fascia with a 4 × 4 sponge and extend the incision medially after the peritoneum has been safely removed from under the remaining musculofascial layers of the abdominal wall.

FIGURE 21G. Identification of the psoas muscle is the key to the retroperitoneal space. Pass indirectly through the retroperitoneal space to the psoas muscle. Avoid opening the retropsoas space, which is a blind pouch. The dissection must proceed medial to the psoas muscle, not laterally. The genitofemoral nerve can be identified coursing on the psoas muscle. The spine is just medial to the psoas and can be partially hidden by it. Palpate the spine medial to the psoas and locate the raised intervertebral disc surface with the finger by slowly moving from left to right across the disc surface.

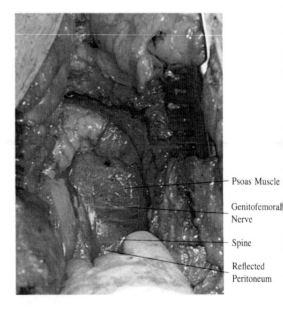

Psoas Muscle

Genitofemoral Nerve

Spine

Reflected Peritoneum

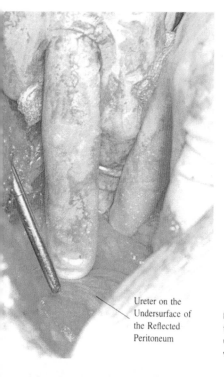

Ureter on the
Undersurface of
the Reflected
Peritoneum

FIGURE 21H. The ureter will be reflected with the peritoneal sac on its undersurface and can be identified when necessary.

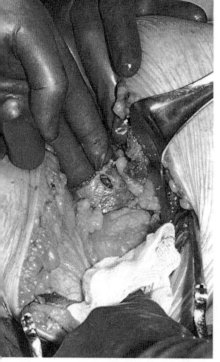

FIGURE 21I. For certain pathologic conditions with a thick-walled, well-defined peritoneal abscess, dissection takes place inside the abscess wall. It is opened in the retroperitoneal space and the bleeding points clamped and ligated in the abscessed wall. Pictured is a well-defined tuberculous retroperitoneal abscess that allows finger penetration in a glove-like manner. Chronic pyogenic infections may give an entirely different picture, that is, one of a diffuse, dense scarring of the peritoneum to the spine.

8. Once the lumbar disc can be identified, use a blunt elevator or a padded small retractor to sweep the soft tissue from left to right across the disc space. The lumbar veins are a horizontal tether. Variations in formation of the inferior cava and lumbar veins are the rule rather than the exception.[2] The most important of these veins is the iliolumbar vein, which crosses the body of L5 from right to left and ascends in the left paraspinous area.[3] This vessel is a direct tether to the left to right retraction of the aorta off the spine and is very vulnerable to avulsion (Fig. 21J).

9. For operations on the L4–L5 disc space, identify the iliolumbar vein early in the dissection. Ligate it after clamping the vein with angled tonsil clamps and passing two or three ligatures around the vein. Do not tie these veins too close to the vena cava, as a possible sidewall injury may result. After permanent ties are on the vein, transect it. Greater mobilization of the vena cava and venous structures, left to right, is obtained.

Lumbar veins of varying sizes at various positions can always be present. Some may be directly posterior to the vena cava and of quite large diameter.

Caution: *The iliolumbar vein is a vein that consistently requires ligation.*

10. Dissection on the anterior spine consists of gentle stretching and pulling of the structures, blunt dissection, direct pressure over many small bleeding areas with a sponge, and a minimum of electrocautery. The paraspinous sympathetic plexus between the spine and psoas muscle varies in size and number of fibers. Branches course between the preaortic and paraspinous chains. Preserve paraspinous sympathetic fibers that do not impede the dissection.

11. Dissect with the fingertip and blunt elevators all the vascular structures from left to right to give adequate visualization of the inplate of the vertebral body above the disc[4] (Fig. 21K).

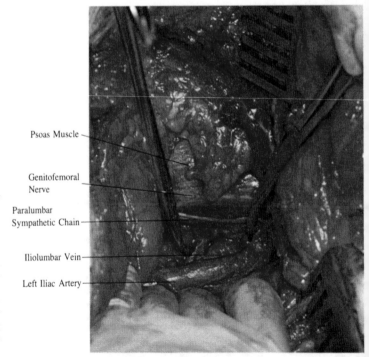

Psoas Muscle

Genitofemoral
Nerve

Paralumbar
Sympathetic Chain

Iliolumbar Vein

Left Iliac Artery

FIGURE 21J. For the lumbar approach to L4–L5 and above, the aorta and vena cava are swept left to right off the spine. The iliolumbar vein is an important direct tether to this left-to-right dissection. This lumbar vein crosses from the vena cava to approximately the level of the L5 body. Any dissection that exposes L4–L5 to the left of the left common iliac and vena cava requires identification, ligation, and division of the iliolumbar vein. Find the L4–L5 disc and dissect distally to the L5 body to identify the iliolumbar vein.

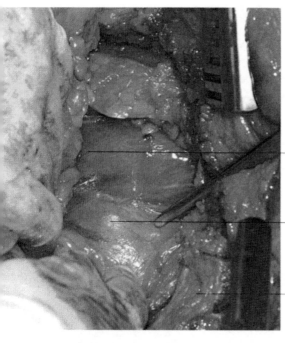

Psoas Muscle

L4-L5
Intervertebral
Disc

Left Iliac Artery
and Vein

FIGURE 21K. Dissection sweeps the prevertebral tissue off the disc space first, as this is a more avascular area. Use a sponge-covered finger or blunt instrument. Always obtain X-ray confirmation of the level.

12. For retraction, position malleable Deaver-type retractors around the disc space. Alternately, prepare four Freebody Steinmann retractors with rubber sleeves and mount in a Steinmann pin holder.[5] Stabilize the pin on the finger and engage the tip into the vertebral body under direct vision (Figs. 21L, 21M, 21N). Inspection and palpation

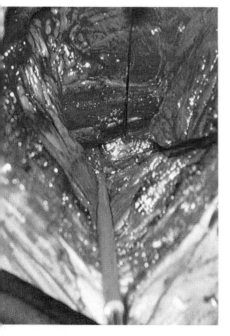

FIGURE 21L. The Freebody Steinmann pin retractor should be loaded in a Steinmann pin holder with an easy release and the pin covered with a red Robinson catheter. Retraction of the vena cava and aorta off the spine allows insertion of the Steinmann pin into the right inferior vertebral body of L4. The tip of the pin should be guarded carefully and held on the finger tip as it is positioned on the spine. The Steinmann pin should be held with two hands by the surgeon while the assistant taps it into place.

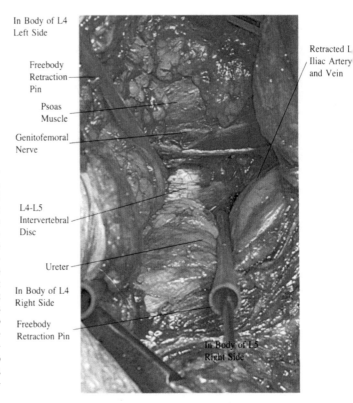

In Body of L4 Left Side

Freebody Retraction Pin

Psoas Muscle

Genitofemoral Nerve

Retracted L Iliac Artery and Vein

L4-L5 Intervertebral Disc

Ureter

In Body of L4 Right Side

Freebody Retraction Pin

In Body of L5 Right Side

FIGURE 21M. Place first the right superior pin, then the right inferior pin. Careful blunt dissection must hold the left common iliac artery and vein retracted to the right while the pin is inserted. The pin holder should be removed carefully. The pins should be checked for stability. These permanent stay retractors will retract the major vessels from the area of the disc excision and grafting, but care must be taken not to dislodge these pins during the procedures, as the sharp point can produce damage if inadvertently extracted. If the pins are angled toward the disc space too acutely, they will enter the disc space, interfere with disc removal, and require repositioning.

should confirm that there is no vascular structure between the tip of the pin and the vertebral body. The assistant taps the pin into the body while the surgeon maintains control of the pin. Remove the pin inserter. Avoid the tendency for the pin to enter the disc space by directing the tip of the pin horizontal to the disc space. Be a sufficient distance away from the end plate to allow work on the disc space without dislodging the pin. The rubber sheath aids in protecting the tip on extraction. Place the superior and inferior right-sided pins before placing the left-sided pins.

13. Expose the annulus of the disc (Fig. 21M). There should have been minimal sharp dissection and cautery in the area. The disc is now prepared for the operative procedure. The vena cava and iliac artery and vein are held by the Freebody retractors.

14. Special curved or malleable retractors can be used instead of the Freebody retractors or between the pins for protection of the vena cava.

15. Closure: Remove the Freebody retractors, allowing the vessels and peritoneum to move back to the left and suturing each muscle layer with a running stitch.

Caution: The retractors must be extracted with the same amount of care as when they were inserted. The sheath and a finger must guard the tip; otherwise, the vena cava will be torn as the sharp tip passes the vessel that is tented around it.

Remember:

1. The incision should follow the skin guidelines for optimum spine exposure.
2. Achieve careful hemostasis in the muscle layers.

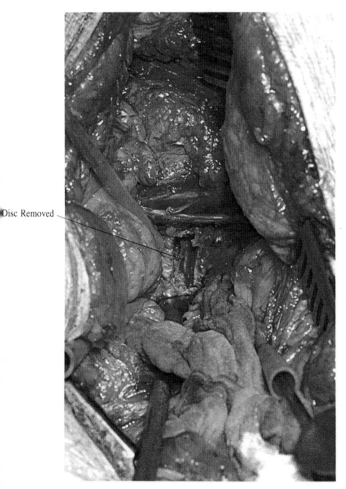

Disc Removed

FIGURE 21N. The annulus of the disc is resected for adequate visualization of the disc space. The Steinmann pins are in place. For removal of the Steinmann pins, the surgeon should place his fingertip on the tip of the pin between the pin and the retracted tissue as it is extracted from the vertebral body. The pin holder should be used for maximum control at this point. The vena cava must be held with the finger, and retracted from the pin as it is extracted. As the tip is pulled out, the vena cava can be torn as it bowstrings across the tip. Many of these problems can be avoided with experienced use of malleable retractors.

3. Incise the transversus abdominis muscle layer and the transversalis fascia in the lateral portion of the wound.
4. Beware of thinning muscle layers and the peritoneum's superficial position medially near the rectus sheaths.
5. Pass directly to the psoas muscle.
6. Identify the raised, soft, white disc.
7. Identify, ligate, and divide the iliolumbar vein.
8. Sweep prevertebral tissue left to right across the disc.
9. Insert the Steinmann pin after placing it directly on bone with the fingertip.
10. Retract the Steinmann pin again with the fingertip preventing the tip of the pin from damaging the left iliac artery and the vena cava.

References

1. Perry J: Surgical approaches to the spine. In Pierce D, Nichol V (eds): The Total Care of Spinal Cord Injuries. Boston, Little, Brown, 1977, pp 53–81.

2. Harmon PH: Anterior extraperitoneal lumbar disc excision and vertebral bone fusion. Clin Orthop 16:169–198, 1963.

3. Hodgson AR, Yau ACMC: Anterior surgical approaches to the spinal column. In Apley AG (ed): Recent Advances in Orthopaedics. Baltimore, Williams & Wilkins, 1964, pp 289–323.

4. Royal ND: A new operative procedure in the treatment of spastic paralysis and its experimental basis. Med J Anat 77:30, 1924.

5. Freebody D, Bedall R, Taylor RD: Anterior transperitoneal lumbar fusion. J Bone Joint Surg 53B:617–627, 1971.

Anterior Retroperitoneal Muscle-Sparing Approach to L2–S1 of the Lumbar Spine

Salvador A. Brau

1. Place the patient in the supine position on a Jackson or other X-ray table with an inflatable bag under the lumbar region. Discretionary inflation of the bag allows extension of the spine at the time of discectomy and graft placement, if needed.

2. The approach surgeon stands on the left and the assistant on the right. The level of the transverse incision in the craniocaudad plane depends on the level of the spine to be approached (Fig. 22A). The incision for L5–S1 is usually placed at the junction of the lower and middle third of the distance between the umbilicus and the symphysis pubis (Fig. 22B). For L4–L5, the incision is placed just below the umbilicus and for L3–L4 just above. For L2–L3, the incision is placed about 5 cm above the umbilicus. The incision, however, should be moved caudad or cephalad depending on the angle of L5–S1 and the relationship of L4–L5 to the iliac crest as seen on a lateral X-ray of the lumbar spine. The information seen on that X-ray allows the surgeon to place the incision precisely by palpating the iliac crest, then moving the incision site accordingly. Because the incision is small, especially when compared to the size of a paramedian incision used for the same levels, optimal placement is crucial for introducing the working sleeves, templates, and inserters at the proper angle, parallel to the vertebral end plates, in a straight anteroposterior (AP) plane. It is usually better to be a little below rather than a little above the disc space; so when in doubt, go lower. The lateral X-ray of the lumbar spine will also show whether there is osteophytic activity or major vessel calcification, or possibly both. These conditions will warn the surgeon that a much more difficult situation is at hand.

3. Begin the incision at the midline and carry it transversely to the lateral edge of the left rectus muscle. For two-level exposure, the incision should be more oblique, starting midline at the level of the lower disc and ending at the level of the upper disc at the lateral edge of the left rectus muscle (Fig. 22C). For three levels, the obliquity increases, but the incision is never vertical or paramedian.

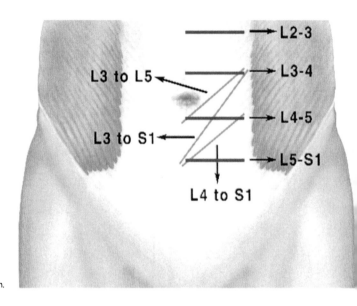

FIGURE 22A. Typical location of incision.

4. Carry the incision to the anterior rectus sheath using electrocautery and carry the subcutaneous portion of the incision beyond the ends of the skin incision both medially and laterally. This technique should expose this fascia from beyond the midline to the external oblique aponeurosis. Incise the rectus fascia from 1 cm to the right of the midline to the edge of the rectus laterally. The anterior rectus sheath is then elevated anteriorly away from the muscle belly for a distance of 4 to 6 cm both superiorly and inferiorly to allow full mobilization of the rectus muscle (Fig. 22D). Medial, lateral, and posterior dissection of the muscle is then carried out both with cautery and with

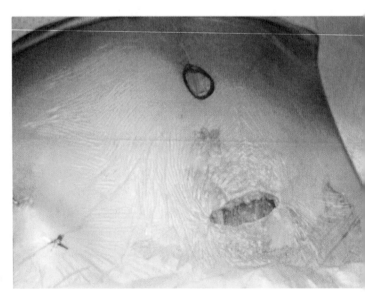

FIGURE 22B. Incision for L5–S1 with a steep angle.

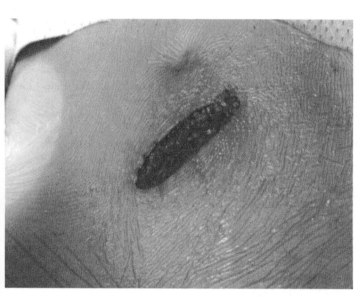

FIGURE 22C. Typical incision for L4–L5, L5–S1 approach in a normal weight patient.

finger dissection, taking great care to avoid injury to the inferior epigastric vessels. The inferior epigastric vessels run along the undersurface of the muscle and must be elevated with the muscle and retracted with it using an appropriate curved retractor. The rectus muscle is now mobilized circumferentially (Fig. 22E) and can easily be retracted both medially and laterally. Lateral mobilization of the rectus should not result in rectus denervation in exposing up to three levels (L3 to S1). In approaching multiple levels that include L2–L3, care must be taken not to injure the intercostal nerve that perforates the posterior rectus sheath and enters the muscle at that level as that trauma may result in rectus muscle paresis.

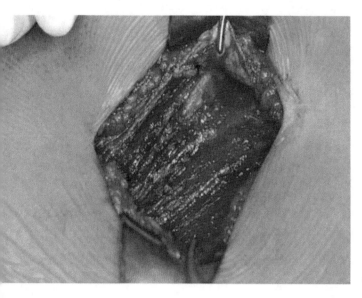

FIGURE 22D. Anterior rectus sheath elevated away from left rectus muscle.

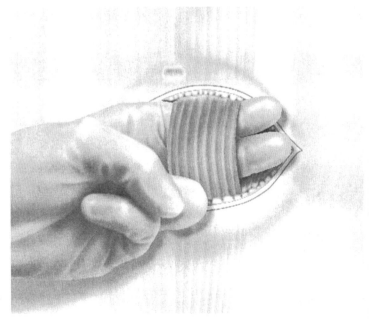

FIGURE 22E. Left rectus muscle mobilized circumferentially.

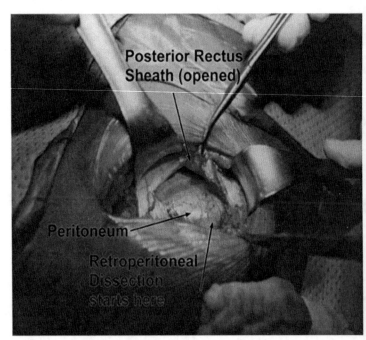

FIGURE 22F. Left rectus muscle elevated away from the posterior rectus sheath.

5. With the rectus muscle initially retracted medially (Fig. 22F), and for level L4–L5 or above, carefully incise the posterior sheath with a knife for 4 to 5 mm until the peritoneum is seen to shine through. Grasp the edges with a hemostat, then lift it away and very carefully dissect it from the peritoneum and incise it with scissors as far inferiorly and superiorly as possible. This layer can be quite tenuous, and care must be exercised to prevent peritoneal lacerations. The peritoneum will now bulge upward (Fig. 22G). Using your index finger, carefully push the peritoneum posteriorly at the edge of the fascial incision and slowly develop a plane between it and the undersurface of the internal oblique and transversus muscles and fascia; this will lead you into the retroperitoneal space (Fig. 22H).

6. Continue careful blunt finger dissection posteriorly and then start pushing medially, trying to elevate the peritoneum away from the psoas muscle. Should the peritoneum be entered, the tear should be repaired with absorbable suture material at that time; delaying this repair will only lead to major peritoneal repairs later on. Be careful not to enter the retropsoas space at this point because this error will lead to unnecessary bleeding in a blind pouch. The genitofemoral nerve can be easily identified over the psoas. The ureter can usually be identified as the peritoneum is lifted away from the psoas. Both these structures should be preserved from injury (Fig. 22I).

7. Once the psoas is identified, palpate medially to feel for the discs and vertebral bodies and the iliac artery. At this point, insert the entire hand (if the size of the incision allows) and make a fist in the retroperitoneal area (Fig. 22J). Sweep with the closed fist up and down to elevate the peritoneum away in all directions. Most single-level incisions are too small to allow a full fist to enter the retroperitoneum, so sweep with individual fingers or a sponge stick. A Harrington retractor is then inserted to elevate the peritoneal contents away from the vessels and allow further dissection. A Balfour retractor with appropriately deep blades is then inserted to keep the incision open

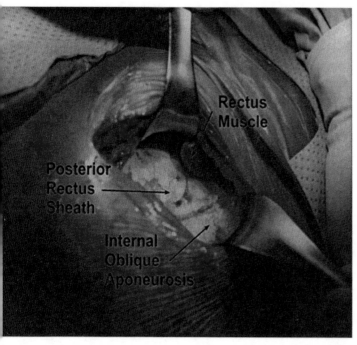

FIGURE 22G. Posterior rectus sheath incised and elevated to expose underlying peritoneum.

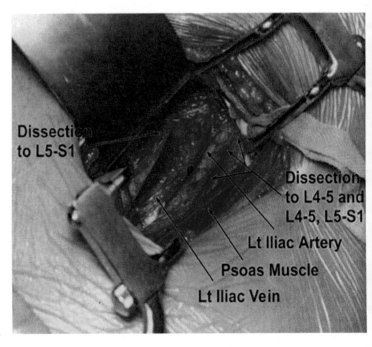

Dissection to L5-S1

Dissection to L4-5 and L4-5, L5-S1

Lt Iliac Artery

Psoas Muscle

Lt Iliac Vein

FIGURE 22H. Path to retroperitoneum.

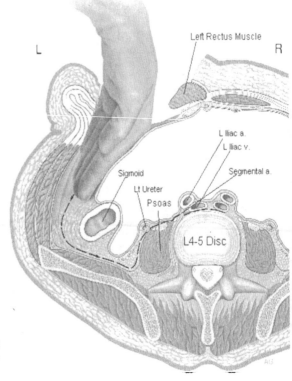

Left Rectus Muscle

L

R

L Iliac a.

L Iliac v.

Segmental a.

Sigmoid

Lt Ureter

Psoas

L4-5 Disc

FIGURE 22I. The ureter is identified above the psoas muscle as the peritoneum is elevated anteriorly.

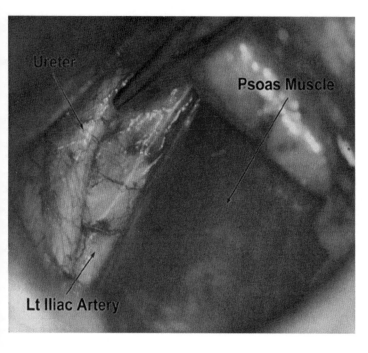

FIGURE 22J. The fist is used to elevate the peritoneum away from retroperitoneal structures.

in the craniocaudad plane. A dry lap sponge tucked superiorly into the space above the psoas before insertion of the Balfour is helpful in keeping retroperitoneal fat from creeping down and obscuring the field.

8. For operations on only L4–L5 or for operations that combine L4–L5 with either L3–L4 or L5–S1, the iliolumbar vein(s) must be ligated and cut because they serve as a tether, preventing mobilization of the iliac vein away from the anterior surface of the spine, and thus prevent proper exposure. With the Harrington–Balfour retractor combination in place, dissect bluntly just above the iliac artery and move the retroperitoneal tissues away from it (Fig. 22K). Expose and skeletonize the entire length of the common and external iliac arteries as far distally as possible (Fig. 22L). This distal mobilization will allow these vessels to be moved to the right for proper exposure of L4–L5. Using a Kittner or peanut sponge, proceed with sweeping blunt dissection along the lateral edge of the artery, going deep; this can usually be done fairly quickly because there are no branches of the iliac artery at this level. The lymphatics present in this area are easily swept away as well, but some hemostasis may be necessary with clips or cautery. This step will expose the left common iliac vein just underneath and medial to the artery. Continue the sweeping blunt dissection posteriorly to identify the iliolumbar vein(s), which crosses the body of L5 and dives into the left paraspinous area. Variations in the formation of the common iliac vein and the iliolumbar veins are common, and great care must be exercised to identify, ligate, and transect these veins and avoid avulsion (Fig. 22M). Ligation should be carried out in place before transection and not too close to the junction to the iliac vein itself to avoid injury to its sidewall. For any operation that involves L4–L5, these maneuvers are mandatory, unless the approach can be done below the bifurcation and between the iliac vessels.

9. The left iliac vein and artery can now be separated away from the spine using gentle, peanut sponge, fingertip, and blunt elevator dissection. In most patients the vein "peels" away from the anterior surface of the spine easily (Fig. 22N). In some patients, however, there is intense inflammatory reaction in the plane between the vein and the

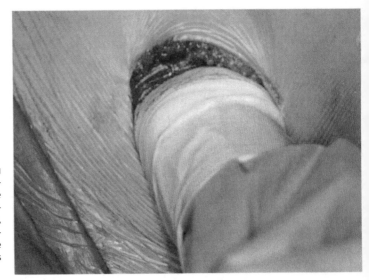

FIGURE 22K. Left iliac artery following the fist dissection. For L5–S1, dissection is carried medial and deep to the artery. For L4–L5, the dissection proceeds lateral and deep to the artery, and the artery is then retracted medially to expose the lateral wall of the vein. Deeper dissection then exposes the iliolumbar vein(s).

anterior longitudinal ligament, especially when osteophytes are present, so the dissection can be quite difficult and tedious. It is much easier to expose toward the right side of the spine from a more lateral aspect while elevating the vessels. This is the reason for going lateral to the left rectus muscle during this part of the approach.

10. All the vascular structures are thus swept from left to right, providing adequate visualization of the disc(s) and vertebral bodies involved. Segmental vessels running across the valleys on the anterior surface of the bodies can be transected between clips and swept to the sides with blunt dissection. Make sure you can get at least one finger between the vein and the ligament so that you can then palpate the right lateral edge of the spine with the vessels above your finger(s) (Figs. 22O, 22P). Be careful not to

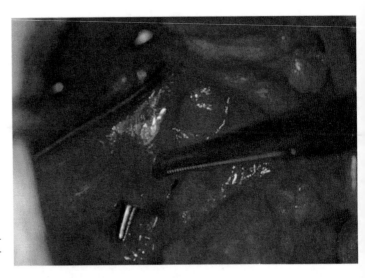

FIGURE 22L. Left iliac artery fully skeletonized from its origin to the distal external iliac.

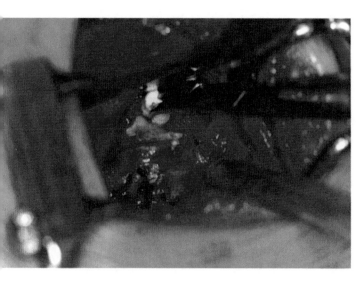

FIGURE 22M. Right-angle clamp under iliolumbar vein in preparation for ligation.

tear tissues that do not give way easily, as in doing this as you may tear lumbar veins coming in from the right side. Once this part of the exposure is completed (Fig. 22Q), the retractors (Balfour and Harrington) are removed.

11. The table-held retractor post and arms or ring are then set up. The surgeon's left hand then reenters the retroperitoneal space with the rectus now moved laterally, and the fingers move to the right side of the spine following the planes previously dissected. A Brau-ALIF radiolucent (Thompson Surgical Instruments, Traverse City, MI), 1- to 1¼-inch-wide blade with a small reverse lip is then placed blindly onto the right side of the spine using the finger(s) as a guide (Fig. 22R). This blade is then attached to table-held retractor system, then pushed to the right to elevate the vascular struc-

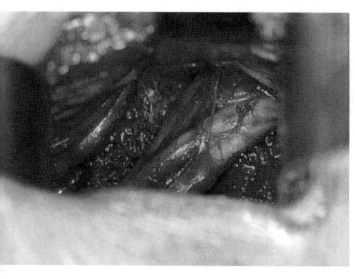

FIGURE 22N. Peanut sponge dissection under the vessels to expose L4–L5. Note metal clip on the iliolumbar vein stump.

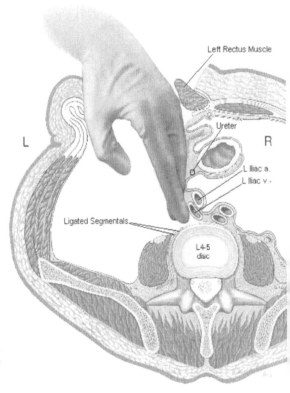

FIGURE 220. Finger dissection under the vessels toward the right side of the disc.

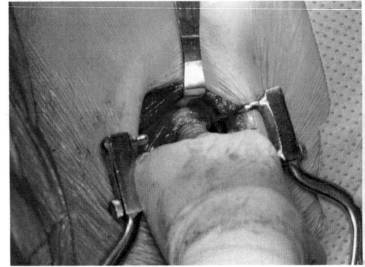

FIGURE 22P. Cross-sectional view shows finger dissection under the vessels going toward the right side of the disc after peanut sponge dissection has been performed. The tip of one finger should eventually reach to touch the right lateral side of the disc to be exposed.

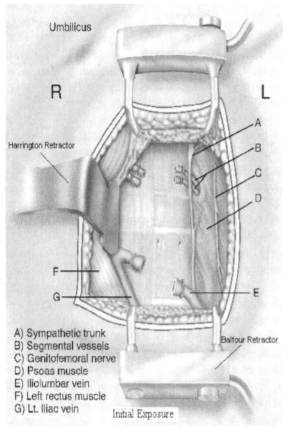

Umbilicus

R   L

Harrington Retractor

A
B
C
D

F
G
E

A) Sympathetic trunk
B) Segmental vessels
C) Genitofemoral nerve
D) Psoas muscle
E) Iliolumbar vein
F) Left rectus muscle
G) Lt. Iliac vein

Balfour Retractor

Initial Exposure

FIGURE 22Q. Overall view of initial exposure at L4–L5 before removal of the Harrington and Balfour retractors.

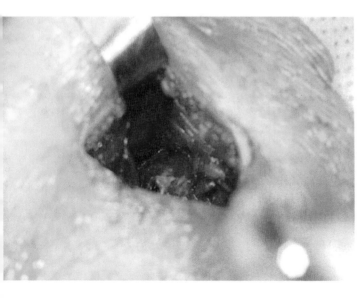

FIGURE 22R. Insertion of first Brau-ALIF blade onto the right side of the disc. The left rectus muscle is now in a lateral position.

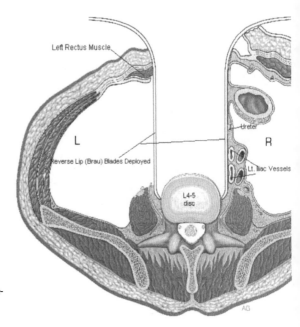

FIGURE 22S. First Brau-ALIF blade deployed on the right.

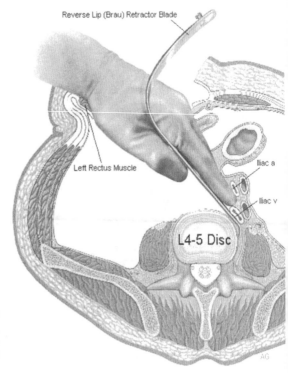

FIGURE 22T. Cross-sectional view of the first Brau-ALIF blade deployed. Note contact of the reverse lip with the disc. Also note compression of the left iliac vessels at L4–L5.

tures and expose the anterior surface of the spine (Figs. 22S, 22T). With a small incision, the left rectus muscle acts as a tether preventing the right retractor blade from achieving a vertical position once engaged to the side of the spine. Going medial to this muscle helps reduce some of this tension and makes it much easier to deploy these blades. Once secured to the table-held retractor system, the reverse-lipped blade will not move. The reverse lip keeps the blade anchored to the edge of the spine and prevents it from slipping anteriorly once tension is applied. Without this reverse lip, the retractor blade will not work effectively and the exposure will not be secure or stable.

12. Place a second such blade on the left side of the spine and attach it to the table-held system to complete the exposure. With the left rectus now retracted laterally, the spine is fully exposed to allow placement of sleeves, distractors, templates, and other devices in a direct AP plane (Figs. 22U, 22V). Additional retractor blades often must be placed superiorly or inferiorly to complete the exposure. X-rays should be taken after the first two blades are placed so as not to obscure the field with too much hardware. With these blades well anchored to the lateral wall of the vertebral column, the spine surgeon and his assistant can now work on the disc without other hands or retractors being in the way and with relative security that vessels will not slip around the retractors and be exposed to injury. Retractor blades that are straight or that curve away from the edge of the spine cannot provide engagement or contact to the spine itself. This engagement, together with the attachment of the retractor to the operating table, provides two-point stability and security to the exposure. In addition, there are no gaps through which the iliac vein can squeeze and intrude into the field of work.

13. For operations on L5–S1, the dissection is carried anterior and medial to the left iliac artery with the Harrington–Balfour retractor combination placed into that plane to elevate the peritoneal contents. The disc is palpated and dissection carried toward it with blunt dissection between the iliac vessels and below the aortic bifurcation. The middle sacral vessels may be taken between clips, ligatures, or cautery. Cautery is kept to a minimum, in males, to avoid injury to the superior hypogastric plexus fibers. The left iliac vein sometimes needs to be widely mobilized to allow placement of the

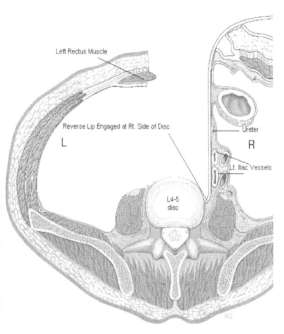

Left Rectus Muscle

Reverse Lip Engaged at Rt. Side of Disc

L

R

Ureter

Lt. Iliac Vessels

L4-5 disc

FIGURE 22U. Cross-sectional view with both Brau-ALIF blades deployed.

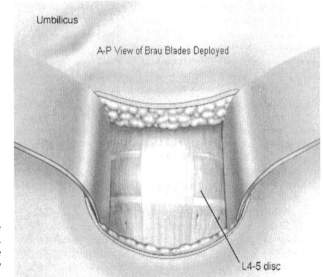

FIGURE 22V. View of the final exposure at L4–L5 in a normal weight patient. In an obese patient, blades may have to be placed superiorly and inferiorly as well.

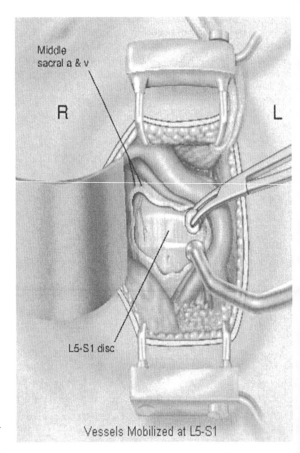

FIGURE 22W. View of the vessels mobilized at L5–S1.

reverse-lipped retractor against the left lateral edge of the spine. This vein is seen deep to the artery and is swept toward the left with a peanut sponge to expose that side of the disc. Dissection toward the right exposes that side of the disc, and a reverse-lipped retractor can again be used to maintain exposure to that side by anchoring the lip on the lateral aspect of the spine. The iliac vessels are not usually visualized on the right side (Fig. 22W). The table-held retractor is again used to keep the two reverse-lipped blades in place with the left rectus muscle again mobilized laterally.

14. For operations of L3–L4 and L2–L3, mobilization of the iliac vessels is usually not necessary with only an occasional need to transect the iliolumbar vein(s) to obtain adequate mobilization. This step makes approaching these two levels somewhat easier, except that L2–L3 is extremely difficult to expose in more obese patients, so it should only be approached this way in thin patients or those of normal weight.

15. When approaching L4–L5 and L5–S1, it is usually necessary to get to L5–S1 between the vessels and to L4–L5 lateral to them. Occasionally, L5–S1 can be exposed via the lateral approach used for L4–L5 if the bifurcation is low. In these cases, you can actually see both levels simultaneously with only minimal adjustment of the retractor and its blades to provide optimal access. In some cases, it is possible to expose L4–L5 by going between the vessels after having completed the exposure of L5–S1. This method requires a high bifurcation, which has been seen only in about 5 percent of our patients.

16. Discectomy and instrumentation are then performed (Figs. 22X, 22Y). Upon completion, remove the retractor blades sequentially, leaving the right-sided blade for last. Check the integrity of the vessels thoroughly, especially looking for arterial thrombosis or injury due to stretching. Remove the lap sponge and allow the tissues to fall back together anatomically. The individual fascial layers are then closed separately with running absorbable sutures, making sure that the anterior rectus sheath is well approximated. The posterior sheath need not be closed if it is tenuous and does not offer any significant strength to the closure. A thick, substantial posterior rectus sheath, however, should be closed. Subcutaneous tissues and skin are then closed according to the surgeon's preference. No Steinman pins or sharp-pointed retractors are ever used for retraction with this approach.

17. The expected complications of this approach, as described in our own clinical study of 386 patients,[1] are shown in Table 22.1. All but two planned levels were suc-

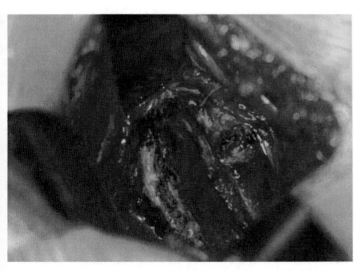

FIGURE 22X. View of final exposure at L5–S1 with disc removed.

FIGURE 22Y. View of instrumentation being carried out at L5–S1.

cessfully exposed (99.5%), and there were no deaths. Patients with calcified vessels have been subjected to this approach with good results. The exposure, however, may need to be limited and may only allow placement of devices that can be deployed from an anterolateral direction, such as a femoral ring graft.

18. In about 60% of patients with exposure at L4–L5, the iliac artery is completely occluded by compression; this, in some difficult cases, has lasted for more than 1 hour. No complications have been identified, however, and we do not recommend releasing the retractors until the arthrodesis is completed at that particular level. If more than one level is approached, the retractors must be redeployed for the additional levels, and during that time flow is restored.

Remember:

1. Plan the incision carefully using the lateral X-ray of the lumbar spine. Start with larger incisions, then use smaller incisions as you become more familiar with the approach. It is usually better for the incision to be a little below the disc rather than above it. Thus, it is better to err "low" rather than "high."

TABLE 22.1 Complications of the Anterior Retroperitoneal Muscle-Sparing Approach to L2–S1

Complication	Percentage of Patients in Study Affected
Myocardial infarction	0.25
Retrograde ejaculation	0
Rectus denervation	0
Arterial thrombosis	1.2
Venous injuries	0.7
DVT	1
Ileus	1
Wound infection (superficial)	0.5
Hernia	0.5
Compartment syndrome	0.25

2. The posterior sheath–transversalis fascia can be very thin and the peritoneum easy to enter, especially at higher levels and closer to the midline, so go as lateral as possible.
3. Mobilize the rectus muscle circumferentially, start the retroperitoneal dissection lateral to it, then place the final retractors medial to it. The initial exposure is easier to perform working lateral to the rectus muscle whereas the final exposure is easier to maintain with the muscle lateral to the retractors.
4. Avoid the retropsoas plane and stay anterior to the psoas muscle.
5. Try to identify the ureter as you elevate the peritoneum anteriorly.
6. Always ligate and transect the iliolumbar vein(s) for L4–L5.
7. Identify the raised soft disc(s) early on by fingertip palpation; this will let you know if the placement of the incision is adequate.
8. Sweep the prevertebral tissues sideways across the disc(s) left to right.
9. Make sure the vessels are mobilized distally as far as possible.
10. Check for vascular injury, bleeding, or thrombosis before closing and check the pedal pulses after closure of the incision.

Reference

1. Brau SA, Watkins RG, Williams LA: Complications of the Approach to Anterior Lumbar Spine Surgery. Poster Presentation, North American Spine Society, Annual Meeting, New Orleans, LA, October 25–28, 2000.

23

Anterior Retroperitoneal Flank Approach to L5–S1

1. For the left retroperitoneal approach to L5-S1, place the patient in the right lateral decubitus position held by either the inflatable "beanbag" or appropriate towel padding. Take care to prevent any degree of left hip flexion, which could permit the thigh to interfere with the exposure.

2. Make the incision from the midaxillary line, midway between the iliac crest and lowest rib, curving in a lazy-S configuration to the lower half of the symphysis-to-umbilicus distance. This point is approximately at the junction of the middle and distal third (Fig. 23A).[1,2]

3. With the electrocautery, divide the fascia and the external oblique and internal oblique muscles in the line of the incision. The transversus abdominis muscle is very thin. Open it in the posterior portions of the incision closer to the midaxillary line. Each of these muscle layers thins out anteriorly, and the peritoneum is very superficial at the edge of the rectus sheath. This is the area where the peritoneum is often inadvertently entered. If this occurs, repair the peritoneum after it has been well exposed and before the spinal work. With identification of the peritoneum and retroperitoneal space in the midaxillary line, bluntly dissect the peritoneum from the undersurface of the transversalis fascia before opening the rest of the abdominal wall incision.

4. For added exposure, bluntly dissect the peritoneum from the posterior aspect of the rectus sheath. The edge of the rectus sheath itself can be opened and the rectus muscle can be partially cut.

5. Proceed directly to the psoas muscle. Identify the genitofemoral nerve running on the surface of this muscle. The spine is medial to the muscle. With identification of the muscle, retract the peritoneal sac and ureter on the undersurface of the peritoneum medially.

6. Palpate the spine with a finger and find a disc for orientation: usually it is the L4–L5 disc (Fig. 23B). With identification of the L4–L5 disc, palpate the pulse of the left common iliac artery and the aortic bifurcation.

7. The bifurcation of the aorta is critical in determining the exact approach from this point. The usual bifurcation at the L4–L5 disc level was present in 69% of anatomical dissections by Harmon, but there is great variation.[3]

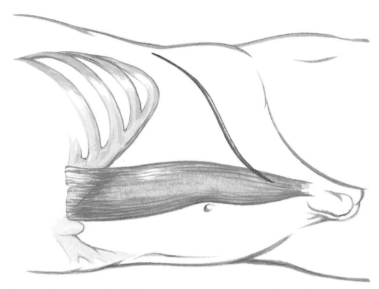

FIGURE 23A. For the left retroperitoneal approach to L5–S1, place the patient in the left lateral decubitus position. Take care to prevent any flexion of the left hip greater than 30 degrees, as the thigh will interfere with the exposure. Incise the skin and subcutaneous tissue from the midaxillary line, midway between the iliac crest and lower rib, curving in a lazy "S" configuration of the lower half of the symphysis-to-umbilicus distance; this is approximately at the junction of the middle and distal third of the distance between the symphysis and umbilicus. Divide with the electrocautery the external oblique, internal oblique, arid transversus abdominis muscles, much as described in Chapter 21. Enter the retroperitoneal space and retract medially the peritoneal sac.

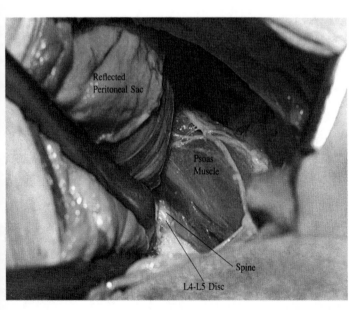

FIGURE 23B. Identify the psoas muscle. The psoas muscle is the key to the retroperitoneal exposure. The genitofemoral nerve on the psoas muscle helps with this identification. Sweep the peritoneal sac from left to right and identify the spine. Find the disc space. Most commonly this is the L4–L5 space or the L3–L4 space. Obtain an identifying X-ray at this point to localize the level. For the approach to L5–S1, after identification of the spine itself, palpate in the midline within the bifurcation to locate the L5–S1 disc.

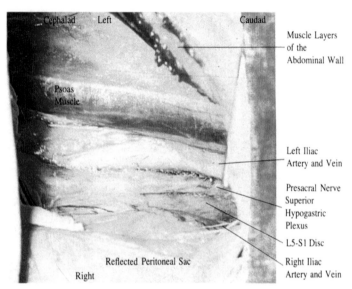

FIGURE 23C. Immediately medial to the psoas muscle is the spine. The approach to L5–S1 differs from the approach described in Chapter 21 in that at this point, the surgeon should pass a finger over the left common iliac artery and palpate the L5–S1 disc in the bifurcation. Three structures may be over the L5–S1 disc at this point, depending on the level of bifurcation of the aorta: (1) the left iliac vein, (2) the middle sacral vein, or (3) the superior hypogastric plexus or presacral nerve. Carefully, with blunt dissection, expose the disc of L5–S1 in this bifurcation. Make no horizontal cuts across the front of L5–S1. At this point, use blunt dissection only. Identify the disc. Retract the left common iliac vein, cephalad and to the left. The middle sacral vein can usually be bluntly dissected longitudinally and horizontally to allow retraction to the right. The superior hypogastric plexus nerve should be retracted and swept off the intervertebral disc, usually from left to right bluntly.

8. Palpate the left common iliac artery and pass over it medially to the L5–S1 disc. By placement of the finger and a subsequent blunt retractor such as a sponge-covered elevator, develop a plane just to the right of the left common iliac artery. (Fig. 23C).

Caution: Remember: The left iliac vein lies within the aortic bifurcation. It often courses directly on the surface of the L5–S1 disc and may be flattened against the disc or L5 body, its venous character obscured. Mobilize it to the left and cephalad with the left iliac artery.

9. The middle sacral artery and veins are present in the bifurcation. The key to handling these structures is blunt dissection just to the right of the left common iliac artery, sweeping from left to right the prevertebral tissue, including the middle sacral vessels and superior hypogastric plexus, off the lumbosacral disc. Occasionally the middle sacral vessels are of formidable size, but seldom do they have to be ligated.[4]

10. An additional structure in the bifurcation is the superior hypogastric sympathetic plexus (Fig. 23D). The key to avoid damaging the superior hypogastric plexus is to avoid transverse cuts on the face of the disc until all the prevertebral tissue has been elevated from the annulus and to avoid electrocautery on the surface of the L5–S1 disc. Small bleeding points are encountered when doing this dissection, but they are usually easily controlled by direct finger pressure or packing with hemostatic gauze. Usually the left iliac artery and vein are retracted to the left but may require retraction to the right on occasion.

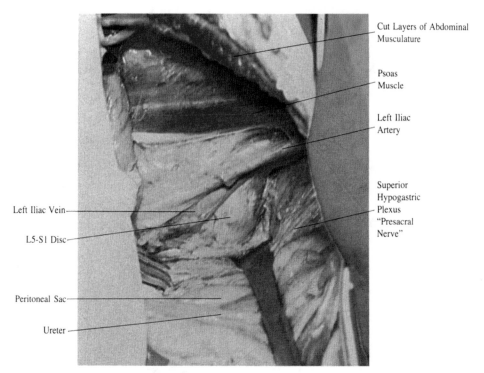

FIGURE 23D. Sweep the prevertebral tissue bluntly off the front of the L5–S1 disc. The superior hypogastric plexus may be a diffuse plexiform nerve formation that is retracted with the other tissue, or it can be a discrete well-defined presacral nerve.

Caution: Locate and ligate the iliolumbar vein before any mobilization of the left iliac artery to the right.

11. Always obtain X-ray confirmation of the level. It can be done easily by insertion of a 22-gauge spinal needle. Because the L5–S1 disc and the sacrum are often angled very horizontally, the body of L5 can be mistaken for the sacrum.

12. Insert the Freebody-type rubber-covered Steinmann pins: the superior right pin first, the lower right pin next. Insertion of these Freebody pins into the sacrum is difficult if there is a marked falloff of the sacrum. Take care not to drive the Steinmann pins too forcefully and skive off the surface of S1 into the pelvic soft tissues.[5] Place the pins between two fingers.

13. Dissect the last of the soft tissue off the spine with the fingers. The tip of the Steinmann pin is set into the bone, well protected by the surgeon's fingers. Tilt it to allow the maximum retraction, but with caution. If the tip of the Steinmann pin enters the disc space, it will loosen as the disc is dissected; therefore, the angle of the pin should be somewhat transverse to the disc space. After placement of the inferior right pin, insert the two left-sided pins. The left iliac vein is usually tented around the left inferior pin (Fig. 23E). Expose the disc between the four pins.

14. Any number of modified curved cobra-type retractors may be used instead of the Freebody pins.

15. Closure: Allow the peritoneal sac to fall into place. Close the muscle layers with running suture. The transversus abdominis and the internal oblique muscles be closed together.

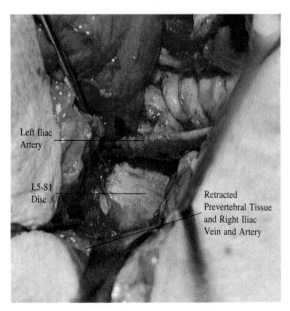

Left Iliac
Artery

L5-S1
Disc

Retracted
Prevertebral Tissue
and Right Iliac
Vein and Artery

FIGURE 23E. Exposure of tile L5–S1 disc and insertion of Steinmann pins should be carried out as described in Chapter 21. There is often great difficulty in placing the Steinmann pin into S1, as there is a marked dropoff of the S1 surface as the spine goes into lordosis. Great care should be taken to avoid allowing the Steinmann pin to slide off the surface of the sacrum into the pelvis. It should be very carefully placed, held by the surgeon with both hands, and tapped into place by the assistant. The superior left pin will be responsible for retracting the left common iliac vein. This vein is often a flat poorly defined structure on the front of the disc and should be very carefully retracted, and the pin inserted with great care. When working on the L5–S1 disc, the slant of the interspace often requires one to work from a caudad to cephalad direction. This restriction again emphasizes the importance of using a skin incision that is low enough to allow work in this area. Removal of the Steinmann pins should be undertaken with extreme care, with the tips protected as they are extracted.

Caution: During closure, protect the tips of the Steinmann pins as they are withdrawn to avoid lacerating the vascular structures being retracted.

Remember:

1. The skin incision should extend midway into the interval between the symphysis and umbilicus.
2. Avoid entering the peritoneum in the anterior aspect of the incision.
3. Identify the retroperitoneal space in the more proximal portion of the incision.
4. Dissect the peritoneum off the undersurface of the transversalis fascia before opening the rest of the abdominal wall.
5. Identify the L4–L5 disc and the left common iliac artery.
6. Identify the iliolumbar vein.
7. Locate the L5–S1 disc in the bifurcation by finger palpation and begin blunt dissection just to the right of the left common iliac artery.
8. Beware of the left common iliac vein crossing on the surface of the L5–S1 disc within the bifurcation.
9. Bluntly mobilize the middle sacral vessels and the superior hypogastric plexus from left to right.
10. Do not allow the Freebody pins to skive off the anterior surface of S1.

References

1. Hodgson AR: Anterior approaches to the spinal column. Clin Orthop 56:1968.
2. Hodgson AR, Yau ACMA: Anterior approaches to the spinal column. In Apley AG (ed): Recent Advances in Orthopaedics. Baltimore, Williams & Wilkins, 1964, pp 289–323.
3. Harmon PH: Anterior extraperitoneal lumbar disc excision and vertebral body fusion. Clin Orthop 16:169–198, 1963.
4. Duncan HMM, Jonck LM: The presacral plexus in anterior lumbar fusion of the lumbar spine. S Afr J Surg 3(2):93–96, 1965.
5. Freebody D, Bedall R, Taylor RD: Anterior transperitoneal lumbar fusion. J Bone Joint Surg. 53B:617–627, 1971.

Anterior Extraperitoneal Midline Incision of L2–S1

1. Position the patient supine on the table, the lower lumbar spine at the level of the kidney rests.

2. Make a lower abdominal pararectus incision through the skin and subcutaneous tissue (Fig. 24A). The most immediate layers are the external oblique with its transition into the linea semilunaris leading to the fascia of the rectus sheath. The linea semilunaris is composed of the aponeurosis of the three layers of the abdominal musculature and their fascia.

3. Incise the fibers of the external oblique, the internal oblique, and the small thin layer of transversus abdominis muscles lateral to the semilunaris in line with the skin incision.

4. Identify the transversalis fascia. The transversalis fascia is the internal investing fascial layer of the abdominal cavity. Dissect on the outer surface of this transversalis fascia to the edge of the rectus sheath. At this point the transversalis fascia splits to form the lamina of the rectus sheath. The posterior lamina of the rectus sheath forms the endoabdominal fascia in this area.

5. Incise the transversalis fascia lateral to the linea semilunaris carefully and identify the peritoneum through the incision (Fig. 24B).

6. Begin the incision in line with the skin incision, dissecting the peritoneum with a sponge or gloved hand off the undersurface of the transversalis fascia. Open the abdominal wall after the peritoneum has been identified and cleared (Fig. 24C).

7. Dissect bluntly the peritoneum from the lateral abdominal wall progressing posteriorly. Identify the psoas muscle, as in any retroperitoneal approach to the spine. Retract the peritoneum off the left iliac artery and vein by use of the surgeon's hand, a padded Deaver retractor, or sponge sticks. Sweep the peritoneum with the ureter from left to right, and expose the left common iliac artery and vein (Figs. 24D, 24E). Insert Freebody pins or special retractors.

8. (See Chapters 21 and 23.) Palpate and identify an intervertebral disc, remembering that this is a relatively avascular area. With any approach to the L4–S1 area, identify the left iliolumbar vein. Ligate it when necessary. Dissection within the bifurcation of the aorta should be blunt and as avascular as possible. Remember the left common iliac vein lying in the bifurcation over the C5–S1 disc (Figs. 24F, 24G, 24H,

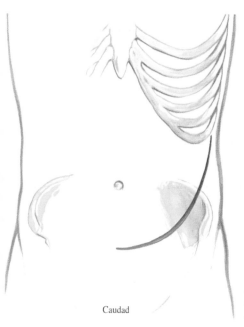

Caudad

FIGURE 24A. Position the patient supine on the table with the lumbar spine over the kidney rests. Make a lower abdominal pararectus incision through the skin and subcutaneous tissue. The most immediate layers are the external oblique with its transition into the linea semilunaris leading to the fascia of the rectus sheath. The linea semilunaris is composed of the aponeurosis of the three muscle layers of the abdominal musculature and their fascia.

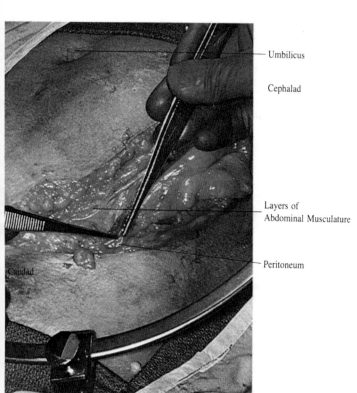

Umbilicus

Cephalad

Layers of
Abdominal Musculature

Peritoneum

Caudad

FIGURE 24B. Incise the external oblique, internal oblique, and transversus abdominis muscles, lateral to the semilunaris in line with the skin incision. Identify the transversalis fascia. Incise the transversalis fascia lateral to the semilunaris and identify the peritoneum through the incision. Dissect the peritoneum with a sponge or gloved hand off the undersurface of the transversalis fascia and open the abdominal wall after the peritoneum has been identified and cleared from the abdominal wall. The left rectus muscle may be divided for increased ease of retraction. Note: The peritoneum may be identified and dissection begun under the rectus sheath, but it is easier to find it laterally.

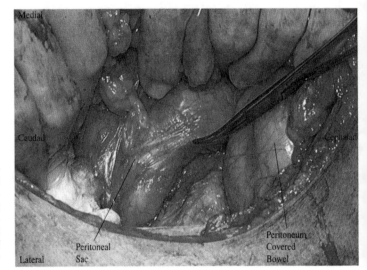

FIGURE 24C. Bluntly dissect the peritoneum from the lateral abdominal wall progressing posteriorly and retract the peritoneum from left to right with the peritoneal sac contents. Dissect the peritoneum medially toward the midline from the undersurface of the abdominal wall to allow extension of the incision medially.

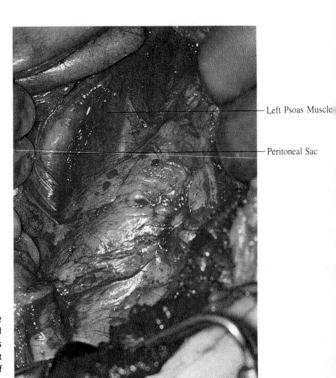

FIGURE 24D. Identify the psoas muscle as the key to the retroperitoneal space. With identification of the psoas muscle, bluntly dissect left to right the peritoneal sac and peritoneum off the major retroperitoneal structures, i.e., the aorta, vena cava, iliac veins, and spine.

Cephalad

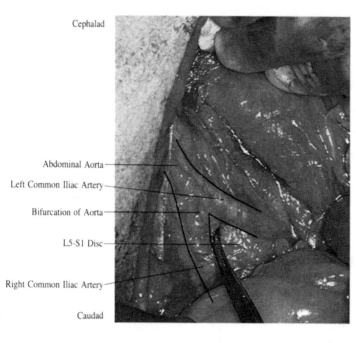

Abdominal Aorta

Left Common Iliac Artery

Bifurcation of Aorta

L5-S1 Disc

Right Common Iliac Artery

Caudad

FIGURE 24E. Sweep the peritoneal sac left to right and identify the bifurcation of the aorta, tile abdominal aorta, and the spine.

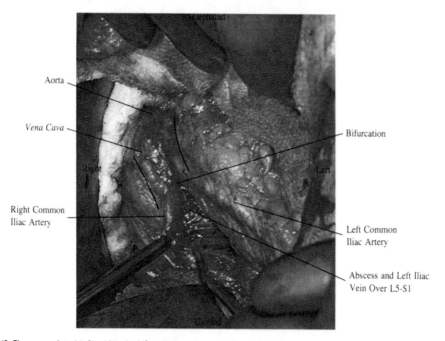

Aorta

Vena Cava

Right Common Iliac Artery

Bifurcation

Left Common Iliac Artery

Abscess and Left Iliac Vein Over L5-S1

FIGURE 24F. The approach to L5–S1 within the bifurcation requires identification of the left iliac vein, as this structure courses right to left through the bifurcation. For approaches to the spine cephalad to L5 the approach should be carried out as described in Chapter 21, with ligation of the iliolumbar vein and left-to-right retraction. Note: There is significant variation of vascular anatomy in this area. The level of aortic bifurcation may be high, necessitating an approach to L4–L5 from within the bifurcation. An anomalous left iliac vein can make exposure of L5–S1 almost impossible, especially with a flank incision.

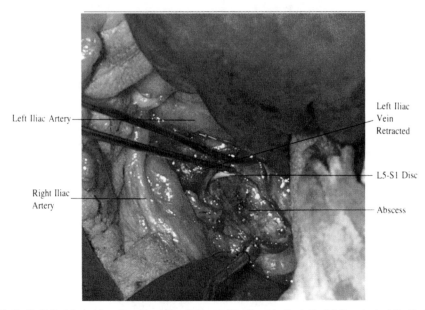

Left Iliac Artery

Right Iliac
Artery

Left Iliac
Vein
Retracted

L5-S1 Disc

Abscess

FIGURE 24G. The L5–S1 disc is in the bifurcation with a darkened abscess of the S1 vertebral body. The left iliac vein should be identified in the prevertebral tissue. The middle sacral vein and superior hypogastric plexus are swept off the front of the L5 disc.

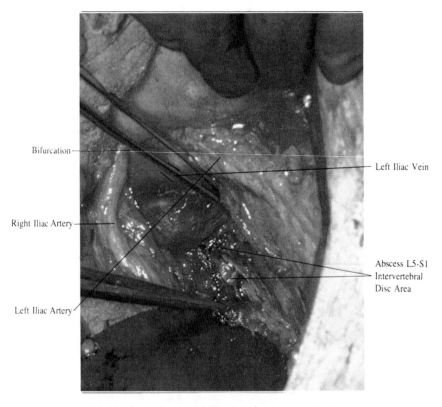

Bifurcation

Right Iliac Artery

Left Iliac Artery

Left Iliac Vein

Abscess L5-S1
Intervertebral
Disc Area

FIGURE 24H. A large, voluminous left iliac vein is often encountered in this area.

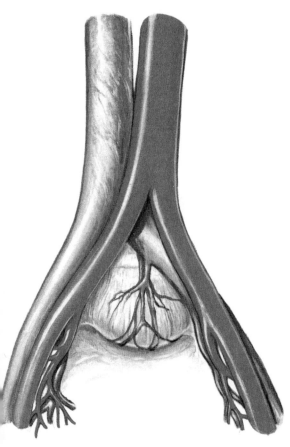

FIGURE 24I. Illustration of the left common iliac vein and the middle sacral vein. The level of bifurcation of the aorta often determines the difficulty in dealing with the left common iliac vein. Often this is a very large structure, 3 cm in diameter, usually passing above the L5–S1 disc with a low bifurcation. It could be quite difficult to retract to the left and may require approach to the L5–S1 disc from the left of the left common iliac artery and vein, retracting both structures to the right.

24I). The variation in inferior vena cava and lumbar veins often dictates the exact approach from this point.

9. Bluntly retract and protect the superior hypogastric plexus.

10. Closure: Allow the peritoneal sac to fall into place. Close the muscle layers with running suture. The transversus abdominis and the internal oblique may be closed together.

Caution: During closure, protect the tips of the Steinmann pins as they are withdrawn to avoid lacerating the vascular structures being retracted.

Remember:

1. Position the patient to allow hyperextension of the lumbar spine.
2. Identify the external oblique, the linea semilunaris, and the edge of the rectus muscle sheath.
3. Identify the transversalis fascia lateral to the rectal sheath.
4. Open the transversalis fascia carefully and identify the peritoneum.
5. Bluntly dissect the peritoneum from the intersurface of the abdominal wall first from medial to lateral anteriorly, then lateral to medial across the spine and large vessels.

6. Identify the psoas muscle.
7. Avoid damaging the iliolumbar vein, and be prepared to manage the venous anomalies present.

Reference

1. Harmon PH: A simplified surgical technic for anterior lumbar diskectomy and fusion; avoidance of complications; anatomy of the retroperitoneal veins. Clin Orthop 37, 1964.

Transperitoneal Midline Approach to L4–S1

1. Position the patient supine over the flexion crease in the table and hyperextend the lumbar spine for greater exposure.

2. Make either a vertical midline incision or the transverse "smile" incision. The "smile" is better cosmetically and gives excellent exposure but requires transection of the rectus abdominis muscle (Figs. 25A, 25B). Identify the rectus sheath; open the anterior portion of the rectus sheath. Transect the rectus abdominis muscle. The posterior rectus sheath, the abdominal fascia, and the peritoneum are conjoined in this area. Incise carefully through the posterior rectus sheath and abdominal fascia to the peritoneum (Fig. 25C).

3. Pick up the peritoneum (Fig. 25D). Open it carefully to avoid bowel damage and extend the opening the length of the wound. Pack off the bowel and identify the posterior peritoneum over the sacral promontory.

4. Palpate the aorta and both iliac vessels through the posterior peritoneum (Figs. 25E, 25F). Identify the softer texture of the L5–S1 disc.

5. Inject the retroperitoneal space with saline to achieve separation of the peritoneum from the vascular structures.

6. Pick up the peritoneum with Adsons and handle it delicately.

7. Make a small incision and extend the opening (Figs. 25E, 25G, 25H).

8. At this point, despite the fact that there may be bleeding in this area, avoid use of the cautery anterior to L5–S1 to prevent damage to the superior hypogastric plexus. Take care to avoid the left common iliac vein crossing over the L5–S1 disc within the aortic bifurcation (see Figs. 24C, 24H). It often lies as a flat, white, bloodless ribbon across the disc.

9. After identification of the left common iliac artery and left common iliac vein, start blunt dissection just to the right of the left iliac artery and carry it left to right across the front of the disc, sweeping the superior hypogastric plexus and soft tissue from left to right (see Figs. 23D, 26A).

10. The middle sacral artery and vein are bluntly dissected from left to right without sacrifice at this point. Longitudinal blunt dissection allows better mobilization of these vascular structures. When bleeding is encountered, use direct finger and sponge pressure for a short time, followed by blunt dissection. Control hemmorhage with packing and pressure. Divide and tie if necessary (Fig. 25I).

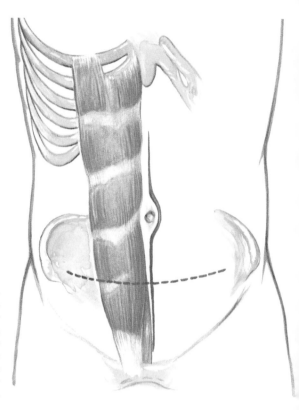

FIGURE 25A. Position the patient supine over the flexion crease in the table and hyperextend the lumbar spine for greater exposure. Make a vertical midline incision or the transverse "smile" incision. The smile incision is better cosmetically, gives excellent exposure, and requires transection of the rectus abdominis muscle.

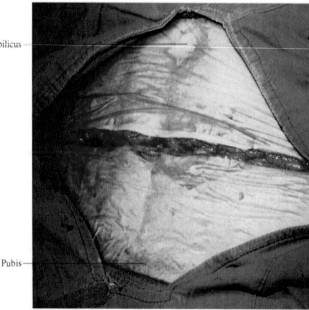

Umbilicus

Pubis

FIGURE 25B. Transverse "smile" incision.

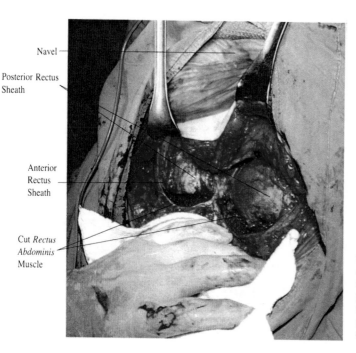

Navel

Posterior Rectus
Sheath

Anterior
Rectus
Sheath

Cut *Rectus
Abdominis*
Muscle

FIGURE 25C. Open the anterior portion of the rectus sheath and transect each rectus abdominis muscle. Identify the posterior rectus sheath. The posterior rectus sheath, abdominal fascia, and peritoneum are conjoined in this area.

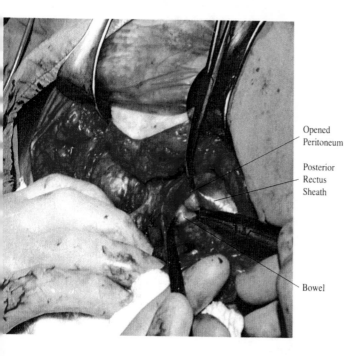

Opened
Peritoneum

Posterior
Rectus
Sheath

Bowel

FIGURE 25D. Incise carefully through the posterior rectus sheath and abdominal fascia and identify the peritoneum. Pick up the peritoneum, carefully open the peritoneum to avoid bowel damage, and extend the peritoneal opening the entire length of the wound. Insert a self-retaining Deaver-type retractor.

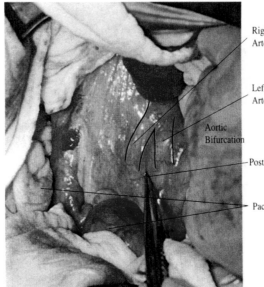

Right Iliac
Artery

Left Iliac
Artery

Aortic
Bifurcation

Posterior Peritoneum

Packed Off Retracted Bowel

FIGURE 25E. Pack off the bowel to allow adequate exposure of the posterior peritoneum over the sacral prominence. Palpate for the aortic pulse and common iliac artery. With identification of the sacral prominence and the bifurcation of the aorta, one may inject the posterior retroperitoneum with saline to allow elevation of the peritoneum off the important vascular structures.

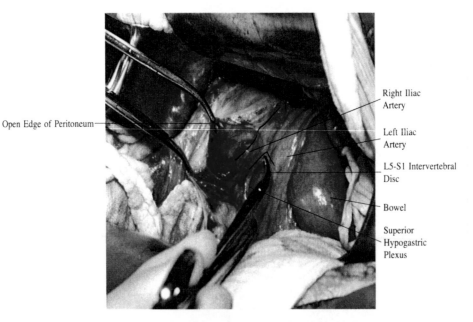

Open Edge of Peritoneum

Right Iliac
Artery

Left Iliac
Artery

L5-S1 Intervertebral
Disc

Bowel

Superior
Hypogastric
Plexus

FIGURE 25F. Open the posterior peritoneum as carefully as one would open the anterior peritoneum. Elevate with Adson forceps and incise. Extend this opening in the posterior peritoneum vertically, retract the peritoneum, and bluntly dissect the peritoneum off the vessels of the bifurcation. After removal of the peritoneum use blunt dissection only. Feel for the prominent softness of the L5–S1 inter- vertebral disc and bluntly dissect the material, usually from left to right, off the face of the L5–S1 disc. Again, one must be very careful to avoid damaging the superior hypogastric plexus at this point in the operation. Likewise, the middle sacral vein and left iliac artery can be atraumatically retracted if careful blunt dissection is carried out.

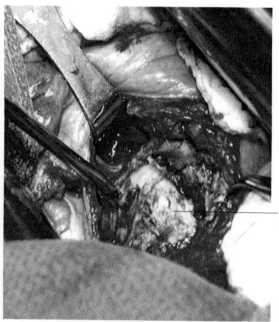

L5-S1
Intervertebral Disc

FIGURE 25G. Exposure of the intervertebral disc of L5–S1 within the bifurcation of the aorta.

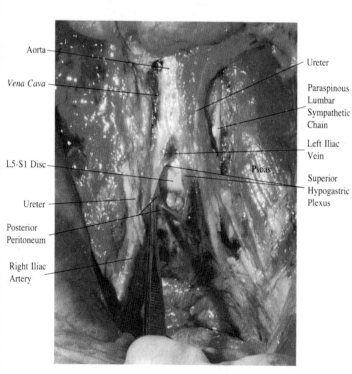

Aorta

Vena Cava

L5-S1 Disc

Ureter

Posterior
Peritoneum

Right Iliac
Artery

Ureter

Paraspinous
Lumbar
Sympathetic
Chain

Left Iliac
Vein

Superior
Hypogastric
Plexus

Psoas

FIGURE 25H. The bifurcation of the aorta with the opening of the posterior peritoneum emphasized.

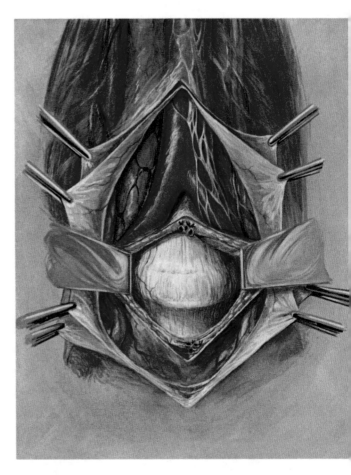

FIGURE 25I. Exposure of the L5–S1 disc with careful opening and retraction of the peritoneum. Identification and retraction of the left iliac vein with the left common iliac artery. This illustration shows ligation of the middle sacral vein and retraction to the left of the plexiform superior hypogastric plexus. One should always employ careful closure of the posterior peritoneum, as well as the standard abdominal closure.

11. Blunt dissection sweeping the material left to right off the front of the disc allows insertion of the four Freebody-type Steinmann pins into the L5 and S1 vertebral bodies (Fig. 25G) or positioning of special Deaver-type retractors. Again, beware of the left common iliac vein when inserting the Steinmann pins.

12. With isolation of the L5–S1 disc and X-ray confirmation of level, disc excision and graft may be done.

13. For additional exposure of L4–L5, the level of the aortic bifurcation and the size of the left iliac vein determine how the vessels are retracted. Always ligate and divide the iliolumbar vein for L4–L5 exposure.

14. Closure: Close each layer from peritoneum to muscle, subcutaneous tissue, and skin.

Remember:

1. The peritoneum is found under the thin posterior rectus sheath.
2. Open the posterior peritoneum over the superior promontory very carefully.
3. Start the dissection to the right of the left iliac artery and sweep from left to right.
4. Use blunt dissection and direct pressure to control retroperitoneal bleeding over the lumbosacral disc.

5. Beware of the left iliac vein in the aortic bifurcation.
6. Divide and ligate the iliolumbar vein for L4–L5 exposure.

References

1. Freebody D, Bendall R, Taylor RD: Anterior transperitoneal lumbar fusion. J Bone Joint Surg 53B(4):617–627, 1971.
2. Hodgson AR, Yau ACMC: Anterior surgical approaches to the spinal column. In Apley AG (ed): Recent Advances in Orthopaedics. Baltimore, Williams & Wilkins, 1964, pp 289–323.
3. Lane J, Moore ES: Transperitoneal approach to the intervertebral disc in the lumbar area. Ann Surg 127:1948.

26

Superior Hypogastric Sympathetic Plexus

The preaortic sympathetic plexus is a continuation of the thoracolumbar sympathetic chain extending down anterior to the aorta and vertebral bodies in the retroperitoneal space (Fig. 26A). The inferior hypogastric plexus is at approximately the L3–L4 level and the superior hypogastric plexus at L4–S1. There is considerable variation in the structure of the superior hypogastric plexus.[1] As the superior hypogastric plexus fibers arch over the L5–S1 disc in the bifurcation of the aorta, the predominance of fibers are usually closer to the left iliac artery. These fibers may have the form of multiple strands or one predominant large simple nerve trunk. The superior hypogastric plexus contains the sympathetic function for the urogenital system.

Parasympathetic function for the urogenital system is supplied by the S1–L4 nerve roots that contribute to the pelvic splenic nerves. Somatic function from S1, S2, S3, and S4 is carried predominantly by the pudendal nerve.

Ejaculation is predominantly a sympathetic function, whereas erection is predominantly a parasympathetic function through control of the vasculature of the penis. Disruption to the sympathetic plexus results in retrograde ejaculation and sterility. Although the sympathetic fibers also have some effect on the motility of the vas deferens, important in transportation of the spermatoza from the epididymis to the seminal vesicle,[2] the main effect of damage to the superior hypogastric plexus is improper closing of the bladder neck, with resultant retrograde ejaculation.[2]

The pathophysiology of retrograde ejaculation is known. The muscle components of the bladder neck–urethral junction are a continuation of the bladder muscle. Emission of seminal fluid from prostatic and ejaculatory ducts into the posterior urethra excites afferently the sacral and lumbar cords, which send efferent motor impulses over autonomic and somatic pathways. Although parasympathetic nerves actively relax the external sphincter and somatic nerves cause the genital and perineal muscles to start involuntary rhythmic contractions, the lack of sympathetic stimulation fails to maintain the involuntary closure of the bladder muscle of the visceral neck. The pressure differential forces the fluid into the bladder. The prognosis for recovery from retrograde ejaculation is good,[3] and bladder aspiration techniques have been used to obtain sperm in refractory cases. Incidence of true sterility without retrograde ejaculation is not known. Impotence or failure of erection should not be produced by damage to the

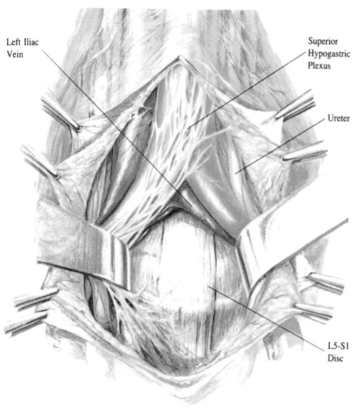

Left Iliac
Vein

Superior
Hypogastric
Plexus

Ureter

L5-S1
Disc

FIGURE 26A. The superior hypogastric plexus within the bifurcation of the aorta. Methods to avoid damaging the hypogastric plexus: (1) Use blunt dissection, retraction, and spreading to remove the prevertebral tissue from the sacral promitory. (2) For the transperitoneal midline approach, very carefully open the posterior peritoneum and bluntly dissect the prevertebral tissue from right to left. (3) With spreading and blunt dissection, attempt to retract the middle sacral vein and artery without electrocautery. Avoid electrocautery on the anterior surface of L5-S1. When this vessel is of considerable size, use vascular clips or ligation. (4) Opening the posterior peritoneum higher over the bifurcation and extending the opening down over the sacral promitory may allow better visualization and retraction of these tissues.

superior hypogastric plexus. Methods to avoid damaging the hypogastric plexus are the following[4]:

1. For the transperitoneal midline approach, very carefully open the posterior peritoneum, and bluntly dissect the prevertebral tissue from right to left.[5]
2. Opening the posterior peritoneum higher over the bifurcation, then extending the opening down over the sacral promontory, may allow one to visualize and retract these tissues more easily.[2–5]
3. Use blunt dissection, retraction, and spreading to remove the prevertebral tissue from the L5–S1 disc.
4. With spreading and blunt dissection, attempt to retract the middle sacral artery and vein without electrocautery. When this vessel is of considerable size, use vascular clips or tie ligation.
5. Make no transverse scalpel cuts on the front of the L5–S1 disc until the annulus of the disc is clearly exposed.
6. Avoid use of electrocautery within the aortic bifurcation.

References

. LaBate JS: The surgical anatomy of the superior hypogastric plexus—"presacral nerve." Surg Gynecol Obstet 67:199, 1938.

2. Johnson RM, McGuire EJ: Urogenital complications of anterior approaches to the lumbar spine. Clin Orthop 154:114–118, 1981.

3. Flynn JC, Hoque A: Anterior fusion of the lumbar spine. J Bone Joint Surg 61A(8):1143–1150, 1979.

4. Duncan HMM, Jonck LM: The presacral plexus in anterior lumbar fusion of the lumbar spine. S Afr J Surg 3(2):93–96, 1965.

5. Freebody D, Bedall R, Taylor RD: Anterior transperitoneal lumbar fusion. J Bone Joint Surg 53B:617–627, 1971.

En Bloc Sacrectomy

Katsuro Tomita • *Hiroyuki Tsuchiya* • *Norio Kawahara* •
Masahiko Hata • *Hideki Murakami*

Sacral tumors may present a difficult problem to the surgeon who desires to obtain a clear margin of excision. Frequently, tumors in this anatomical location are of a low grade biologically, such as chordomas or chondrosarcomas, and therefore unlikely to result in metastatic disease even though they are locally aggressive. Curative ablation of sacral tumors may be considered difficult because of the relationship between the anatomical location of the sacrum and the plexus of the lumbosacral nerves and vessels on the one hand and intrapelvic organs on the other. It is also difficult to reconstruct the continuity between pelvis and spine. However, en bloc sacrectomy may well be oncologically indicated, even for sacral tumors, to reduce the incidence of local tumor recurrence leading to fatal disease. In this chapter, we introduce the surgical classification of sacral tumors and the method of total or partial (segmental) en bloc sacrectomy with a T-saw.[1,2]

Surgical Staging of Sacral Tumors

Although extensive wide excision is generally desirable for malignant sacral tumors, inadequate tumor excision is sometimes performed to prevent bladder–bowel dysfunction and loss of spinopelvic stability after sacrectomy. Because insufficient tumor ablation may cause local tumor recurrence, jeopardizing the patient's life, complete excision of sacral tumors should be performed even though stability and the lumbosacral nerves are sacrificed.

The surgical staging system for musculoskeletal tumors was developed by Enneking.[3] Stage 3 benign aggressive tumors, such as giant cell tumors of bone, can be treated by intracapsular excision or marginal excision. Low-grade malignant tumors, such as chordomas and chondrosarcomas, should ideally be treated with wide excision; however, at the very least, marginal excision should be performed, because an intralesional excision of those tumors will surely result in local recurrence leading to treatment failure or fatal disease.[4] High-grade tumors, such as osteosarcomas, malignant fibrous histiocytomas, and Ewing's sarcomas, should be excised with a more radical margin beyond the reactive zone, if feasible, and treatment should include chemotherapy and/or radiotherapy.

Dysfunction After Sacrectomy

Depending on the level of sacral resection, various degrees of neurologic dysfunction and loss of stability of the sacroiliac joint will occur after the excision of sacral tumors (Fig. 27A).

1. Neurologic Deficits

Sacral amputation between S2 and S3 causes sexual dysfunction because the sacral nerves below S3 are sacrificed, and sacral amputation between S1 and S2 causes bladder–bowel dysfunction because the sacral nerves below S2 are sacrificed. Total sacrectomy with the dissection between L5 and S1 leads to total loss of sacral nerve function, although ambulation can be preserved when the lumbar nerves are preserved above L5. Division of the sacrum just below the lower border of the S3 vertebra does not result in disturbance of the sphincteric function, but bilateral sacrifice of the S2, S3, and S4 nerve roots leads to urinary and fecal incontinence, and impotence for males. Patients about to undergo high sacral amputation should be apprised of this risk. Preservation of only one S2 root leads to a weakened but present sphincter control[5,6] whereas unilateral preservation of the S2 and S3 roots apparently has no such effect.[7,8] However, it is possible for patients to control urination by self-catheterization or by increasing abdominal pressure and evacuation by using an enema. The exact nature of these deficits remains controversial, however, because some authors contend that unilateral preservation of the S2 root can maintain complete anorectal continence[9] whereas others hold that when both S2 roots are preserved sphincter problems are mild and reversible.[10] Finally, it appears that early rehabilitative treatment for 1 year after surgery may restore normal bladder function.[11]

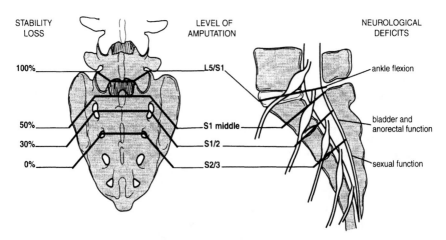

STABILITY LOSS	LEVEL OF AMPUTATION	NEUROLOGICAL DEFICITS
100%	L5/S1	ankle flexion
50%	S1 middle	bladder and anorectal function
30%	S1/2	
0%	S2/3	sexual function

FIGURE 27A. Level of sacrectomy and dysfunction.

2. Stability Loss

Reconstruction should be performed depending on the degree of stability loss between pelvis and spine. Preservation of the sacroiliac joint has a great impact on the stability between spine and pelvis. In a study using cadavers by Gunterberg et al., the weakening of the posterior arch of the pelvis after sacral resection below S1 was found to be approximately 30% and after resection through S1 approximately 50%.[12] Native stability of the posterior arch of the pelvis is preserved, however, when sacrectomy is performed below S2. In our experience, augmentation with bone grafts and sacral rods is advisable after sacrectomy through S1 to prevent fracture of the sacral body by shearing force. After total en bloc sacrectomy, the stability between pelvis and spine should be reconstructed in combination with spinal instrumentation and bone grafts.

Surgical Classification of Sacral Tumors (Fig. 27B)

We classified surgical procedures for sacral tumors into four types on the basis of the extension of tumors and the level of sacral resection (sacrectomy).

1. Type I, low sacral amputation: tumor is excised by sacrectomy below S2.
2. Type II, high sacral amputation: tumor is excised by sacrectomy through S1 or S1–S2.
3. Type III, total sacrectomy: tumor involving S1 is excised by sacrectomy through L5–S1.
4. Type IV, extended sacrectomy: tumor extending beyond the sacroiliac joint or toward the lumbar spine is excised by total sacrectomy combined with excision of the ilium, vertebra, or intrapelvic organs.

Surgical Techniques

There are two major approaches for en bloc sacrectomy: the posterior approach and the combined anteroposterior approach. The posterior approach is indicated for types I and II and the anteroposterior approach for types III and IV.

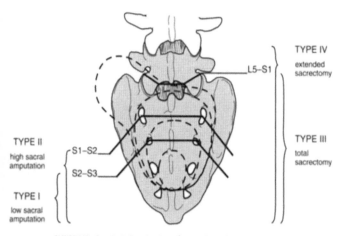

FIGURE 27B. Surgical classification of procedures for sacral tumors.

1. Type I: Low Sacral Amputation

A Mercedes star incision (reversed Y) or a midline longitudinal skin incision is made on the lower back of the patient in a prone position (Fig. 27C).The levator ani muscle and anococcygeal ligament are cut in the area around the coccyx and around the sacrum. The insertion of the bilateral gluteus maximus muscles is cut up to the edge of the sacroiliac joint. Below this, the piriformis muscle, sacrotuberous ligament, and sacrospinous ligament are cut by means of electric cauterization. The peritoneum with presacral membranous tissue is then exposed and manually separated from the presacral surface. The sacrum below the sacroiliac joints becomes free after the completion of these procedures. Laminectomy at S1, S2 is performed, and the dura mater or cauda equina is ligated and severed. A T-saw is guided from the S2 neural foramen to the greater sciatic notch, and each of the lateral wings of the sacrum is osteotomized bilaterally. Next, the T-saw is guided in front of the S2 vertebral body through the already osteotomized lines, and the S2 vertebral body is osteotomized from ventral to dorsal. For a lesion below S2, a simple transverse osteotomy with the T-saw can be conducted. In these types of cases, reconstruction is not necessary because the sacroiliac joints are not excised. However, sexual function or, rarely, bladder function is disturbed to some extent when the sacral nerves below S3 are sacrificed.

2. Type II: High Sacral Amputation (Fig. 27D)

Wide exposure of the posterior aspect is achieved by the posterior approach with a Mercedes star incision or a longitudinal incision. The T-saw is guided from the S1 neural foramen to the greater sciatic notch by using the T-saw guide (Fig. 27E), after which the lateral part and iliac wing are osteotomized by a sawing motion of the T-saw

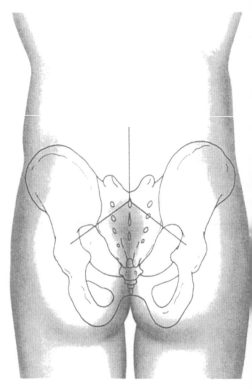

FIGURE 27C. Skin incision for posterior approach (Mercedes star incision).

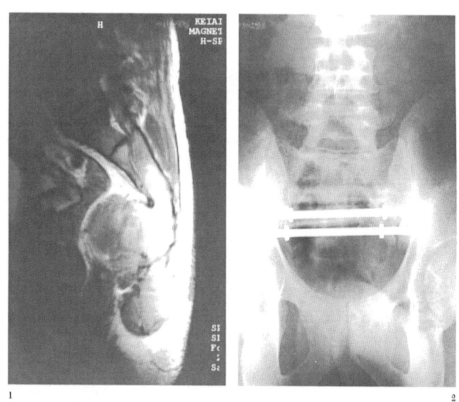

FIGURE 27D. High sacral amputation. (1) Magnetic resonance imaging (MRI) shows a chordoma extending anteriorly and into the spinal canal. (2) Postoperative radiograph shows the reconstruction using autogenous fibula in conjunction with sacral bars.

(Fig. 27F). Careful attention should be paid to the superior gluteal vessels, which can be ligated if necessary. After manual dissection of the anterior aspect of the sacrum from the presacral membrane and the peritoneum, the disc between S1 and S2 is cut with the T-saw, which has been placed at the presacral surface, through the S1 foramina, with the aid of the T-saw guide. After these procedures, the sacrum is amputated at the level of S1–S2. As we have experienced stress fracture of the S1 vertebral body following sacral amputation below S1, we usually perform dual fibulae grafts with sacral rod reinforcement between the posterior iliac wings (Fig. 27G).

3. Type III: Total Sacrectomy[8] (Fig. 27H)

Total sacrectomy is a most difficult and challenging operation, as it demands advanced and integrated skills in the techniques of tumor surgery, pelvic surgery, and spinal surgery. Total sacrectomy consists of three steps: (1) the anterior procedure; (2) the posterior procedure, to remove the sacrum en bloc; and (3) the reconstruction of the pelvic ring and spinal continuity.

We usually reach the tumor extraperitoneally with bilateral, para-abdominal incisions beside the rectus abdominis muscles, for which a longitudinal midline skin incision or an arched transverse incision can be used (Fig 27I). The median sacral artery and both internal iliac arteries are ligated, and, if necessary, the tumor vessels from the lumbar segmental arteries also are ligated. However, the internal iliac vein should not be ligated, if possible, to avoid congestive bleeding during the second step, the poste-

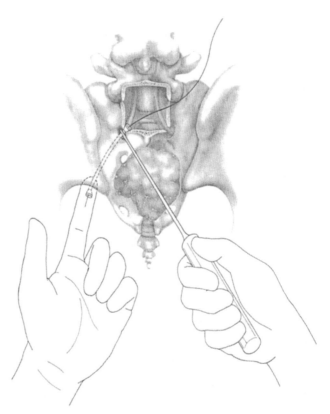

FIGURE 27E. Introduction of T-saw from the first sacral foramen to the sciatic notch for the amputation between S1 and S2.

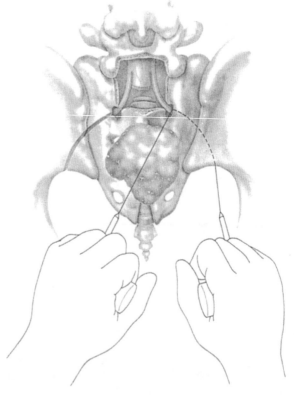

FIGURE 27F. Cutting the sacrum and posterior iliac wing by T-saw.

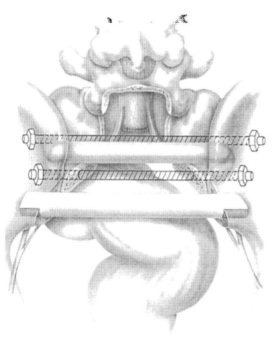

FIGURE 27G. Augmentation of pelvic ring using fibula combined with sacral bars after high sacral amputation.

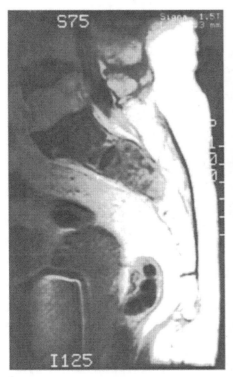

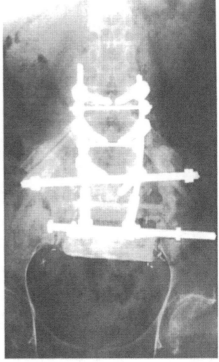

1

2

FIGURE 27H. Total sacrectomy. (1) Magnetic resonance imaging (MRI) shows a chondrosarcoma involving S1 and S2 vertebral bodies. (2) Postoperative radiograph shows the reconstruction using massive autogenous bone graft and spinal instrumentation.

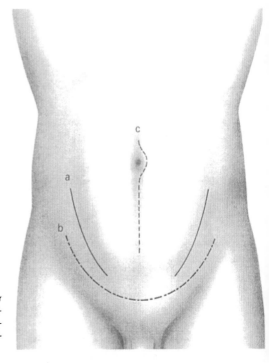

FIGURE 27I. Skin incision for anterior approach: (*a*) bilateral para-abdominal incision; (*b*) arched transverse incision; (*c*) longitudinal midline incision.

rior approach. The anterior sacroiliac ligament, anterior longitudinal ligament, and intervertebral disc (L5–S1) are cut by electric cauterization (Fig. 27J). If feasible, the S1 and S2 nerves are severed at the level of the anterior foramen. The T-saw is then placed on the slit of the L5–S1 disc and on the sacroiliac joints or the osteotomy lines of the ilium. Each end of the T-saw can be easily found during the posterior surgical process.

The second step is the posterior approach, which is started by a Mercedes star incision to obtain broad posterior exposure of the whole sacrum. After laminectomy and double ligation of the dural sac at the level of L5–S1, all the ligaments connected to the sacrum are divided. The top end of the T-saw is found and pulled, and the sacroiliac joints or ilium are osteotomized with a sawing motion of the T-saw from inside to outside (Fig. 27K). The L5–S1 disc is also cut with the T-saw (Fig. 27L). By lifting the sacrum, all connecting tissues can be cut by cauterization. At this time, laceration of the common iliac veins and venous plexus should be avoided. With these procedures, the whole sacrum with the tumor is removed en bloc from the back.

The reconstruction between the spine and the pelvis is performed on the basis of triangular frame (pyramid) reconstruction. After the placement of pedicle screws into the L3–L5 vertebral bodies, the spinal column is pulled down and L5 is affixed to the bilateral ilium with sacral rods into the L5 vertebral body and by spinal instrumentation connecting the spine and the pelvis. This phase is followed by massive bone grafts, using autogenous fibulae and bone chips or cancellous allografts (Fig. 27M).

4. Type IV: Extended Sacrectomy

When the tumor develops outside the sacrum, such as the L5 vertebra or ilium, this type of surgery becomes necessary. Although the surgical technique is similar to type III, it is a more aggressive, destructive, and demanding operation. The sacrum with the ilium and intrapelvic organs are excised to obtain a tumor-free margin. For some cases, a stoma is constructed by an abdominal surgeon.

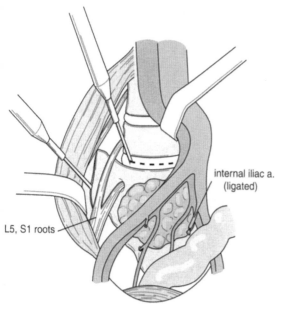

internal iliac a.
(ligated)

L5, S1 roots

FIGURE 27J. Surgical exposure of the presacral area.

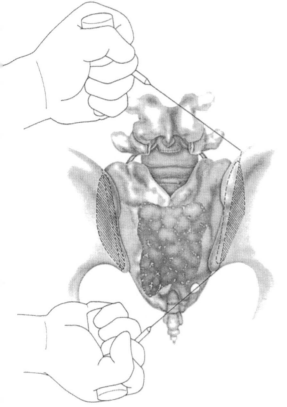

FIGURE 27K. Cutting the sacroiliac joints by T-saw for total sacrectomy.

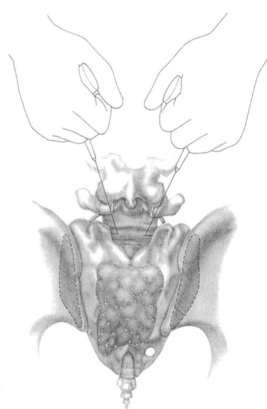

FIGURE 27L. Cutting the intervertebral disc between L5 and S1 by T-saw.

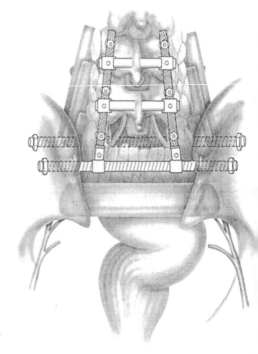

FIGURE 27M. Pyramid frame reconstruction.

Operating Time, Bleeding, and Disinfection

Operating time for low sacral amputation is about 2 to 3 hours whereas high sacral amputation requires about 3 to 6 hours. The total sacrectomy usually takes about 6 to 12 hours because each step (anterior procedure, posterior procedure, and reconstruction) takes about 2 to 4 hours. Although the amount of bleeding varies depending on tumor histology, vascularity, and tumor size, that for high sacral amputation is roughly 1500 to 3000 mL and that for total sacrectomy 5000 to 8000 mL. For some cases, postoperative management in the intensive care unit is necessary.

After sacral tumor resection, the wound is highly susceptible to postoperative infection, because this operation takes a long time, a large dead space develops, massive metallic implants are put in place, and the wound is very close to the anus and perineum. Therefore, suction drains (usually two tubes on either side inserted from the back) should be left in place until the discharge diminishes to less than 50 mL per day (usually 10 to 14 days after the operation). Strict attention should be paid to avoiding wound contamination by urine or stool.

Results

Between 1986 and 1996, we have treated 13 patients with en bloc sacrectomy. The mean age of the patients was 51 years, ranging from 29 to 72 years. Of the 13 patients with a sacral tumor, 7 had a chordoma, 2 a chondrosarcoma, and 1 each a giant cell tumor of bone, a malignant fibrous histiocytoma, an osteosarcoma, and a leiomyosarcoma. The type I procedure was performed on 2, type II on 4, type III on 5, and type IV on 2 patients. A marginal or wide tumor-free margin was obtained in all cases. During the follow-up period from 6 months to 10 years (mean, 45 months), there has been no local tumor recurrence and all patients are still free of disease.

Discussion

Intralesional excision of a sacral tumor (aggressively benign, low-grade or high-grade tumors) has been found to result in a local tumor recurrence rate of almost 100%. We established a surgical classification of sacral tumors based on the extent of the tumor and the size of the sacral resection. As the L5–S1 disc and sacroiliac joint are strong barriers, total sacrectomy or extended total sacrectomy is sometimes indicated. In such a case, reconstruction to stabilize the continuity between spine and pelvis is essential, but the most effective reconstruction procedure has yet not been established. We introduced the pyramid frame reconstruction, which represents a step to establishing an ideal reconstruction.

Excessive bleeding is also a problem to be controlled. As a method to control the bleeding from the pelvic venous plexus, ligation of the internal iliac veins has been believed to be mandatory. However, we have considered that ligation of the internal iliac veins may have an opposite effect for hemostasis, because it may lead to congestion of the pelvic and the epidural venous plexus. Therefore, we studied the effect of ligation of the internal iliac vein on these venous plexuses experimentally.[13] We found that pressure of both the internal iliac vein and the epidural vein increases right after ligation of the internal iliac vein. Currently, we do ligate the internal iliac arteries but we avoid ligating the internal iliac veins based on this study. Instead, if possible we ligate the segmental veins entering the sacral foramina while exposing the anterior surface of the sacrum.

With the advent of the T-saw, osteotomy at the sacroiliac joints, L5–S1, or ilium became easy to perform, because the osteotomy can be performed from inside to outside (from spinal canal to lamina, from the abdominal side to the back) in contrast to conventional osteotomy using a osteotome. With the use of the T-saw, osteotomy can thus be performed safely and correctly.[1]

Resections below the body of the S3 vertebra do not endanger continence of the anal and bladder functions. On the other hand, total sacrectomy sacrifices all bilateral nerve roots below S1. However, despite sensory disturbance below S1, inability to flex the ankles, and bladder–bowel dysfunction, patients can walk with the aid of a short leg splint, control urination by self-catheter or manual abdominal pressure, and control their defecation by using an enema.

Although sacral resection is a large-scale operation requiring considerable time and surgical skill, sacral tumors should be treated on the basis of oncologic principles to avoid local tumor recurrence and to save the patient's life. Adequate resection of sacral tumors results in good prognosis and good quality of life for the patient. Consequently, every effort should be made to improve surgical procedures, reconstruction methods, and management of neurologic dysfunction for this rare tumor.

References

1. Tomita K, Kawahara N: The threadwire saw—a new device for cutting bones. J Bone Joint Surg 78A:1915–1917, 1996.
2. Tomita K, Kawahara N, Baba H, et al: Total en bloc spondylectomy for solitary spinal metastases. Int Orthop 18:291–298, 1994.
3. Enneking WF: A system of staging musculoskeletal neoplasms. Clin Orthop 204:9–24, 1986.
4. Kaiser TE, et al: Clinicopathologic study of sacrococcygeal chordoma. Cancer 54:2574–2578, 1984.
5. Gunterberg B, Kewenter J, Peterson I, et al: Anorectal function after major resections of the sacrum with bilateral or unilateral sacrifice of sacral nerves. Br J Surg 63:546–554, 1976.
6. Stener B, Gunterberg B: High amputation of the sacrum for extirpation of tumors, principles and technique. Spine 3:351–366, 1978.
7. Shikata J, Yamamuro T, Kotoura Y, et al. Total sacrectomy and reconstruction for primary tumors. J Bone Joint Surg 70A:122–125, 1988.
8. Tomita K, Tsuchiya H: Total sacrectomy and reconstruction for huge sacral tumors. Spine 15:1223–1227, 1990.
9. Andreoli F, Balloni F, Bigiotti A, et al: Anorectal continence and bladder function. Effects of major sacral resection. Dis Colon Rec 29:647–652, 1986.
10. Gennari L, Azzarelli A, Quagliuolo V: A posterior approach for the excision of sacral chordoma. J Bone Joint Surg 69:565–568, 1987.
11. Torelli T, Campo B, Ordesi G, et al: Sacral chordoma and rehabilitative treatment of urinary disorders. Tumori 74:475–478, 1988.
12. Gunterberg B, Romanus B, Stener B: Pelvic strength after major amputation of the sacrum. Acta Orthop Scand 47:635–642, 1976.
13. Hata M, Kawahara N, Tomita K: Prevention of excessive hemorrhage from venous plexus during total sacrectomy [abstract]. J Jpn Spine Res Soc 8:274, 1997.

Approach to the Posterior Aspect of C1–C2

1. Position the patient's head in the self-retaining neurosurgical head fixation device that is attached to the table. Attach the drapes to the patient's neck with stay sutures. Neck flexion will increase exposure, but flexion is limited by the type of pathology present, usually to a neutral, slightly flexed position. With instability problems, confirm the position of the spine with X-ray.

2. Incise the midline skin and subcutaneous to fascia and obtain hemostasis with rapid application of hemostats and electrocautery. Insert self-retaining retractors.

3. Deepen the incision with the cautery knife, staying in the thin white median raphe, and avoid cutting muscle tissue. The median raphe of the cervical spine is a tortuous structure; it does not follow a straight midline incision. Open the median raphe to the spinous processes of C2 and C3 and the occiput. In children, to avoid spontaneous fusion at adjacent levels, including the occiput, expose no spinal levels unnecessarily.

4. Expose the spinous processes with a #15 blade or cutting cautery on their bulbous bifid tips. The ligamentous attachments to C2 are very prominent. Identify any spina bifida of the cervical spine on the preoperative X-ray and at surgery. Insert the Cobb elevator, first facing up to elevate the tip subperiosteally, then facing down to complete the subperiosteal elevation medial to lateral approximately 1 inch at each level. At levels below C2, identify the medial edge of the facet joint at the base of the lamina and pack at each level as it is exposed. When necessary, expose the occiput with elevators. Insert self-retaining retractors to expose the base of the skull and the dorsal spine of C2. The area in between will contain the ring of C1. Many times this is very deep compared with C2.

5. Maintain firm lateral traction on the wound. With a sharp Cobb elevator, feel for and identify the posterior tubercle of C1 longitudinally in the midline. Begin the subperiosteal dissection to bone.

Caution: Often C1 is very thin, and direct pressure can fracture it or cause the surgeon to slip off the ring and penetrate the atlanto-occipital membrane. Elevation on this ring can be very dangerous if there is subluxation with constriction of the posterior dura under this ring. The dura may be vulnerable on both the superior and inferior edges of the ring of C1.

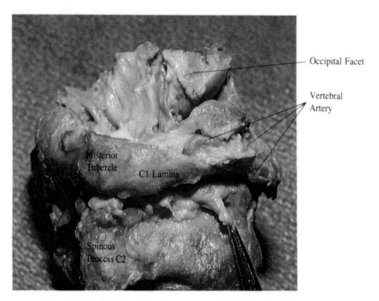

FIGURE 28A. A dissected specimen of the C1–C2 articulation emphasizes the two potential areas of damage to the vertebral artery in this area. One is between the C1–C2 articulation in an exposed, posterior lateral position; the other is on the superior ring of C1. This specimen has a bone encasing the vertebral artery. A portion of much of the roof of the tunnel has been removed, emphasizing that when dissecting on the ring of C1, identification of the edge of the groove immediately preceding the vertebral artery allows one to locate the artery before any damage. The specimen does not show the bluish hue of the vessels usually encountered operatively. In the forceps is the posterior ganglion and ramus of C2, which is the warning landmark one reaches laterally before the vertebral artery between C1 and C2.

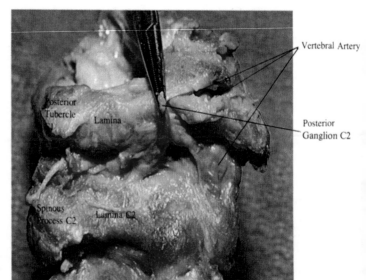

FIGURE 28B. The usual location of the second cervical ganglion medial to the vertebral artery.

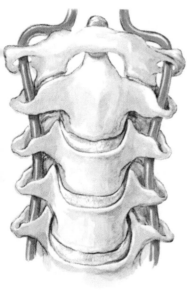

FIGURE 28C. The vertebral artery enters the foramen transversarium of C6, and courses through each foramen transversarium anterior to the spinal nerve. The foramen transversarium of C1 is in a relatively more posterior position than that of the lower cervical vertebrae. After passing through the foramen transversarium of C1, the vertebral artery courses posteromedially to enter the spinal canal and the foramen magnum.

6. Dissect laterally only approximately 1.5 cm. An important landmark on the ring of C1 laterally is the second cervical ganglion, which lies at approximately 1.5 cm on the lamina of C1 in the area of the groove for the vertebral artery (Figs. 28A, 28B). Carefully identify the most medial aspect of the groove for the vertebral artery and vein on the superior border of the C1 ring.[1] The bluish color of the vein is visualized first (Fig. 28C). By seeing the initial ridge or the vein one can avoid damaging the artery. There is seldom any indication for dissection lateral to the groove of the vertebral artery on C1. The vertebral artery and vein not only are vulnerable in the groove, but as the artery passes from the foramen transversarium of C2 to that of C1, it is in close lateral and posterior proximity to the joint (Figs. 28D, 28E).[2]

7. The vertebral artery enters the foramen transversarium at the sixth vertebra and progresses cephalad. It exits through the foramen transversarium of C1 and progresses posteriorly as well as medially in the groove of the superior border of C1 toward the midline, then turns cephalad along the spinal cord to enter the foramen magnum (Figs. 28F, 28G). The vertebral artery can be damaged by penetrating the atlanto-occipital membrane of the superior border of the ring of C1 more medial than the usually safe 1.5 cm from the midline (Figs. 28E, 28H).

8. With exposure of the ring of C1 and exposure to bone of the posterior occiput, different operative procedures require exposure of the dura under the edge of the foramen magnum.[3–5] No attempt should be made to decompress the posterior fossa under the edge of the foramen magnum without sufficient visualization of the area cephalad to the foramen. This step is best accomplished by placement of two bur holes just off the midline of each side of the skull. The caudal extent of the holes is usually determined by the angle of the drill on the skull as limited by the shoulders.

9. Penetrate to the inner periosteum and the bone edge with a small dissector.

10. Expand the hole caudally to the foramen with rongeurs. The edge itself curves under and projects anteriorly. Periosteum of the skull at this point is often conjoined with the dura of the spinal cord (Fig. 28I). There is a median venous sinus in the midline, and the fascial attachment of the periosteum of the skull to the dura often contains a transverse sinus as well.

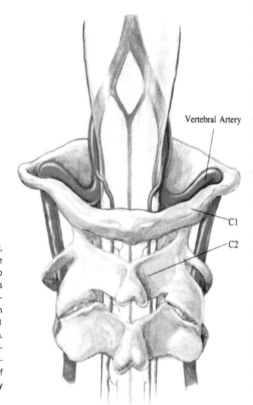

Vertebral Artery

C1

C2

FIGURE 28D. From the posterior view, the relatively exposed position of the vertebral artery is seen just lateral to the C1–C2 articulation. Also seen is the course of the vertebral artery posteromedially on the ring of C1. Often it is encased in bone on the ring of C1 or has a very prominent bony trough. The atlanto-occipital membrane covers the vertebral artery on the superior ring of C1. The posterior ramus of C2 is the guide to the vertebral artery between C1 and C2.

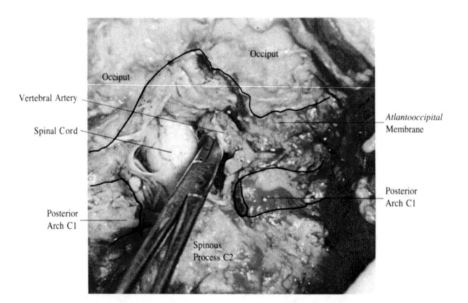

Occiput

Occiput

Vertebral Artery

Spinal Cord

Atlantooccipital Membrane

Posterior Arch C1

Posterior Arch C1

Spinous Process C2

FIGURE 28E. A slightly different view. The bluish hue of the vertebral artery on the superior portion of the posterior ring of C1 is easily seen. The course of the vertebral artery medially to enter the fora-men magnum beside the spinal cord emphasizes the potential danger of damage to the vertebral artery by penetration of the atlanto-occipital membrane.

Under the
Atlantooccipital
Membrane

Exposed Vertebral
Artery on Superior
Aspect of the
Ring of C1

Foramen
Transversarium
C1

Foramen
Transversarium
C2

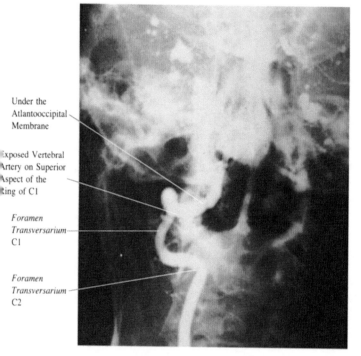

FIGURE 28F. The course of the vertebral artery at the C1–C2 articulation is posterolateral after leaving the foramen transversarium of C2 and posteromedial after leaving the foramen of C1.

Vertebral Artery
on the posterior
arch of C1

C1

Foramen
Transversarium C1

Vertebral Body C2

Foramen
Transversarium C2

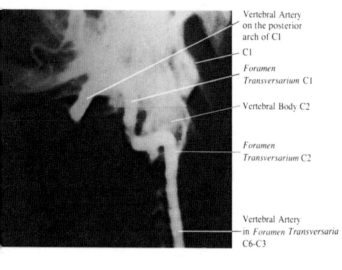

Vertebral Artery
in *Foramen Transversaria*
C6-C3

FIGURE 28G. The course of the vertebral artery is from the foramen transversarium of C1 posteriorly in the region of the C1–C2 articulation through the transversarium of C1, then posteromedially in the posterior rim of C1.

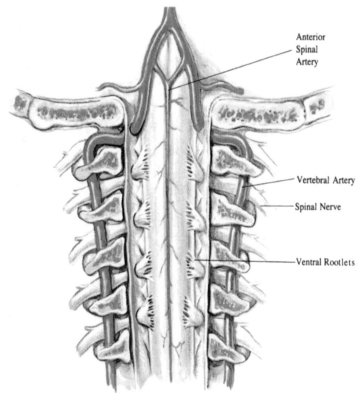

Anterior
Spinal
Artery

Vertebral Artery

Spinal Nerve

Ventral Rootlets

FIGURE 28H. The anterior view without vertebral bodies emphasizes the formation of the anterior spinal artery. There are numerous variations in this formation, ranging from a unilateral vertebral artery contribution to no contribution.

11. Passing instruments under the edge of the foramen can produce dangerous bleeding in the posterior fossa with no means of control. Therefore, resect down to the edge from above.

12. For the more lateral approach to the C1–C2 facet joint, the vertebral artery between C1 and C2 must be identified. In rotatory dislocations of C1–C2, the artery is stretched tightly across the joint on the side that C1 is anterior to C2 and is easily damaged.

13. Closure: Remove retractors, allow muscle to fall together, and close the fascia, subcutaneous tissue, and skin.

Remember:

1. Keep the incision in the winding, shifting median raphe to decrease bleeding.
2. Identify the large, prominent spinous process of C2.
3. Identify the posterior tubercle of C1 deep in the wound.
4. Dissect laterally on CI no more than $1^1/_2$ inches, or look for the bluish tinge of the vertebral artery and veins on the superior border of C1, or look for the edge of the vertebral artery notch on the superior border of C1, or stay medial to the dorsal ramus of C2.
5. Beware of the vertebral artery with any exposure of the C1–C2 facet joint.
6. Beware of dural penetration from slipping off or breaking through C1.
7. Do not approach the foramen magnum from under the edge of the foramen.
8. Make drill holes above and remove bone distally.

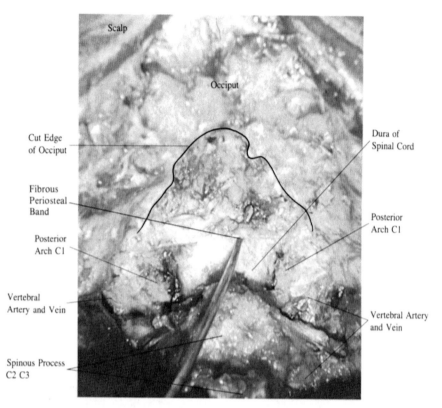

FIGURE 28I. In the posterior approach to the foramen magnum, one must first place bur holes in the occiput above the foramen magnum. Two parasagittal holes allow removal of bone from the dura with a Harrison-type rongeur. Careful dissection medially from the bur holes protects one from the often significant fragile sinus, and dissection caudally approaches the foramen magnum. After removal of the occiput including the bony rim of the foramen magnum, which is a sharp-lipped structure projecting directly anterior in the transverse plane, one encounters the fibrous attachment of the inner periosteum of the skull to the dura at the rim of the foramen magnum. There is sometimes a transverse venous sinus in this area that produces bleeding, which can be significant, when torn. Attachment to the dura in this area may produce a dural leak unless the area is carefully dissected.

9. Beware of attachments of venous sinus, periosteum, and dura at the tip of the posterior edge of the foramen magnum.

References

1. Fielding JW: Personal communication.
2. Watkins RG, O'Brien JP: Anatomy of the cervical spine. Sound Slide Program, American Academy of Orthopaedic Surgeons, Atlanta, GA, 1980.
3. Robinson RA, Southwick WO: Surgical approaches to the cervical spine. American Academy of Orthopaedic Surgeons: Instructional Course Lectures, Vol. XVII. St. Louis, Mosby, 1960.
4. Rothman R: The Spine, Vol. I. Philadelphia, Saunders, 1975, pp 124–125.
5. Logue V: Compressive lesions at the foramen magnum. In Ruge D, Wiltse L (eds): Spinal Disorders: Diagnosis and Treatment. Philadelphia, Lea & Febiger, 1977, pp 249–273.

Posterior Approach to the C1–C2 Joints

Bernard Jeanneret

The posterior exposure of the atlantoaxial joints may be indicated for insertion of transarticular screws at C1–C2 for bone grafting of the joints themselves, for exact evaluation of the congruency of the atlantoaxial joints (e.g., for reduction of a rotatory dislocation or an unstable Jefferson fracture), or for the resection of small tumors of the lateral mass of the atlas.

This chapter describes the exposure of the atlantoaxial joints and the posterior aspect of the lateral masses of the atlas. We present the transarticular screw fixation technique for C1–C2 as described by Magerl et al.,[1] and use the example of an open reduction and internal fixation of a Jefferson fracture to illustrate the possibilities of this approach.

Positioning the Patient

The patient is intubated using the endoscopic technique and placed prone on the operating table, with the head positioned in a head holder (Fig. 29A). Halo traction may be used to allow easier open reduction of a Jefferson fracture or to stabilize an unstable situation; however, the author does not use halo traction. Using lateral image intensifier control immediately after positioning the patient in the prone position, the atlantoaxial reduction is checked. If anterior subluxation of C1 on C2 has occurred during positioning, the head is lifted together with the head holder, using fluoroscopic control to monitor reduction. This maneuver will reduce C1 on C2. The upper cervical spine is then flexed as much as possible by tilting the head holder, still under lateral fluoroscopic control, while the lower cervical spine is only slightly flexed. Flexion of the upper cervical spine is important to allow correct placement of the transarticular screws for C1–C2.

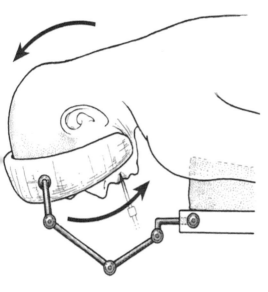

FIGURE 29A. The patient is placed prone on the operating table, the head maintained in a head holder. The occipitocervical joints are flexed as much as possible but the lower cervical spine is only slightly flexed.

Surgical Exposure

Approach (Figs. 29B, 29C)

A midline incision is performed from the protuberantia occipitalis externa to the tip of the spinous process of C5. The musculature is divided in the midline down to the tips of the spinous processes and down to the occiput. The spinous process of C2 is prominent and easy to find. The musculature attached to it is cut at its insertion with electrocautery. To allow adequate exposure of the atlas, the musculature attached to the occiput must be retracted laterally, from the protuberantia occipitalis externa down to the vicinity of the foramen magnum; this is done using a Cobb elevator while an assistant is holding the head to prevent undue motion at C1–C2. Bleeding from the bone is controlled with bone wax. Spreading of the musculature with sharp retractors allows for best visualization and also minimizes blood loss. The posterior arch of the atlas is located in the depth between the occiput and the spinous process of C2, both of which are already exposed. The posterior arch of C1 is found by gently dividing the soft tissues between the occiput and the spinous process of C2 until bony contact is obtained. Starting in the midline, the muscle attachments to the posterior arch of the atlas are gently cut directly on the bone using either a knife or electrocautery. The posterior arch of the atlas is exposed subperiosteally on a width of approximatively 2 cm. Although careful exposure of the midportion of the posterior arch is without danger, care must be taken when reaching the lateral part because the vertebral artery runs over the cranial part of the arch and enters the spinal canal behind the lateral mass of the atlas. The superior part of the posterior arch is therefore only prepared in the midportion and only if a wire loop must be passed around it later in the procedure.

The spinous processes, the laminae, and the articular processes of C2 and C3 are now exposed subperiosteally without destroying the joint capsules of C2–C3. Consequent soft tissue retraction helps for adequate exposure; the muscles are meticulously retracted with sharp retractors to allow for best visualization of the operative field.

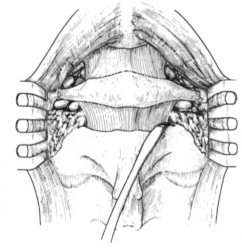

FIGURE 29B. After subperiosteal exposure of the occiput, posterior arch of the atlas, and posterior elements (spinous process, lamina, and articular masses) of C2 and C3, the cranial part of the lamina of C2 is exposed and followed subperiosteally toward the isthmus, staying on the crest of the lamina.

Subperiosteal Dissection of the Atlantoaxial Joints

Using a small sharp elevator (4 to 5 mm wide), the cranial surface of the lamina of C2 is exposed (Fig. 29B). Along this crest, the elevator is gently brought anteriorly and the soft tissues detached, still staying strictly subperiosteally and exposing the isthmus of C2. The soft tissues located cranial to the elevator contain the nerve root C2 as well as the surrounding venous plexus. These structures are gently retracted with a slightly curved dissector exposing the isthmus, while dissection is carried on further anteriorly, still remaining strictly on the crest and subperiosteally. In the anterior part of the isthmus, an upward step is felt corresponding to the slope located just behind the superior articular facet of C2. The joint capsules are thin and can be opened using the elevator. By turning the elevator upward, the posterior aspect of the lateral mass of the atlas can be exposed subperiosteally by slightly scratching the bone with the sharp elevator. The capsule can be elevated with a dissector, exposing the joint (Fig. 29C). If desired, a

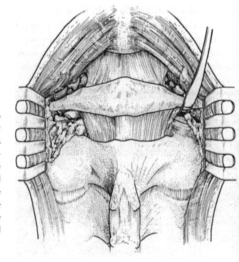

FIGURE 29C. The soft tissues cranial to the elevator contain the nerve root C2 as well as its surrounding venous plexus. These elements are gently retracted with a dissector. Once the posterior aspect of the atlantoaxial joint has been reached, the capsule can be opened and retracted with the same dissector, exposing parts of the posterior aspect of the atlantoaxial joint.

K-wire can be inserted into the posterior aspect of the lateral mass of the atlas under direct vision (Fig. 29D1). The K-wire should be slightly flexible, for example, 1.6 mm in diameter. When retracting the soft tissues with this K-wire, the cartilage of the atlantoaxial joints can be seen (Fig. 29D2). A small dissector can also be placed lateral to the lateral mass, remaining inside the joint capsule and exposing the posterolateral aspect of the joint.

During exposure of the isthmus, the venous plexus surrounding the nerve root of C2 may be damaged with venous bleeding as a consequence. This hemorrhage may be stopped by introducing a small amount of collagen between the venous plexus and the isthmus of C2; however, care must be taken not to exert pressure on the dura. The best prophylaxis for such a bleeding is to stay subperiosteally during the preparation and to retract the nerve root of C2 with the surrounding plexus using great care.

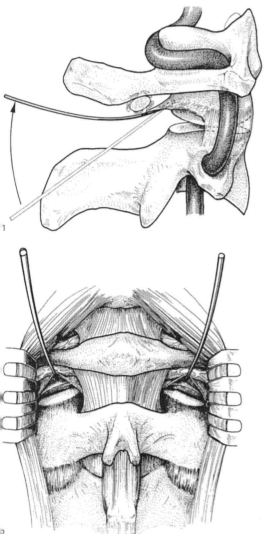

FIGURE 29D. (1) To allow better visualization of the atlantoaxial joint, a K-wire may be driven into the posterior aspect of the lateral mass, the K-wire being inserted underneath the joint capsule. By elevating the K-wire, the soft tissues containing the nerve root C2 are retracted cranially, allowing visualization of the joints. (2) Posterior view of both atlantoaxial joints after the K-wires are retracted cranially.

Exposure of the Posterior Aspect of the Lateral Masses of C1

For better visualization of the posterior aspect of the lateral masses of C1, it may sometimes be necessary to also expose it cranially, starting from the posterior arch of the atlas (for example, for removal of a small tumor in the posterior part of lateral mass or for reducing an unstable Jefferson fracture). The caudal aspect of the posterior arch of the atlas is then exposed subperiosteally on both sides until the junction to the lateral masses is reached, using sharp dissectors or an elevator. Care is taken not to expose the cranial aspect of the arch where the vertebral artery could be damaged. Once the posterior aspect of the lateral mass has been reached, the nerve root of C2 is completely freed from its attachments to the lateral mass, allowing visualization of the posterior aspect of the lateral masses and of the atlantoaxial joint both cranially and caudally. Theoretically, the nerve root C2 could be cut and ligated, if absolutely necessary for adequate exposure.

Transarticular Screw Fixation of C1–C2

Indications

Transarticular screw fixation of C1–C2 (Fig. 29E) is always used in combination with a fusion (see following) and may be indicated in the following situations:

1. Painful osteoarthritis of the atlantoaxial joints.
2. Acute or chronic atlantoaxial instability caused by
   - Developmental abnormalities [e.g., os odontoideum (Fig. 29F); hypoplasia of the dens axis, cranial assimilation of the atlas]
   - Trauma (e.g., dens fracture or dens pseudoarthrosis, tear of the transverse ligament, Jefferson fracture)
   - Aseptic inflammatory processes (rheumatoid arthritis, psoriasis)
   - Infection (e.g., tuberculosis)
   - Tumor
3. In combination with plate or rod fixation for occipitocervical fusion

Contraindications

The technique should not be used in cases of collapse of C2 caused by massive destruction of the lateral masses of C2 as can be seen in late cases of rheumatoid arthritis or other rare circumstances. In such cases, introduction of the drill aiming toward the anterior arch of the atlas could result in a perforation of the vertebral artery traversing its sinus at the level of C2.

Advantages

The technique has been shown to be very effective and versatile. Compared to a Gallie or Brooks fusion, transarticular screw fixation has been shown to be more stable,[2–4] to allow retention in reduced position in almost all circumstances, and to be possible even when the posterior arch of the atlas is broken or absent.[5–8]

Technique of Insertion of Transarticular Screws at C1–C2

For performing the transarticular screw fixation at C1–C2, it is usually not necessary to expose the atlantoaxial joints or the posterior aspect of the lateral mass of the atlas. It is sufficient to expose the isthmus, which must be very well visualized to allow correct insertion of the screw. If the posterior arch of C1 is intact and a posterior fu-

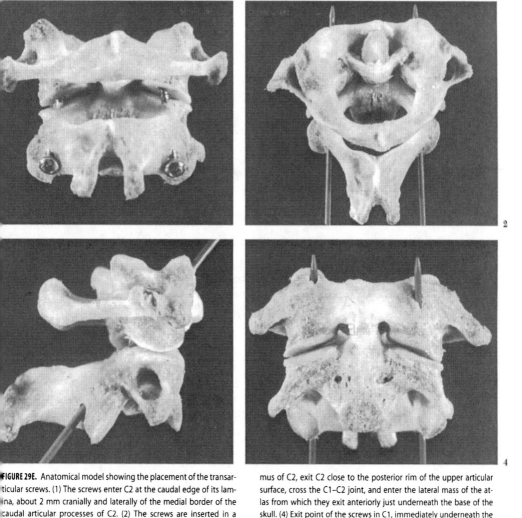

FIGURE 29E. Anatomical model showing the placement of the transarticular screws. (1) The screws enter C2 at the caudal edge of its lamina, about 2 mm cranially and laterally of the medial border of the caudal articular processes of C2. (2) The screws are inserted in a straight sagittal fashion. (3) The screws aim cranially toward the isthmus of C2, exit C2 close to the posterior rim of the upper articular surface, cross the C1–C2 joint, and enter the lateral mass of the atlas from which they exit anteriorly just underneath the base of the skull. (4) Exit point of the screws in C1, immediately underneath the base of the skull.

sion using the Gallie technique is planned (see bone grafting), the wire loop should be inserted around it before the screw fixation itself is performed, because insertion of this wire could be more dangerous or even impossible afterward.

When the wire loop has been passed around the posterior arch of the atlas (Fig. 29G) and the isthmus on both sides has been identified, atlantoaxial reduction is again checked under lateral image intensifier control. Persistent anterior dislocation of C1 on C2 may be reduced by pushing on the spinous process of C2 with a Kocher clamp or by pulling gently on the wire loop passed around the posterior arch of C1. Posterior dislocation of C1 on C2, on the other hand, may be reduced by pulling on the spinous process of C2 or by pushing on the intact posterior arch of C1. The drillholes for the 3.5-mm titanium screws are now prepared using a 2.5-mm drill bit and lateral image intensifier control. The drill's entering point is found on a straight sagittal line passing through the medial aspect of the isthmus and is located at the caudal edge of the lam-

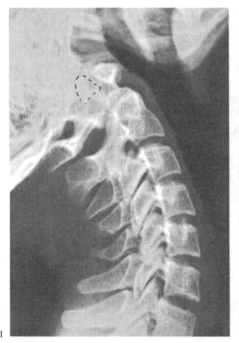
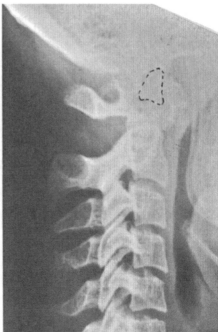

1

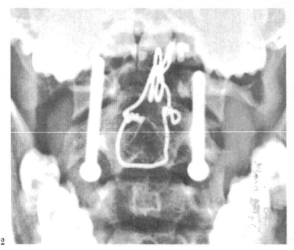
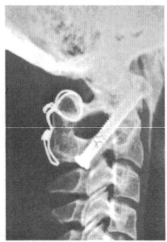

2

FIGURE 29F. A 21-year-old woman with chronic neck pain. (1) Flexion/extension views show a massive instability C1–C2 resulting from an osodontoideum. (2) Transarticular screw fixation C1–C2 with posterior bone grafting according to Gallie was performed. At follow-up, 24 months after surgery, the fusion is healed.

ina of C2, about 2 mm cranial and lateral of the medial border of the caudal articular process of C2. The drill aims straight sagittally forward, toward the medial aspect of the isthmus and the posterior part of the atlantoaxial joint. The adequate caudocranial inclination is found with the image intensifier; the drill must aim toward the middle or cranial portion of the anterior arch of the atlas. Accurate caudocranial drilling may sometimes be difficult because the neck muscles and the shoulders may prevent correct

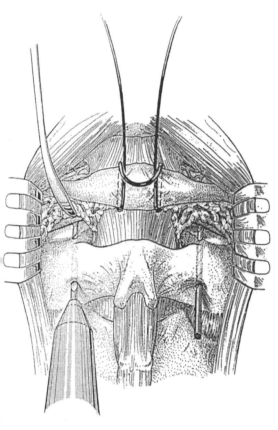

FIGURE 29G. After a cerclage wire has been passed around the posterior arch of C1, the screw holes are prepared as described in the text. In this figure, the right hole has been prepared first: this drill bit is left in place to prevent redislocation of C1 on C2 while the hole on the left side is being drilled. The soft tissues containing the greater occipital nerve and the surrounding blood vessels are retracted by a curved dissector to allow the vision on the isthmus of C2, permitting correct drilling.

placement of the drill. This problem can be corrected either by gently pulling the spinous process of C2 cranially using a towel clamp, thus allowing a better drill angle, or by inserting the drill percutaneously through the paravertebral neck muscles.

The so-called tap-drilling method is always used for safer drilling of the screw holes. On its way, the drill passes the isthmus of C2 close to its posterior surface, exits C2 at the posterior rim of the upper articular surface, crosses the C1–C2 joint, and enters the lateral mass of the atlas from which it exits anteriorly immediately underneath the base of the skull. After having drilled the first hole, this drill bit is left in place to stabilize C1–C2 and prevent redislocation of C1 on C2 while drilling the opposite hole. One 3.5-mm AO titanium cortex screw is inserted while the drill on the opposite side is still in place; the screw length is measured; and tapping is performed using image intensifier control. The tap must cross the C1–C2 joint and enter the lateral mass of the atlas to prevent possible redislocation while inserting the screw.

Bone Grafting

There are three different methods of bone grafting.

1. When the posterior arch of the atlas is intact, a regular Gallie fusion may be performed (Fig. 29H). The wire, however, must be passed around the arch of C1 before transarticular screw fixation is performed; otherwise, passage of the wire around the posterior arch of C1 may be very difficult, dangerous, or even

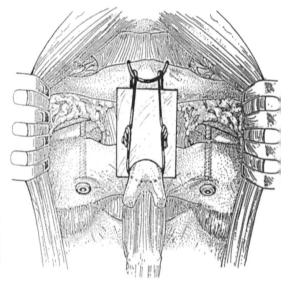

FIGURE 29H. After insertion of both screws, a corticocancellous bone graft is placed posteriorly according to the technique described by Gallie and fixed with the wire loop.

impossible. To allow magnetic resonance imaging (MRI) postoperatively, if necessary, a titanium wire is preferred.

2. In cases of hypoplasia or absence of the posterior arch of the atlas, the atlantoaxial joints themselves are bone grafted (Fig. 29I). For this purpose, the atlantoaxial must be exposed as described previously. After the joints are exposed, the cartilage is removed with either a small curette, a chisel, or a bur. The space is packed with bone graft after having prepared the drillhole for the C1–C2 screw fixation, just before inserting the screw itself.

3. In the presence of a fracture of the posterior arch of the atlas, bone graft chips can be positioned over the posterior arch of the atlas and over the lamina of C2.

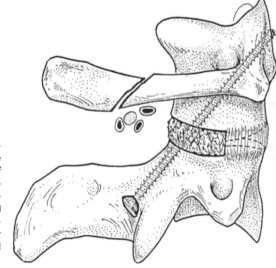

FIGURE 29I. Bone grafting of the atlantoaxial joints themselves may be performed if necessary as in cases of hypoplasia, bilateral fracture, or absence of the posterior arch of the atlas. The cartilage and the subchondral bone of the atlantoaxial joints are removed either with a small curette or a bur, and the bone graft is positioned once the screws have been inserted.

This bone graft is stabilized by the soft tissues when the wound is closed and will give a solid fusion mass that will stabilize C1 on C2 once the fracture of the atlas has also healed. Of course, bone grafts can also be inserted in the atlantoaxial joints themselves; however, this makes exposure more difficult because the joints must be exposed.

Postoperative Care

The patient is allowed to ambulate the first or second day after surgery. A Philadelphia-type collar is worn for 6 weeks if a Gallie-type fusion has been added. The collar is removed in bed as well as for daily care. If no Gallie fusion has been added, the period is extended to 12 weeks and a soft collar is worn in bed.

Open Reduction and Stabilization of an Unstable Jefferson Fracture

Rationale for Surgical Treatment

Unstable Jefferson fractures (by definition, with rupture of the transverse ligament) are a therapeutic quandary. Closed reduction by halo traction is rarely possible and, if successful, maintenance of the reduction achieved is very difficult. Anterior open reduction and internal fixation of the fracture itself are possible; this technique, however, only addresses the bony fracture without addressing the life-threatening atlantoaxial instability resulting from the tear or avulsion of the transverse ligament. Some authors, therefore, advocated a primary occipitocervical or an atlantoaxial fusion to also treat the atlantoaxial instability. Although the occipitocervical fusion definitively blocks motion at both the C0–C1 and the C1–C2 level, the technique presented here combining open fracture reduction with transarticular screw fixation C1–C2 has the advantage of preserving the motion at the level CO–C1.

Exposure

To allow open reduction of the Jefferson fracture, the posterior aspect of the lateral masses must be exposed on both sides to allow exact evaluation of the lateral drift and reduction of the lateral masses under direct visual control.

Open Reduction of the Lateral Masses

After subperiosteal dissection of the posterior aspect of the lateral masses has been performed on both sides as just described, reduction of the lateral masses is performed using a specially designed clamp (Fig. 29J), which is gently inserted around the posterolateral corner of the lateral masses of the atlas; each arm of the clamp is inserted separately 1 cm deep, taking care to stay subperiosteally. Immediately adjacent to the clamp runs the vertebral artery, which enters the transverse process of C1. Therefore, very careful subperiosteal dissection is mandatory. After both arms of the clamp have been inserted, the arms are connected and compression is applied on the lateral masses (Fig. 29K), resulting in a compression of the C1 ring and therefore reduction of the dislocated lateral masses. Reduction is performed under visual control of the position of the lateral border of the lateral masses of C1 relatively to the lateral border of the superior articular processes of C2; both should be flush.

Alternatively, another reduction method uses two stiff K-wires driven straight posteriorly into the lateral masses of the atlas. Reduction may be performed by applying compression forces using, for example, an external fixator as used for fingers.

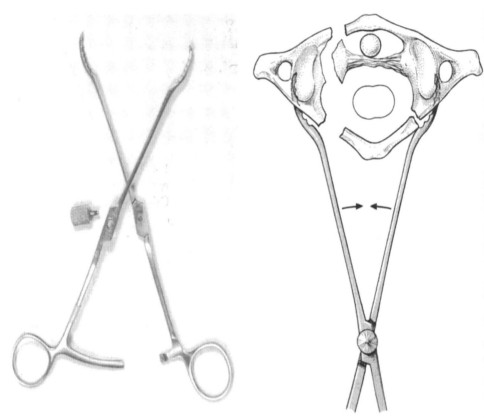

FIGURE 29J. Reduction clamp. This prototype has been produced by Ull-rich, St. Gallen, Switzerland.

FIGURE 29K. Technique of open reduction of Jefferson fractures using the clamp described in Figure 29J. Both arms of the clamp are introduced separately around the lateral masses of C1 and connected when they have been introduced. The nerve roots of C2 run caudally of the clamp, the vertebral artery laterally of it. Reduction is achieved by applying anterior compression and is monitored under direct visual control, as described in the text.

Stabilization of C1 on C2

Once the lateral masses are reduced, a transarticular screw fixation at C1–C2 is performed on both sides, using the technique just described (Fig. 29L).

Bone Grafting

Bone graft chips can be positioned over the fractured posterior arch of the atlas and over the lamina of C2. This bone graft is stabilized by the soft tissues when the wound is closed and provides a solid fusion mass that will stabilize C1 on C2 when the fracture of the atlas has also healed.

Postoperative Care

The patient is allowed to get up the first or second day after surgery. A four-poster type brace is worn for 12 weeks. The collar is removed for daily care. During the night, a soft collar may be worn.

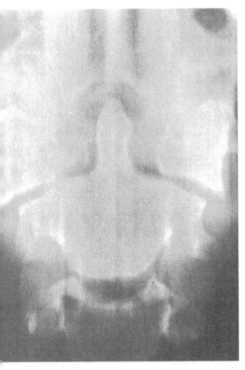
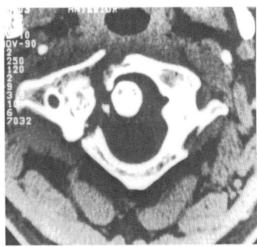
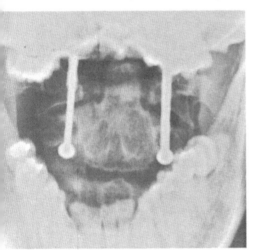
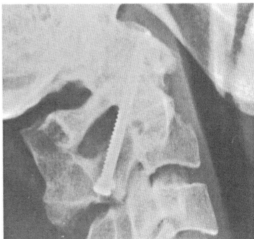

FIGURE 29L. A 34-year-old man with unstable Jefferson fracture after a fall on his head during an explosion of a gas tank. The AP view shows lateral dislocation of the lateral masses of the atlas and the CT scan shows bony avulsion of the transverse ligament. (2) Open reduction and stabilization were performed 2 weeks after the accident. Bone graft chips were positioned over the posterior arch of C1 and C2, with- out stabilizing them. Postoperative immobilization was in a four-poster brace for 3 months; 30 months later, the posterior fusion is solid. The patient complains about some neck pain but also about difficul- ties in concentrating as a result of the brain concussion sustained at the time of injury.

References

1. Magerl F, Seemann P-S: Stable posterior fusion of the atlas and axis by transarticular screw fixation. In Kehr P, Weidner A (eds): Cervical Spine, Vol. I. Springer, Wien, 1987.
2. Grob D, Crisco J, Panjabi M, Dvorak J: Biomechanical evaluation of four different posterior atlantoaxial fixation techniques. Spine 17:480–490, 1992.
3. Hanson PB, Montesano PX, Sharkey N, Rauschning W: Anatomic and biomechanical assessment of transarticular screw fixation for atlantoaxial instability. Spine 16:1141–1145, 1991.
4. Wilke H-J, Fischer K, Kuger A, Magerl F, Claes L, Wörsdörfer O: In vitro investigations of internal fixation systems of the upper cervical spine. Stability of posterior atlanto-axial fixation techniques. Eur Spine J 1:191–199, 1992.
5. Jeanneret B: Posterior transarticular screw fixation of C1–C2. Tech Orthop 9:49–59, 1994.
6. Grob D, Jeanneret B, Aebi M, Markwalder T: Atlanto-axial fusion with transarticular screw fixation. J Bone Joint Surg 73B:972–976, 1991.
7. Müller ME, Allgöwer M, Schneider R, Willenegger H: Manual of Internal Fixation. Techniques Recommended by the AO-ASIF Group. Springer, Berlin, 1991.
8. Jeanneret B, Magerl F: Primary posterior fusion C1/2 in odontoid fractures. Indications, technique and results of transarticular screw fixation. J Spinal Disord 5:464–475, 1992.

Cervical Foraminotomy: Indications and Technique

Peter Dyck

Several terms that reappear throughout this chapter are first defined: neural foramen, nerve root, and foraminotomy.

When two contiguous vertebrae are apposed, a lateral, somewhat cylindrical tunnel is formed that serves as an exit for segmental nerve roots. From the standpoint of surgical importance, the ventral floor is made up of the disc space and the adjacent joint of Luschka. The roof is formed by the overlapping inferior and superior zygapophyseal joints. Superiorly and inferiorly, the pedicles of the respective vertebrae form the bony limits; this constitutes the neural foramen.

The nerve root is the most important structure that passes through this foramen. It is invested by surrounding fat and accompanied by epidural veins (Fig. 30A). This nerve root is composed of a sensory ganglion and its proximal preganglionic axons and postganglionic motor axons arising from the anterior horn cells within the spinal cord and terminating in the muscle fiber they innervate. These sensory and motor structures are bathed by cerebrospinal fluid and invested by an outpouching of the common dural sac referred to as the dural root sleeve. It is this structure that is seen at the time of surgical exposure.

The C5 nerve root forms a 45-degree angle with the spinal cord as it traverses its foramen, and this angle increases as one descends; so that C8 is essentially at right angles as it enters the spinal canal outlet.

Foraminotomy is decompression of a nerve root by removal of offending pathologic material within and in the proximity of a neural foramen. Ventrally, disc material or osteophytic bone may be removed. The latter is particularly true of the joint of Luschka, whose hypertrophic excrescences usually encroach on the nerve root within its axilla. Dorsally decompression is accomplished by resection of the medial aspect of the superior and inferior facets; this is performed with a high-speed drill.

It is imperative to determine preoperatively the extent of neck flexion tolerated by the patient without aggravating neurologic symptoms.

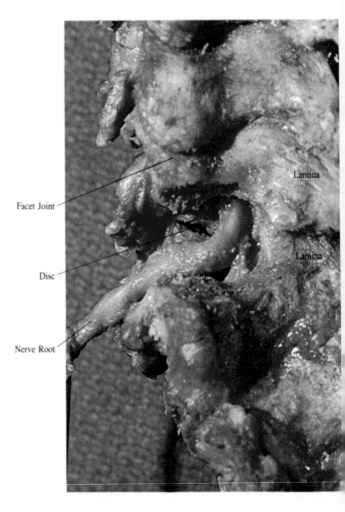

Facet Joint

Disc

Nerve Root

Lamina

Lamina

FIGURE 30A. Ventral retraction of the nerve root shows the intervertebral disc.

1. In spite of the inherent dangers of air embolism, I prefer the upright position to the prone (Fig. 30B).[1,2] The Mayfield headrest is used. Skeletal pin fixation remains an option, but I prefer the "horseshoe" headrest. The suboccipital scalp is shaved sufficiently to tape the head in place and to allow operative preparation of the surgical field. Flexion of the neck distracts the facets and facilitates exposure, as does slight lateral flexion contralateral to the lesion.

2. The level and length of the midline posterior cervical incision are determined by external landmarks, for example, a prominent C7 spinous process. Meticulous attention to hemostasis is essential. To accommodate the application of hemostatic Raney clips, the subcutaneous tissue may be slightly undercut.

3. A self-retaining retractor is placed and the trapezius fascia incised, allowing retraction of the muscle mass on the side of the lesion.

4. Then, the splenius and semispinalis capita, the lower semispinalis cervicis, and the multifidus muscles are separated from the spinous processes and contiguous laminae by subperiosteal dissection with a periosteal elevator or Bovie "cutting" electrocautery.

5. The wound is repeatedly irrigated with a sterile saline or comparable solution to cool the operative field when the electrocautery is used; this helps prevent potential

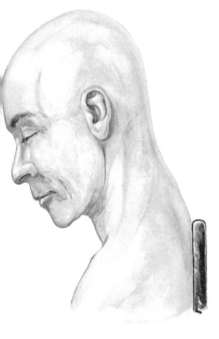

FIGURE 30B. The upright position is used in preference to the prone position. The Mayfield headrest supports the head. Skeletal pin fixation remains an option, but the horseshoe headrest is preferred. The occipital scalp is shaven sufficiently to tape the head in place and to allow operative preparation of the surgical field. Flexion of the neck distracts the facets and facilitates the exposure, as does slight lateral flexion contralateral to the lesion. There is some inherent danger of air embolus in the upright position.

air embolism. Muscle stripping is greatly facilitated when the bony projection of a bifid spinous process is resected on the side of the exposure (Fig. 30C).

6. Having exposed the lamina at the level of interest, radiologic corroboration is obtained. While roentgenograms are being developed, the lateral dissection is continued

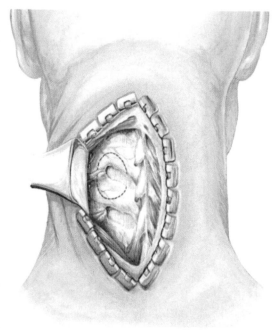

FIGURE 30C. The incision should extend two spinous processes above and two below the desired level. Open the skin and subcutaneous tissue. Slightly undercut the subcutaneous tissue and apply hemostatic Raney clips. Place the self-retaining retractor and incise the trapezius fascia. Retract the muscle mass on either side of the lesion. Use either a periosteal elevator or the cutting electrocautery to remove the paraspinous musculature from the spinous process and the lamina of the involved side. Beginning at the tip of the spinous process, obtain the subperiosteal plane before sweeping out on the lamina. Resection of the bifid spinous process may aid greatly in the muscle stripping exposure. Irrigate repeatedly with saline. Maintain meticulous hemostasis.

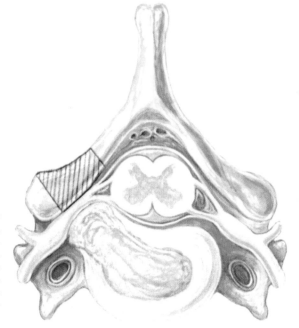

FIGURE 30D. After X-ray confirmation of the level, expose the medial two-thirds of the zygapophyseal joint and maintain retraction with a handheld Meyerding retractor. For exposure of a specific disc space such as C5–C6, remove the overlying inferior articular process of CS and, to a lesser extent, the superior articular process of C6.

so as to expose the medial two-thirds of the zygapophyseal joints in question. Although difficult for the assistant, a handheld Meyerding retractor maintains this exposure best.

7. A high-speed drill is utilized in the removal of overlying superior and to a lesser extent the inferior facets. Part of the inferior and lateral lamina of the vertebra above

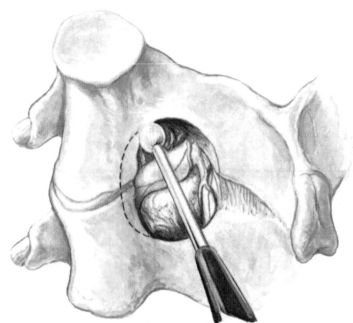

FIGURE 30E. With the bur, remove the inferior, lateral lamina of the vertebra above and the superior, lateral lamina of the vertebra below. The interposed ligamentum flavum comes away with the bony removal. Be very cautious.

and the superior and lateral lamina of the vertebra below are also drilled away (Figs. 30D, 30E, 30F). The interposed ligamentum flavum comes away with the bony removal. It is a very precarious structure in the neck, in contradistinction to the low back. Bone wax is used to stop intramedullary bleeding.

8. Cautious dissection of the structures within the neural foramen separates the fat and exposes the root sleeve and the ever-present extradural veins (Fig. 30G). When these veins rupture, bleeding may be disconcerting, but should not present a serious problem. Hemostasis may be obtained by packing with a small cotton pledget or preferably with a bipolar coagulator.

9. When soft disc protrusion is encountered, it is usually an extrusion of a substantial part of the nucleus pulposus. The extruded disc and the easily accessible intradiscal material are removed, but no endeavor is made to perform a complete discectomy. A more aggressive discectomy only promotes myelopathy (Figs. 30H, 30I).

10. When a so-called hard disc is encountered, the small, curved, and straight Cloward curettes are employed to remove osteophytes arising from the intervertebral disc space and the axillary osteophytes emanating from the joint of Luschka (Fig. 30J).

11. A blunt nerve hook may be employed to guide the extent of bony resection, thus achieving adequate neural decompression without undue bony removal (Figs. 30H, 30I, 30J, 30K, 30L).

12. Closure: Having assured oneself of complete hemostasis, absorbable gelatin foam is placed within the foraminotomy and the wound closed in layers without a drain. The fascia is approximated with nonabsorbable suture, the subcutaneous tissue with resorbable synthetic suture material, and the skin closed with a nylon suture.

13. When radicular pain is disabling, 20 mg of epidural methyl prednisone acetate may be applied, soaked in gelatin foam, directly to the exposed nerve root. This step reduces pain but potentially promotes local infection. Hence, I employ a prophylactic antibiotic intraoperatively in such instances. I have never encountered a local infection as a result of such practice, be it in the neck or the low back.

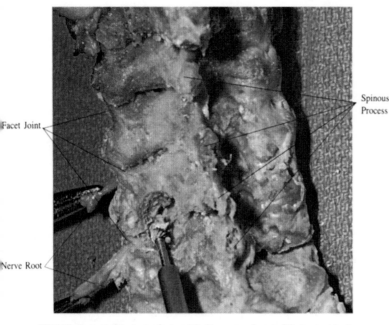

Facet Joint

Spinous Process

Nerve Root

FIGURE 30F. Removal of the lamina facet and the ligamentum flavum of the involved level.

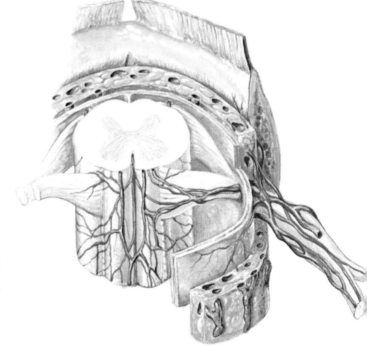

FIGURE 30G. Cautiously dissect the structures within the neural foramen. Separate the fat and expose the nerve root. Beware of the ever-present epidural veins covering the nerve root. Hemostasis after rupture of these veins should be obtained with a small cottonoid pledget or with a bipolar coagulator. Surgicil and packing may be needed.

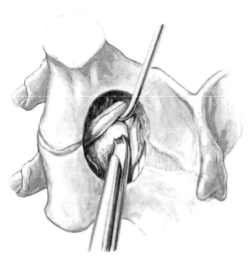

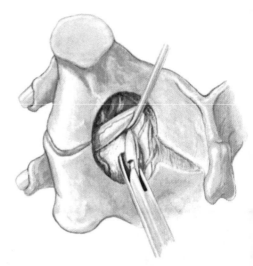

FIGURE 30H. A blunt nerve hook is used to guide the extent of the bony resection. Removal of hard disc material from the intervertebral space may be accomplished after retraction of the nerve root with the kerasin punch.

FIGURE 30I. The pituitary rongeur may be used to retract this material.

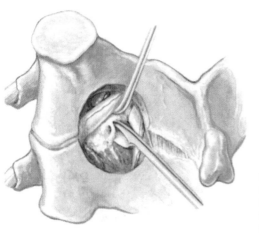

FIGURE 30J. Chisels and curettes may be used to remove osteophytes arising in the vertebral disc space and osteophytes emanating from the joint of Luschka.

14. Postoperatively, the patient is cared for in a 40-degree semi-Fowler position to reduce venostasis at the operative site. No external neck support is necessary, but the patient frequently feels more confident with a soft cervical collar.

A vast literature addresses the surgical treatment of cervical radiculopathy. It is hard to say if one method is superior to another. I have always employed posterior

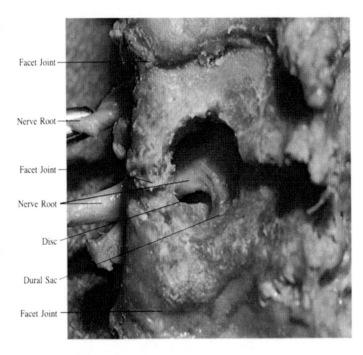

Facet Joint

Nerve Root

Facet Joint

Nerve Root

Disc

Dural Sac

Facet Joint

FIGURE 30K. The nerve root and disc space in the intervertebral foramen without the veins seen in Figure 30G.

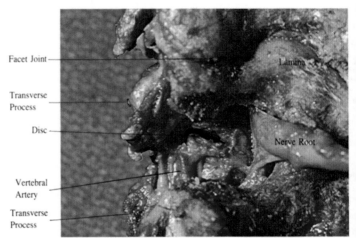

FIGURE 30L. With an unanatomical removal of the nerve root from the intervertebral foramen, one clearly visualizes the joint of Luschka and the intervertebral disc.

Facet Joint

Transverse Process

Disc

Lamina

Nerve Root

Vertebral Artery

Transverse Process

decompression of a nerve root in preference to anterior decompression and interbody fusion. Although the morbidity might be greater during the first few days, posterior decompression does not immobilize a motion segment, allows one to operate at more than one level, and offers adequate decompression of an injured nerve root. There is no need for protracted neck immobilization, and one avoids iliac crest graft site pain.

In experienced hands, the operation can be carried out in less than an hour, even if two foraminotomies are performed.

Remember:

1. Preoperatively check the amount of neck flexion possible without producing severe radiculopathy.
2. Accompany electrocautery dissection with frequent irrigation.
3. Dissect laterally to the medial two-thirds of the facet joint.
4. With the bur, fashion a hole removing more of the cephalad facet.
5. Extract soft tissue fragments without a radical excision of disc contents.
6. Guide the dissection with a nerve hook.
7. Control bleeding with packing, bipolar cautery, and hemostatic material.
8. Understand the anatomy of the intervertebral foramen completely.

References

1. Brain WR, Wilkinson M: Cervical Spondylosis and Other Disorders of the Cervical Spine. Philadelphia, Saunders, 1967.
2. Bucy PC, Chenault H: Compression of the seventh cervical root by herniation of an intervertebral disc. JAMA 126:26–27, 1944.
3. Lee CK, Weiss AB: Isolated congenital cervical block vertebrae below the axis with neurological symptoms. Spine 6:118–124, 1981.
4. Semmes RE, Murphey F: Syndrome of unilateral rupture of the sixth cervical intervertebral disc, with compression of the seventh nerve root. JAMA 121:1209–1214, 1943.
5. Spurling RG: Lesions of the Cervical Intervertebral Discs. Springfield, Thomas, 1956.
6. Tisovec L, Hamilton W: Newer considerations in air embolism during operation. JAMA 201:376–377, 1967.

Microcervical Foraminotomy: An Alternative Posterior Technique for Intractable Radicular Pain

Robert Warren Williams

Microcervical foraminotomy (MCF) is the term used by this author to specifically define a posterior microsurgical technique that has proven extremely successful for the resolution of intractable cervical radicular pain.[1] The procedure was developed in 1972 and absolutely minimizes any degree of laminectomy or facet trauma while allowing for a thorough neurolysis and bony foraminal decompression along the posterior and inferior aspect of symptomatic cervical nerve roots. As many as six foramina have been treated at one sitting. The intervertebral disc, stabilizing bony structures, and any foraminal pathology anterior to the root are not disturbed during this operation. Although primarily indicated for the treatment of intractable pain and neurologic deficit of a radicular distribution, the operation has proven to be just as successful in those individuals with persistent radicular symptoms unresponsive to previous anterior cervical or laminectomy techniques.

Clinical Rationale for This Alternative Approach

A disappointing 5-year personal experience in the consistency with which cervical radicular pain responded to accepted surgical techniques prompted this author to reassess his surgical failures in 1971. In the absence of intrinsic neural disease, persisting foraminal pathology either unrecognized or unreachable during a previous surgical operation seemed the most probable etiology. Because anterior foraminal pathology was protected by the vertebral artery and even the anterior foramen entrance could not be surgically reached without inflicting serious morbidity on the intervertebral disc, a conservative microsurgical technique was developed that allows neurolysis and decompression of any posterior irritative foraminal pathology. This technique is termed microcervical foraminotomy (MCF).

Patient Selection

Since 1972, 574 patients with 1571 symptomatic cervical nerve roots have been treated by this conservative posterior surgical approach. As many as six roots from C4 to C8 have been treated at one sitting. In the absence of intrinsic neural disease, preoperative correlation between abnormal radiodiagnostic studies and symptomatic nerve root levels has become minimally important because foraminal pathology treatable by this operation lies largely outside the spinal canal. Surgical indications for MCF are intractable pain or neurologic deficit of a radicular distribution unresponsive to either exhaustive conservative management or previous cervical operations. Regardless of any preoperative structural radiographic pathology, this operation is only applied to those foraminal levels with clinical radicular symptoms. A expert knowledge of cervical radicular neuroanatomy including dermatonal, myotomal, and reflex distributions seems all that is necessary to localize a clinically symptomatic cervical nerve root and thus its associated neural foramen.[2]

Instrumentation, Anesthesia, and Positioning

Surgical Microscope and Instrumentation

A Zeiss Opmi 1 surgical microscope with straight binoculars and 300-mm lens provides excellent visibility and surgical mobility. Medium to high magnification is used. A self-retaining retractor with lateral blade (1 cm width, 5 cm depth) and dull medial hook is applied for unilateral wound retraction (Williams' Microlumbar Discectomy Retractor; Codman and Shurtleff, Randolph, MA). Other than scalpel and electrocoagulator, instruments required are a blunt 90-degree microhook, a 45-degree, 1.5-mm rongeur, 45- and 90-degree, 1-mm rongeurs, and microcurettes (Fig. 31A). The microcurettes

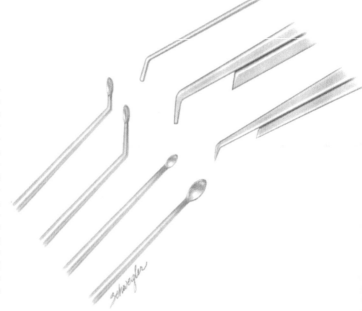

FIGURE 31A. Instrumentation for microcervical foraminotomy (MCF) is minimal. Pictured from *top left clockwise* are a 90-degree microhook, a 45-degree, 1.5-mm rongeur, a straight microcurette, a 90-degree, 1-mm rongeur, and a 45-degree, 1-mm rongeur. Additional instruments not pictured are scalpel, electrocoagulator, electrocutting blade, small periosteal elevator, and the author's 15- and 30-degree-angle microcurettes made by smoothly bending straight microcurettes 1 cm from the cup. (Redrawn with permission from Williams RW. Microcervical foraminotomy: a surgical alternative for intractable radicular pain. Spine 1983;8(7):708–716.)

best suited are one that is straight and two additional that have been smoothly angled by the author to 15 and 30 degrees, respectively. These curvatures should be placed approximately 1 cm from the tip.

Patient Preparation, Anesthesia, and Positioning

Patients receive a complete medical and pulmonary assessment. Antiseptic sponges are provided for home showers and shampoos before hospital admission. The operation is carried out with the patient in the sitting position utilizing a Mayfield pin-type head holder. The chin is slightly flexed to reduce cervical lordosis. General endotracheal anesthesia with mechanical ventilation is applied along with cardiac doppler and central venous pressure monitor for the detection and treatment of possible air emboli. The legs are wrapped, and systolic blood pressure is maintained above 120 mmHg with vasopressor as needed.

Operating Time

Wound entrance, closure, and a one-side, one-level foraminotomy require 1 hour. Each additional foraminotomy adds approximately 0.5 hour to the operating time.

Incision Placement

Accurate placement of the skin incision is paramount to ensure minimal operating time and maximal hemostasis. After palpation of a familiar spinous process, a 1-inch needle is inserted well lateral to the midline and localized by lateral radiogram. A 1.5-inch skin incision is then marked in the midline after reviewing the anatomical placement of the needle. Once the wound is open, a visible spinous process is then notched with a rongeur for future identification and grasped on its tip with a metallic clamp. A second lateral cervical X-ray is then obtained to accurately identify the vertebral level. Once the metallic clamp has been removed, the notched spinous process can be followed inward on its lateral surface by finger palpation to locate the symptomatic interlaminar level. A self-retaining retractor is then applied for direct visualization of the deeper anatomy.

This technique has proven absolutely necessary for the exact localization of foraminal levels, because it is extremely easy for even the most experienced spinal surgeon to become disorientated in the depths of a microsurgical cervical wound. If there is any doubt as to the location, check and recheck again until the appropriate interlaminar level is without question. This operation is so successful for the relief of radicular pain that any persistence in its intensity for even 24 hours following surgery likely indicates that the surgeon was in the wrong place.

Surgical Technique

Dissection to the Lamina

A 1.5-inch posterior midline wound is generous for a two-level foraminotomy. If work is to be done bilaterally, expose only one side at a time as this will ensure minimal blood loss from venous oozing in what sometimes can be a lengthy operation. Unless open veins are unattended with the patient in the sitting position, air emboli will not occur.

The technique of foraminotomy presented here is much more difficult for the surgeon when working on a foramen toward the same side as that of the surgeon's dominant hand. That is, right-side foraminotomies are technically the most difficult for the right-handed surgeon. When working toward the dominant side, tedious wrist extension movements are required while utilizing rongeurs and microcurettes. Such maneuvers are not the case when resculpting a foramen toward the surgeon's nondominant side. Initially, therefore, always treat those foramina that will be technically the most difficult. Proceeding in this manner will markedly reduce the surgeon's fatigue and thus further minimize blood loss and operating time.

Once the wound is open, an electrocutting knife is applied to unilaterally separate the paravertebral fascia from the spinous processes. The lamina and ligamentum flavum are often quite superficial, so use extreme caution with the cutting current. The index finger can then be inserted through the fascia opening, applying gentle inward pressures to displace the paravertebral muscles laterally. Periosteal elevators are seldom necessary. Finger palpation allows for accurate anatomical localization of the deeper interlaminar space when correlated with the previously notched spinous process. Meticulous hemostasis is accomplished by electrocoagulation. Care is taken to avoid electrical instrument contact with the ligamentum flavum, thus preventing potential burn injury to the deeper neural structures. A unilateral self-retaining retractor, as previously described, is then inserted to maintain surgical exposure.

Foraminotomy

Once the interlaminar space associated with the symptomatic root has been accurately identified, the ligamentum flavum is separated from its most lateral attachment to the upper lamina using a straight microcurette. This area of separation is usually no more than 1 cm lateral to the midline. If the interlaminar space is quite narrow or the opposing lamina borders are indistinct as a result of osteoarthritic disease, a power bur can be applied to carefully reestablish the tissue planes.

Once the ligamentum flavum is separated, an appropriate rongeur is inserted under the lateral laminar shelf and small bites of bone are removed in an upward direction (Fig. 31B) until the foramen entrance can be identified by blunt microhook palpation (Fig. 31C). Ligamentum flavum is never intentionally removed during this

FIGURE 31B. Utilizing microcervical foraminotomy (MCF) technique, foraminotomy is initiated by the minimal removal of bone from the most lateral portion of the superior lamina (*arrow*). Do not turn the mouth of the rongeur laterally as it will fracture the facet injuring the synovium. Care is taken not to sacrifice the ligamentum flavum during this minimal laminectomy as the ligament offers excellent protection for the underlying dura and spinal fluid space. (Redrawn with permission from Williams RW. Microcervical foraminotomy: a surgical alternative for intractable radicular pain. Spine 1983;8(7):708–716.)

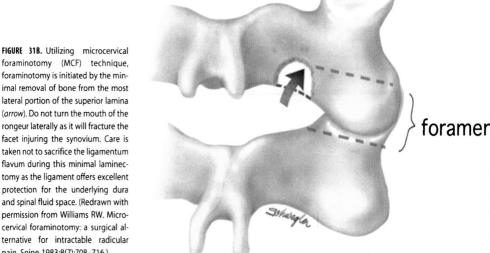

foramen

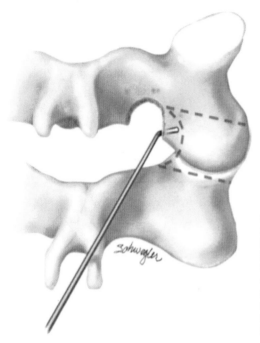

FIGURE 31C. With an area of minimal upward laminectomy completed, a blunt 90-degree microhook is used to locate and explore the foramen entrance. Although this is a blind surgical maneuver, the operator soon learns to estimate the degree of stenosis and perineural adhesion density that will be encountered during posterior foraminal resculpting.

operation because it provides great protection to the underlying dura and neural elements. Most important, during laminar bone removal, do not turn the mouth of the rongeur laterally into the facet or its synovium.

Mastering the technique of locating the posterior foramen entrance and evaluating its probable pathology by blunt microhook palpation will yield invaluable information to the surgeon. The degree of osteoarthritic stenosis, density of posterior and inferior perineural adhesions, and angle with which the foraminal tube exits the spinal canal can all be assessed by this blind surgical maneuver. When strictly adhering to MCF technique, the perineural soft tissues and cervical root will be maximally protected.

After microhook location of the foramen entrance and evaluation of posterior root adhesion density, the angled microcurettes are used with gentle outward pushing movements both laterally and ventrally to progressively separate perineural tissues from the posterior foraminal wall (Fig. 31D). Again, this is a blind surgical maneuver and must be done very carefully, especially when adhesions are dense between the root dura and bone. A thorough restoration of perineural tissue planes is critical, however, and must be accomplished throughout the entire posterior aspect of the foraminal tube including its outlet. Then and only then will the surgeon clearly visualize arterial-type pulsations in the nerve root sleeve. Such pulsations are the absolute key indicator that perineural tissues are adequately separated from the periosteum of the posterior foraminal wall.

With perineural tissue planes reestablished, blind resculpting of the posterior and inferior foraminal bone can be accomplished with angled microcurettes and a 1-mm, 45-degree-angle rongeur) (Figs. 31E, 31F). Proceed tediously outward from the foramen entrance while avoiding mechanical pressures against the root. Motor responses are uncommon unless the surgeon is traumatizing the nerve. Be very cautious during resculpting as postoperative increases in motor deficit, although usually transient, most often belong to the surgeon.

Stenotic lesions in the elderly may be of extremely hard bone, or soft osteoarthritic bone at any age. In either case, tedious bony decompression utilizing microcurettes has

FIGURE 31D. Microcurettes of varying angles are passed through the posterior aspect of the foramen entrance with the sharp cup against bone. Gentle pressures are applied laterally with the smooth backside of the curette toward the nerve, allowing a progressive separation of perineural tissues from the posterior and inferior foraminal wall while protecting the root from sharp instrumentation. Because the inside of the foramen is blind surgical territory, do not pull the curette medially while attempting to resculpt bone until absolutely sure the posterior root dura has been widely separated from the foramen periosteum.

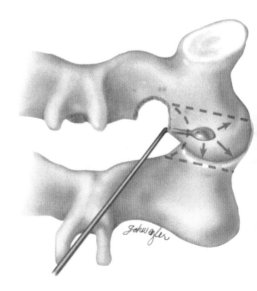

proven the safest method of protecting the nerve while relieving stenosis. Once stenotic pressures have been significantly reduced by microcurette, it will be safe to begin resculpturing the posterior foraminal wall with a 1-mm, 45-degree-angle rongeur. Osteophytes in the root axilla are removed by a similar technique. For the foraminotomy to be considered complete, the perineural tissue planes must be fully reestablished, the nerve root clearly pulsatile, and all posterior stenotic pressure points relieved.

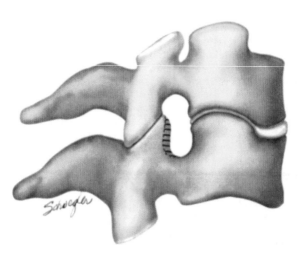

FIGURE 31E. The author's lateral view concept of a foramen stenosed by osteoarthritic disease and what needs to be accomplished during microcervical foraminotomy (MCF) resculpting. The peri-neural tissues are separated from the posterior and inferior foraminal wall using *outward* or lateral pushing movements with the smooth backside of the microcurettes against the root dura. Once perineural tissues have been freed from the bony wall, gentle *inward* curetting is applied to decompress the posterior and inferior stenosing pathology and smooth the foraminal bone. (Redrawn with permission from Williams RW. Microcervical foraminatomy: a surgical alternative for intractable radicular pain. Spine 1983;8(7):708–716.)

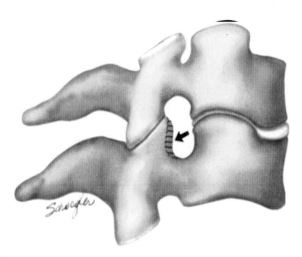

FIGURE 31F. On completion of resculpting, the posterior and inferior foraminal wall should feel widely decompressed to the surgeon when palpated with a blunt microhook (*arrow*). Note that no attempt was made to correct pathology in the anterior foramen. When stenotic pressures and perineural adhesions have been thoroughly released, arterial-type pulsations of the nerve root become visible under magnification. Until these pulsations are clearly present, the surgeon must suspect persisting areas of dural adhesions or osteophytosis along the posterior foraminal wall. The one exception to this observation is, however, the rare bright red edematous nerve roots, as discussed in the text. (Redrawn with permission from Williams RW. Microcervical foraminatomy: a surgical alternative for intractable radicular pain. Spine 1983;8(7):708–716.)

When foramina must be treated bilaterally, complete all work on one side before proceeding to the opposite side. Remove the retractor, place a moist sponge in the unilateral wound to displace air, and only then expose the opposite interlaminar anatomy. Spinal fluid leaks have not occurred following MCF, and potential surgical injuries to the facet and its synovium should be minimal. Blood loss rarely exceeds 100 mL. At wound closure, do not place sutures in the paravertebral muscles; this precaution will markedly reduce postoperative morbidity from muscle spasm.

Postoperative Care

Cervical ice packs are the mainstay during convalescence. The patient ambulates as desired with hospital and discharge medications consisting of oral muscle relaxants, antiinflammatories, and nonnarcotic pain medication. For the first 24 hours following surgery, systemic antiinflammatories may be used. Discharge usually occurs on the third postoperative day unless numerous foramina have been resculpted.

Technical Observations

1. Always obtain two lateral cervical spine X-rays to localize the deeper cervical anatomy. The first, taken with a needle as a marker, is used to place the midline skin mark in reference to superficial landmarks. The second lateral X-ray is then obtained after the wound has been opened. The surgeon should position a mechanical film holder and X-ray tube during initial surgical preparation. Obtain the first lateral X-ray before draping and leave both the X-ray tube and film holder in their exact positions for inclusion under the final surgical drapes. The second X-ray is then obtained after the wound has been opened. I cannot stress strongly enough how important X-ray localization of the deeper cervical anatomy will prove as the operation progresses.

2. The volume of upper lateral lamina removed for identification of the foramen entrance should be kept to a minimum; this is best achieved with a 1.5-mm, 45-degree-angle rongeur. Larger instruments will fracture the facet plates and markedly increase long-term postsurgical muscle spasm. Additionally, ligamentum flavum is not removed during MCF to provide maximal protection to the underlying dura and spinal fluid space.

3. The foramen entrance rarely lies more than 1 cm lateral to the midline. Be very precise in its location, because surgical disorientation at this stage of the operation can lead to disaster.

4. Perineural soft tissues vary greatly in color, texture, and volume, depending on the chronicity and degree of inflammation that have occurred along the posterior foraminal wall. Perineural tissues are hereby defined to include dura, fat, connective, and vascular tissue. Under magnification within a normal foramen, the dura appears yellowish-gray with a wrinkled wet texture, fat is bright yellow and globular, connective tissue is white with a fishnet appearance, and the capillary vasculature is easily visible on the dural sleeve and throughout the other perineural tissues.

In patients with radicular pain only, one can expect a white glistening vascular dura beginning to stick to the foraminal periosteum. Fat and connective tissue will be present but sparse. As the clinical severity of symptoms evolve from only that of radicular pain to those of radicular pain associated with radiculopathies (increasing degrees of motor paresis, sensory loss, and ultimately muscle atrophy), the appearance of perineural tissues changes dramatically. In mild chronic radiculopathies, the dura appears bluish, puckered, and hypovascular whereas the perineural fat and connective tissue begin to atrophy and fibrose. In severe radiculopathies, the perineural fat and connective tissue will have totally disappeared and the dura will appear purplish, shriveled, avascular, and densely adherent to the foraminal wall.

The only exception to these scenarios is the rare patient with acute severe burning radicular pain unresponsive to any type of conservative management. These patients usually have a nontraumatic onset of symptoms, hold the affected arm motionless in their lap, exhibit motor weakness without atrophy, and experience severe burning paresthesias. Almost 50% of these patients are latent diabetics, and this syndrome has never occurred bilaterally. At surgery, the symptomatic nerve roots are visibly bright red and swell dramatically as foraminal pressures are released. These are the only patients in whom arterial-type root pulsations may not become visible following completion of MCF. Always inform the patient with burning radicular pain that their symptoms will require some weeks to resolve.

5. The angles with which the foramina exit the spine may vary greatly from patient to patient. Such variations may lead to technical difficulties when trying to use a 1-mm, 45-degree-angle rongeur to resculpt a foramen that exits anterolaterally at 30 degrees. In such cases, direct mechanical trauma to the root or fracture into the facet can easily occur during use of a rongeur. This is the most important technical reason to initially utilize microcurettes when reestablishing perineural tissue planes and resculpting stenotic foramina. There is one good trade-off, however. Foramina angled laterally at only 20 to 30 degrees provide a spectacular "gun barrel" view of all posterior foraminal pathology. It is here that confidence can be gained in performing those technical maneuvers that most often are blind to the surgeon.

6. The only significant technical complication that has occurred with MCF is when a patient awakens with dense radicular paresis, the degree of which was not present preoperatively (2%). The C5 root is by far the most sensitive to foraminal decompression, especially in latent diabetics and those patients with long-standing radiculopathies clinically manifested by chronic pain, marked weakness with muscular atrophy, and sensory loss. At surgery these nerve roots appear withered, purplish, and may visibly expand dramatically following decompression. Although the postoperative paresis may be dense, it will recover to a minimum of its preoperative status within a maximum of 4 months. Radicular pain, however, clears immediately. The physiologic mechanisms of this phenomena remain speculative. With honest preoperative counseling and the dramatic resolution of their radicular pain, however, all patients experiencing this complication ultimately expressed satisfaction with their surgical result. Always inform the patient with chronic CS radiculopathy of this potential complication.

Conclusion

Intractable cervical radicular pain is a common and often severely disabling clinical problem. In this 22-year surgical experience with 574 patients and 1571 symptomatic nerve roots, radicular pain was usually insidious in onset (60%), with measurable neurologic deficit occurring at more than one root level. For 15%, neural decompensation had occurred to the point of myotomal atrophy. The textbook neuroanatomy of cervical radicular functions has proved reliable for allowing clinical examination to detect specific root levels generating radicular pain and neurologic dysfunction.[2]

Mastering use of the surgical microscope and microsurgical instrumentation has allowed investigation of the posterior anatomy of the cervical nerve roots as they traverse the bony foramina. A variety of structural pathology has been observed that leads to the inadequacy of these neural passages. Most often partially calcified deposits termed osteophytes are present associated with foraminal adhesions. Although radicular pain resolves after MCF, the reversibility of objective neurologic deficit associated with such pathology seems directly related to the degree of neural irritation that these deposits cause in relation to time. As the chronicity of symptoms increase, so also will the degree of perineural tissue atrophy and withering discoloration of the nerve root. In the most severe cases, neurologic deficits may only be stabilized by this procedure or only slightly improved over a period of months.

The relief of radicular pain by this technique speaks strongly for extraneural pathology as its primary etiology. Because the operation does not alter the cervical disc or anterior foraminal anatomy, the resolution of pain must result from relief of root irritative lesions lying posteriorly while allowing relaxation of the root away from similar pathology that exists anteriorly. Whatever the mechanism, the root can be observed to develop rhythmic arterial timed pulsations following wide resculpting of a foramen. Perhaps these pulsations are transmitted via previously ischemic vasonervorum, or from the vertebral artery that lies anteriorly. Cerebrospinal fluid pulsations would not appear to be the mechanism, however, because myelographic flow patterns in the root sleeve seem unchanged following foraminal decompression by MCF, and there have been no spinal fluid leaks.

A considerable number of patients (40%) manifest discogenic pain syndrome[3] in association with radicular pain. These symptoms have also resolved following MCF. Because the cervical disc is never altered by this technique, the pathophysiology of discogenic pain would seem speculative. In addition, preoperative radiodiagnostic studies of all types correlated with clinical examination have only been of value in diagnosing the occasional patient with spinal cord disease not suited for this operation. When radicular pain is the prominent presenting symptom, however, foraminal pathology outside the realm of radiologic diagnosis is most often the etiology.

Most radicular pain will radiate over the C6 and C7 root distributions unilaterally. Because 40% of all patients have asymptomatic preoperative myelographic defects and only 7% of these become symptomatic, never operate on a clinically asymptomatic foramen. For those readers who desire further detailed statistics on MCF, refer to the original 10-year surgical series published in 1983.[1] Although an additional 339 patients have been subsequently treated during the past 12 years, the comprehensive presentation and statistical analysis of the original MCF surgical series remains essentially unchanged.

Acknowledgment

The author thanks publisher J.B. Lippincott of Philadelphia, PA, for their release of copyrighted material previously published in *Spine* 1983;8(7):708–716.

References

1. Williams RW: Microcervical foraminotomy: a surgical alternative for intractable radicular pain. Spine 8(7):708–716, 1983.
2. Chusid JG: Correlative neuroanatomy and functional neurology. In Cutaneous Innervation, 17th edn. Los Altos, Lange, 1979, pp 204–210.
3. Cloward RB: New method of diagnosis and treatment of cervical disc disease. In Clinical Neurosurgery, Vol. 8. Baltimore, Williams & Wilkins, 1957, pp 93–127.

Costotransversectomy

The costotransversectomy is a thoracic spine approach that can be made in one of two positions: prone[1,2] or in the lateral decubitus position tilted anteriorly 20 degrees.[3] Either of two skin incisions, midline or paraspinous, and one of three fascial incisions, midline, longitudinal paraspinous or transverse paraspinous, can be used. The pathology determines the exact approach. For biopsy and exposure of an intervertebral disc or vertebral body, position the patient prone, make a midline incision, and retract the paraspinous muscle mass laterally (Fig. 32A). A transverse incision in the paraspinous fascia and muscle may be necessary. For decompression after Harrington rod insertion, a long midline incision allows adequate lateral retraction to expose the costotransverse joint. Resect the transverse process, resect the pedicle, and decompress the spinal canal.[4] Adequate interbody fusion can be most difficult with the prone position, midline incision approach. Optimum exposure for resection of an entire vertebral body and two intervertebral discs followed by a strut graft is through a semilateral decubitus position, a paraspinous skin incision, and a paraspinous fascial incision.[3]

1. Position the patient prone on the operating table on a suitable frame. The horseshoe-shaped cushion with two chest pads or a four-poster operating frame made of radiolucent material allows excellent chest excursion and support during the operation. For approaches in the upper thoracic spine, the patient's arms are at the side and the head should be carefully positioned on the well-padded cervical headrest with careful padding of the forehead and malar eminences. Pay particular attention to the eyes and allow no pressure on them. Securely anchor the endotracheal tube. For approaches to the lower thoracic spine, position the arms at 90 degrees to the chest, the elbows well padded such as for a lumbar operation. The patient's head can be turned.

2. After prepping and draping, make a midline incision of sufficient length to allow retraction of paraspinous musculature for work lateral to the costotransverse joint (Fig. 32A). *Alternately, a curvilinear skin incision with its midportion 6 cm from the midline and the two ends of the incision approximately 3 cm from the midline can be used to expose directly the lateral outer border of the paraspinous musculature.*

3. Extend the midline incision as in any posterior spinal dissection, cutting with cautery to the spinous processes and removing muscle attachments from the lamina with a sharp periosteal elevator (Fig. 32B). Continue this subperiosteal removal of mus-

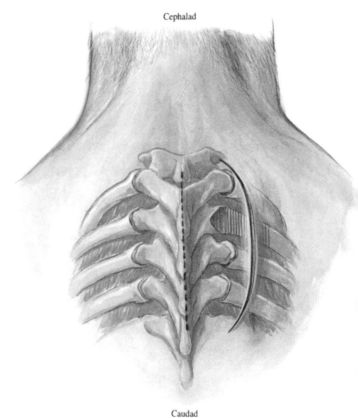

Cephalad

Caudad

FIGURE 32A. Costotransversectomy approach. Position the patient prone. Make a midline incision and retract the paraspinous muscle mass laterally. A transverse incision of the paraspinous fascia and muscle may be needed. Make the incision of sufficient length to allow this lateral retraction. Alternatively, a curvilinear skin incision, its midportion 6 cm from the midline and the end approximately 3 cm from the midline, may be used to expose directly the lateral border of the paraspinous musculature. For the more lateral incision, the paraspinous musculature is dissected from lateral to medial toward the midline. For the midline incision, the paraspinous musculature is elevated from the posterior elements medial to lateral.

culature and fascia laterally onto the rib beyond the costovertebral joint. For unilateral retraction use the single-tooth self-retaining lamina retractor, with the single-tooth edge in the spinous process and the wide retractor blade beneath the paraspinous musculature. *The paraspinous incision cuts through the thoracolumbar fascia laterally and elevates the paraspinous muscle mass medially.*

4. With sharp periosteal dissection, remove the periosteum from the rib, the capsule of the costotransverse joint, and the muscle and fascial tissue covering of the transverse process (Fig. 32B).

5. Incise the costotransverse joint. Rongeur the tip of the transverse process back to the level of its junction with the pedicle, lamina, and superior articular process (Fig. 32C).

6. Identify the neurovascular bundle in the inferior portion of the field as it crosses to the lower edge of the rib (Figs. 32D, 32E, 32F). It should be remembered that the neurovascular bundle courses on the lower edge of the rib. These vessels leave the intervertebral foramen, which is just caudad to the base of the transverse process, and cross to the lower edge of the rib. The ribs are angled caudally from medial to lateral. The articulation of the rib to the spine is in the cephalad portion of the vertebral body at the disc above. At the level of the angle of the rib, the rib is at the midvertebral body level. Therefore, the neurovascular bundle courses exposed in this area between the intervertebral foramen and the inferior border of the rib.

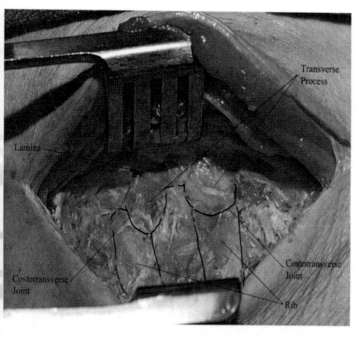

FIGURE 32B. With sharp dissection, remove the periosteum from the rib and the capsule of the costotransverse process. Open the costotransverse joint.

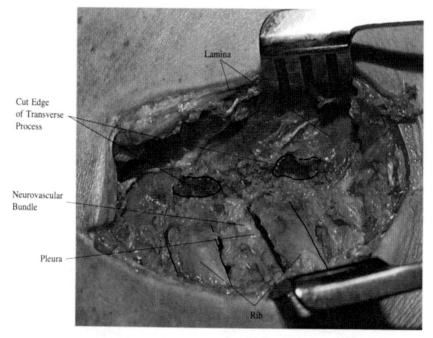

FIGURE 32C. Rongeur the tip of the transverse process back to the level of its junction with the pedicle and periarticular process. Identify the neurovascular bundle on the inferior surface of the rib. Open the periosteum on the outer surface of the rib with the electrocautery. Elevate the posterior periosteum of the rib subperi- ostally to the costal–vertebral articulation. Remove the periosteum circumferentially from the rib. Take care when removing the anterior periosteum of the rib to avoid damaging the pleura immediately beneath the rib bed.

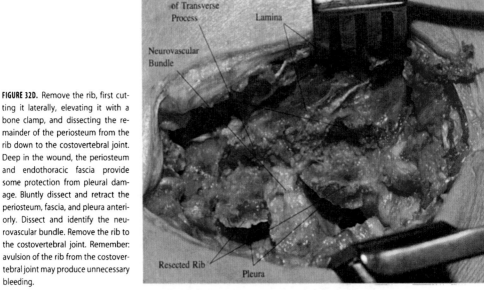

FIGURE 32D. Remove the rib, first cutting it laterally, elevating it with a bone clamp, and dissecting the remainder of the periosteum from the rib down to the costovertebral joint. Deep in the wound, the periosteum and endothoracic fascia provide some protection from pleural damage. Bluntly dissect and retract the periosteum, fascia, and pleura anteriorly. Dissect and identify the neurovascular bundle. Remove the rib to the costovertebral joint. Remember: avulsion of the rib from the costovertebral joint may produce unnecessary bleeding.

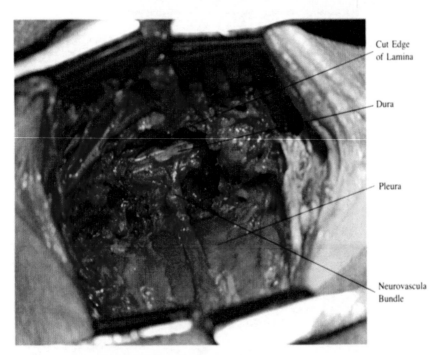

FIGURE 32E. Remove the remainder of the transverse process and the pedicle after dissecting each clear of soft tissue and carefully cutting only on bone. Identify the disc space and vertebral body deep in the wound. Isolate the neurovascular bundle. A costotransversectomy can be done at two levels to allow exposure of two neurovascular bundles. The disc between any two neurovascular bundles can be exposed. After identification of the nerve and neurovascular bundle, traction on the nerve allows identification of the dura and the spinal canal. Keeping the dura in view prevents damage during canal decompression.

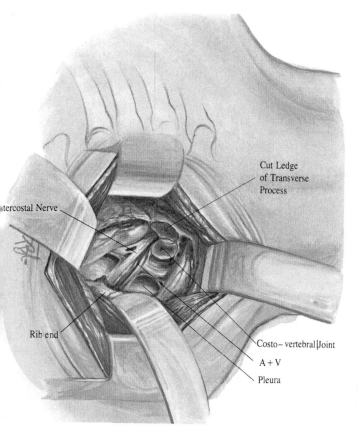

Cut Ledge
of Transverse
Process

tercostal Nerve

Rib end

Costo – vertebral |Joint

A + V

Pleura

FIGURE 32F. Composite view of the neurovascular bundle, pleura, and resected transverse process and rib.

7. Open the periosteum on the outer surface of the rib with the electrocautery. Open the wound with a deep self-retaining retractor. The Cloward self-retaining or Beckman-type retractor enhances the exposure.

8. Elevate the posterior periosteum of the rib subperiosteally to the costovertebral articulation. Remove the periosteum circumferentially from the rib. Take care when removing the anterior periosteum from the rib to avoid damaging the pleura, which lies immediately under the rib bed.

9. Cut the rib lateral at the angle of the rib (Fig. 32D).

10. Elevate the rib with a bone clamp to dissect the anterior surface of the rib under direct vision with less chance of damage to the pleura. Dissect the pleura and the endothoracic fascia off the spine at the costovertebral joint with careful blunt dissection. Avulsing the rib from the vertebral body frequently leads to bleeding from the articulation. Completely remove the rib with a rongeur into the joint (Fig. 32C); this requires time but produces less bleeding than avulsion.

11. Remove the rib to the costovertebral joint (Fig. 32D). Deep in the wound, the periosteum and endothoracic fascia provide protection from damaging the next deepest layer, the pleura. Dissect and identify the neurovascular bundle.

12. Dissect sharply at the base of the transverse process directly down the pedicle onto the vertebral body. Dissect clear the area between the base of the transverse process, the pedicle, and the costovertebral articulations. Identify the vertebral body and the disc space above (Fig. 32E).

13. Take care to avoid the next most cephalad neurovascular bundle. By performing this resection at two levels, that is, resecting two rib beds and two transverse processes, the neurovascular bundle between the two levels is clearly identified. The neurovascular bundle contents can then be separated to identify the nerve.

14. Dissect medially on the nerve, with gentle pulling control the nerve, and then identify the dural sleeve and posterior and anterior dura in the intervertebral foramen. After identification and retraction of the dura, the pedicle, lamina, and articular process can be resected if necessary with the Kerrison rongeur. The key is using the nerve to find the dura and cord.

15. To dissect on the front of the spine, be careful to elevate the prevertebral fascia. Fractures may be exposed with visualization of the posterior body wall as well as the disc and anterior structures. Vertebral body biopsies may be carried out with this incision.

16. It is strongly recommended that any operation in this area have definite X-ray confirmation of level.

17. Closure: Close fascia, subcutaneous tissue, and skin.

Remember:

1. Identify the costotransverse joint.
2. Dissect the transverse process.
3. Identify the neurovascular bundle caudad to the transverse process and rib.
4. Remove the interior periosteum and pleura from the rib laterally.
5. Avoid avulsion of the rib bed.
6. Beware of the neurovascular bundle above.
7. Use the neurovascular bundle to proceed into the spinal canal.

References

1. Cloward R: Hyperhidrosis. J Neurol 30(5):545–551, 1969.
2. Capner N: Evolution of a lateral rizotomy. J Bone Joint Surg 36B(2):173–179, 1954.
3. Bohlman H, Eismont F: Surgical techniques of anterior decompression and fusion for spinal cord injuries. Clin Orthop 154:57–73, 1981.
4. Fiesch JR, Lemer LL, Erickson DL, Chou SN, Bradford DS: Harrington instrumentation and spine fusion for thoracic and lumbar spine fractures. J Bone Joint Surg 59A:143, 1977.

Posterior and Posterolateral
Approaches to the Thoracic Disc

Paul H. Young

Posterior and posterolateral approaches for thoracic disc herniations include (1) laminotomy-facetotomy, (2) transpedicular; and (3) limited costotransversotomy (Fig. 33A).[1–21]

Caution: *Clinically significant thoracic disc herniation is a rare entity (comprising only 0.15% to 0.8% of all disc procedures). Degenerative thoracic discs have a tendency to protrude in the midline (or paracentrally) more often than laterally, and the displaced discal material is frequently calcified and adherent to the dura. As a consequence, symptomatic thoracic discs most often place the spinal cord at risk through a combination of acute and chronic compression, dynamic mechanical injury, and intrinsic or radicular vascular insufficiency. As a result, an approach for a specific thoracic disc herniation should be carefully planned so that it is carried out from a direction that accomplishes, for that particular anatomical setting, adequate thecal sac decompression with minimal risk of injury to the spinal cord (Fig. 33B).*

Procedure

1. Under general endotracheal anesthesia, the patient is positioned prone on padded chest rolls, rolled blanket bolsters, or a Wilson spinal frame to provide adequate cushioning for the chest and abdomen while allowing vacant space under these areas (thereby promoting epidural venous drainage and adequate pulmonary exchange). The operating table (or Wilson frame) is slightly flexed, thereby widening the thoracic interlaminar and interpedicular spaces. The knees are placed in 30 degrees of flexion, and support stockings are used to promote venous drainage. Soft foam padding is placed at all pressure points, and special care is taken to avoid pressure on the lateral femoral cutaneous and common peroneal nerves. The head is turned sideways on a foam cushion, with special caution to prevent compression upon the globes. The arms are positioned upward in a relaxed manner with slight shoulder and elbow flexion (care is taken to avoid any traction on the brachial

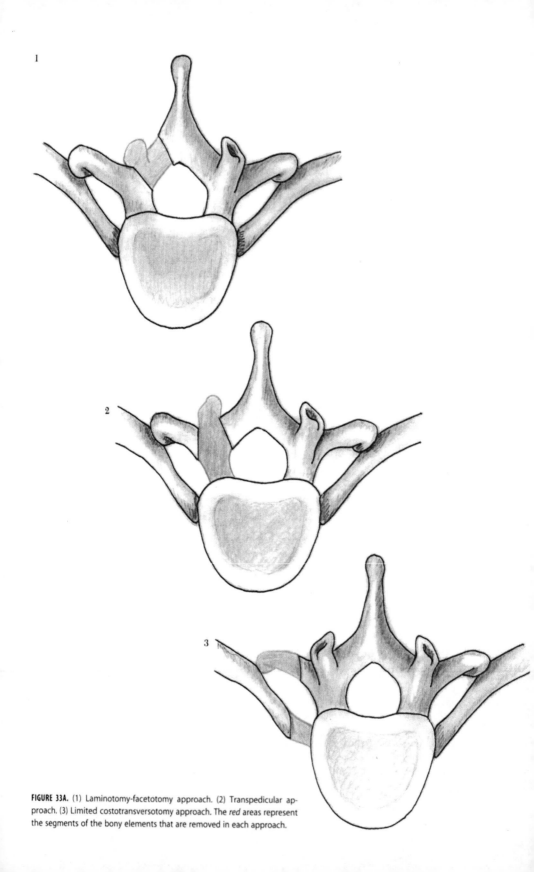

FIGURE 33A. (1) Laminotomy-facetotomy approach. (2) Transpedicular approach. (3) Limited costotransversotomy approach. The *red* areas represent the segments of the bony elements that are removed in each approach.

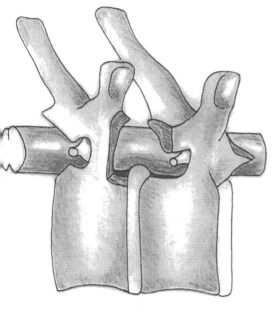

FIGURE 33B. Potential exposure of the spinal canal and disc space afforded by posterior and posterolateral approaches.

plexus). Padding is placed under the elbows to protect the ulnar nerves in the olecranon grooves. The breasts and genitalia are carefully checked for undue pressure points.

Caution: *Appropriate additional support of the patient should be provided so that a small amount of lateral tilt in the operating table away from the surgeon may safely be applied at any point during the procedure. In addition, it is important that the anesthetist be prepared to inflate the lung should the pleura be inadvertently compromised.*

2. The spinous processes, transverse processes, and associated posterior rib tubercles provide helpful superficial landmarks for localization. Using a fingernail (or a marking pen), the surgeon gently indents (or marks) the skin to delineate the intended spinous processes and associated transverse processes and rib tubercles.

Note that heads of the 1st, 11th, and 12th ribs articulate only with their own vertebra whereas the heads of all the other ribs possess two facets and articulate with their own vertebra and the one above (i.e., the 8th rib articulates with both the T7 and T8 vertebrae and crosses the T7–T8 disc space) (Fig. 33C).

An appropriate Betadine skin prep is applied, and 1 g cephalosporin (or when indicated by hypersensitivity, 80 mg gentamicin) is administered intravenously. An 18-gauge spinal needle is inserted off the midline at the suspected appropriate interspinous space, and a lateral radiograph is obtained to confirm the deeper levels of anatomy; this permits the skin incision to be precisely located in relation to the surgical pathology and overlying bony elements. A large percentage of thoracic disc protrusions occur along the lower four thoracic disc spaces (easy to localize); the middle third of the thoracic spine ranks next in frequency; clinically relevant herniations in the upper thoracic spine (where radiographic confirmation of level is often tedious) are fortunately quite rare.

3. A midline or paramedian incision (3–5 cm in length) centered at the level of the appropriate disc space is utilized medial to or along the paravertebral muscle mass. A symptomatic disc is approached from the side of lateralizing signs or symptoms or from the site of greatest protrusion. In the absence of such indications, a left-sided approach (for the right-handed surgeon) is employed.

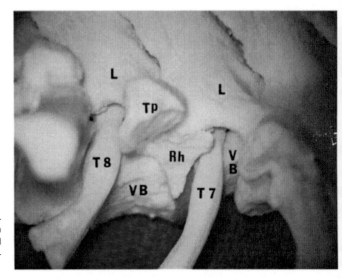

FIGURE 33C. Anatomical relationships. The 8th rib (*RH*) articulates with both the *T7* and *T8* vertebrae (*VB*) and crosses the T7–T8 disc space. (*L,* lamina; *TP,* transverse process.

Once the incision is made, hemostasis is obtained with bipolar coagulation. A small self-retaining retractor is placed, and the subcutaneous tissues are incised with electrocautery.

Laminotomy-Facetotomy Approach

4. A curvilinear incision is made in the thoracolumbar fascia 1 cm off the midline and roughly parallel to the supraspinous ligament. A subperiosteal dissection of the paraspinous musculature and tendinous attachments is carried out using a combination of curved periosteal elevators and small Cobb elevators. An open gauze sponge is gently pushed along the spinous processes and laminae to assist in this dissection. The dissection is carried as far lateral as the facet joint. Use caution to avoid penetration of the interspinous or interlaminar ligaments or injury to the facet (especially its synovial

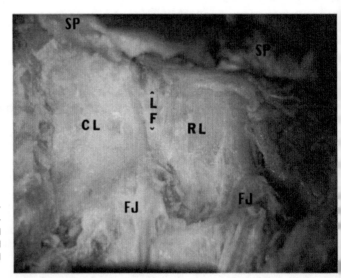

FIGURE 33D. Initial exposure of the interlaminar interval shows the ligamentum flavum (*LF*), rostral (*RL*) and caudal-bordering lamina (*CL*), medial spinous processes (*SP*), and lateral facet joint complex (*FJ*).

membrane) by too vigorous and forceful dissection with periosteal elevators. A self-retaining McCulloch microdiscectomy retractor is inserted.

Caution: The medial prong of the retractor should be positioned carefully between the interspinous ligaments to promote adequate visualization of the interlaminar space.

Caution: Soft tissue remnants overlying the base of the spinous processes, the ligamentum flavum, and laminae are removed when necessary (Fig. 33D).

5. The initial exposure of the spinal canal is guided by posterior spinal element landmarks, especially the laminae and their relationship to underlying structures (notably the disc space and associated nerve root of interest). The rostral bordering lamina at each level of the thoracic spine overlies the disc space for that respective motion segment. As a result, it is the rostrally bordering lamina at each interlaminar interval that requires removal for exposure of that respective disc space. Adequate exposure of the T7–T8 disc space requires partial or complete removal of the T7 hemilamina. The laminotomy is accomplished (under magnification) with a high-speed bur or rongeur (Fig. 33E).

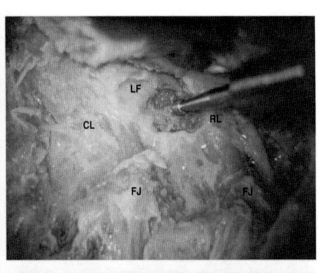

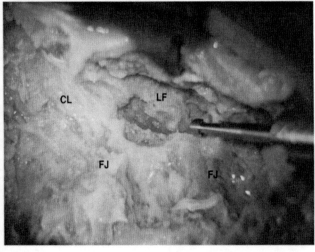

FIGURE 33E. (1) The rostrally bordering lamina (*RL*) is progressively removed with a high-speed bur. (2) Uncovering the underlying ligamentum flavum (*LF*).

Caution: Exercise care in the use of the high-speed bur to avoid the presence of any gauze or cottonoids in the wound that may inadvertently catch on the spinning bur and cause a severe whipping injury to surrounding tissues.

6. The initial removal of the ligament is easiest along its thinner medial aspect. A scalpel can be used to incise the ligament at its apex, and an angled Kerrison rongeur can then be carefully inserted beneath the ligament for removal. On the other hand, enough lamina can be removed such that the rostral margin of the underlying ligamentum flavum is detached, a maneuver that will permit easy access into the epidural space. In this setting, an angled Kerrison rongeur (2 or 3 mm) can be simply utilized to resect the ligament from rostral to caudal (Fig. 33F). Note that the ligamentum flavum consists of both a horizontal and vertical shelf, such that the ligament thickens as it extends from medial to lateral.

7. Adequate decompression of the thoracic spinal canal always involves the removal of the medial portion of the facet joint. The inferior articular facet is usually removed together with the adjoining lamina. The superior articular facet, on the other hand, is usually removed in conjunction with the vertical shelf of the ligamentum flavum (Fig. 33G). Adequate removal of the lateral portion of the ligamentum flavum and the medial aspects of the facet joint (particularly the superior articular facet) should permit full visualization (without overhang) of the medial portion of the appropriate pedicle(s) (Fig. 33H).

Caution: It is particularly important, in the removal of the vertical shelf of the ligamentum flavum and the medial portion of the facet, to proceed with utmost care so as to avoid any compression of the thecal sac contents. Use of the operating microscope (for better lighting, variable magnification, and improved stereoscopic vision) can be quite beneficial in this regard.

8. Following adequate translaminar facet exposure, adequate working space lateral to the thecal sac and between adjoining pedicles (into the foramen) is created to identify laterally placed discal pathology without the need for thecal sac retraction. The

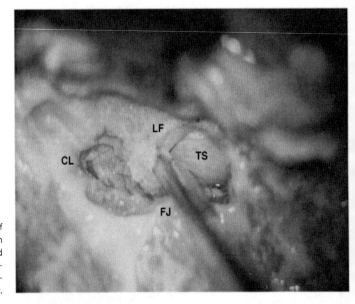

FIGURE 33F. Once the rostral end of the segmental ligamentum flavum (*LF*) has been unroofed, an angled Kerrison rongeur can be used to progressively resect the ligament in a rostral to caudal direction. *TS*, thecal sac.

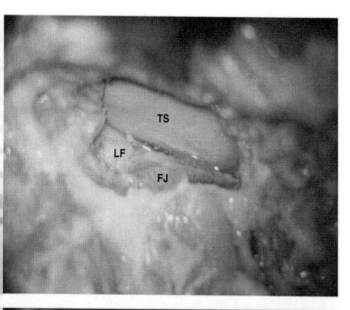

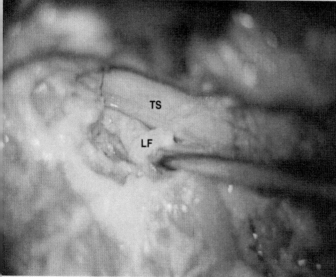

FIGURE 33G. (1) The vertical shelf of the ligamentum flavum (*LF*) is removed in conjunction with the medial portion of the facet joint (*FJ*). (2) This step can be accomplished utilizing either a high-speed bur or an angled Kerrison rongeur.

ateral spinal canal epidural space (subarticular zone) is thoroughly explored to ascertain the position and status of the exiting nerve root (Fig. 33H), the location and relationships of the disc protrusion, and the possibility of associated pathology (such as sequestered fragments, facet or uncinate spurs, or unexpected foraminal masses). Hemostasis in the lateral recess is maintained using bipolar cautery.

Caution: Through this approach, it is very difficult to identify or deal with paracentral or central discal pathology, and no attempt should be made to retract an already compressed thecal sac in these endeavors.

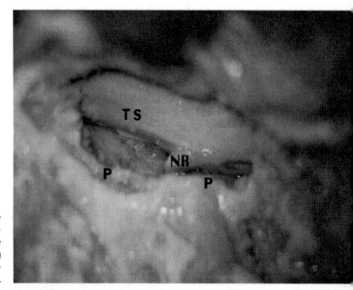

FIGURE 33H. Following adequate translaminar facet resection, adequate working space lateral to the thecal sac (*TS*) and between adjoining pedicles (*P*) is created. Note the exposure of the exiting nerve root (*NR*).

9. The portion of the disc space lateral to the thecal sac is identified and entered (Fig. 33I).

Caution: Operative results following laminotomy-facetotomy approaches for the removal of central and paracentral thoracic disc herniations have traditionally been dismal, likely a result of the degree of spinal cord retraction that is required to resect discal pathology that lies anterior to the thecal sac.

10. The wound is closed in layers (deep fascia, superficial fascia, and subcutaneous tissue with absorbable sutures; skin with staples).

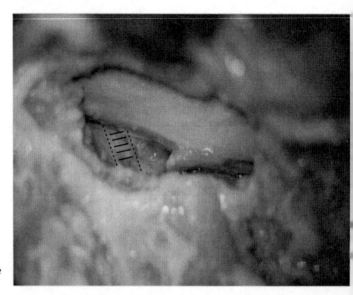

FIGURE 33I. The lateral portion of the disc space is well visualized.

Transpedicular Approach

Repeat steps 1–3 to prep the patient.

4. The paraspinous muscles are dissected subperiosteally from the spinous processes, laminae, and facet joints to the tips of the transverse processes (beyond the lateral border of the facet capsules) (Fig. 33J).

5. Using the high-speed bur, the facet joint posterior to the appropriate disc space is progressively removed. The inferior articular facet is removed flush to the caudal margin of the pedicle above (Fig. 33K1). The superior articular facet and its pedicle are removed flush to the cephalad portion of the inferior bordering vertebral body; this generally requires removing approximately the cephalad one-third of this pedicle (Fig. 33K2).

Caution: *When performed unilaterally, this pedicular facetotomy will not result in destabilization of the involved motion segment.*

6. Following removal of the inferior articular facet, the foramen is completely unroofed and the appropriate nerve root can be readily identified as it exits just beneath its respective pedicle (Fig. 33K). The nerve root should be followed medially and laterally to ensure free passage from the subarticular zone of the spinal canal into the foramen and then out into the extraforaminal zone in relation to the rib head. Blunt nerve hooks of various lengths and angles are helpful in these maneuvers.

7. Following the pediculotomy, adequate lateral exposure to the disc space is created (a 1.5- to 2.5-cm working space), and a clear view of offending disc fragments as well as the paracentral aspects of the thecal sac is thereby obtained (Fig. 33K).

8. The soft central portion of the intervertebral disc is entered, and degenerative disc material is first removed from the core portions of the disc (Fig. 33L). After an adequate cavity has been created in the center portion of the disc, posterior disc material is then progressively removed, beginning at the more lateral aspects and proceeding toward the midline (Fig. 33M). A downward-acting curette is helpful in this maneuver to push firmer disc material from the more posterior aspects into the empty central cavity.

9. The most posteriorly displaced portions of disc and associated posterior longitudinal ligament (especially when calcified or adherent to the dura) are delivered last into the cavity created by the removal of more anterior and central discal components.

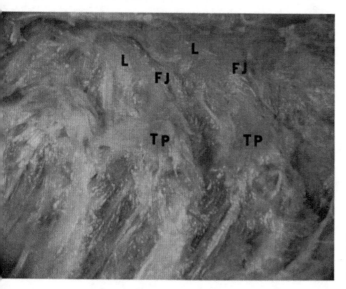

FIGURE 33J. Exposure of the laminae (*L*), facet joints (*FJ*), and transverse processes (*TP*) in preparation for the transpedicular approach.

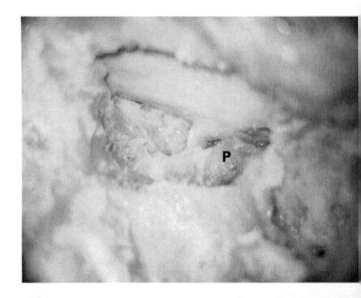

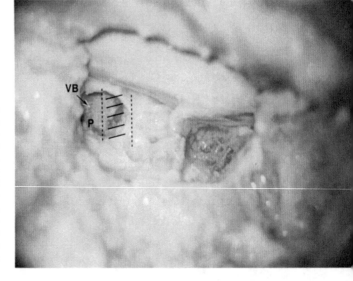

FIGURE 33K. (1) A facet joint posterior to the appropriate disc space has been progressively removed using the high-speed bur. The pedicle (*P*) for that motion segment is well visualized. (2) The superior articular facet and its pedicle (*P*) have been removed flush to the cephalad border of the inferior bordering vertebral body (*VB*) to fully expose the disc space. The foramen has also been completely unroofed, and the exiting nerve root is readily identified passing just beneath its respective pedicle.

Caution: *The limitations of this approach relate to the difficulty in visualizing, without thecal sac retraction, severely protruding midline calcified discs or osteophytes.*

10. The wound is closed in layers.

Limited Costotransversotomy Approach

Repeat steps 1–3 to prep the patient.

4. The paraspinous muscles are incised and reflected to expose the tubercle and neck of the appropriate rib, the entire adjoining transverse process, and the lateral margins of the facet joint capsule (lateral pars interarticularis) (Fig. 33N).

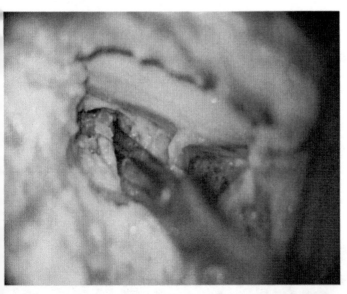

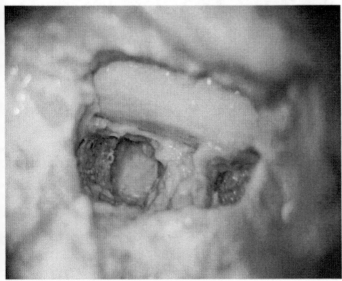

FIGURE 33L. (1) The center part of the disc is entered. (2) Soft disc remnants are removed.

5. The transverse process, associated intertransverse muscles, and costotransverse joint are progressively removed using a high-speed bur or rongeurs until flush with the lateral pars (Fig. 33O).

6. Following division of the costotransverse and capsule ligaments, the rib head is progressively removed using the high-speed bur in a lateral to medial direction until its attachment at the adjoining vertebral bodies and appropriate disc space is identified (Fig. 33P).

Caution: Particular care is taken in this maneuver to preserve the intercostal nerve, segmental artery, and underlying pleura. An operating microscope may be quite helpful.

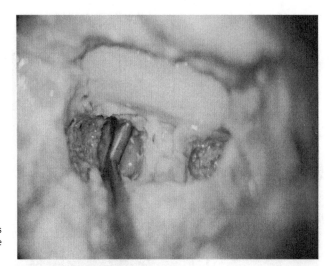

FIGURE 33M. Posterior disc material is progressively displaced into the empty central cavity.

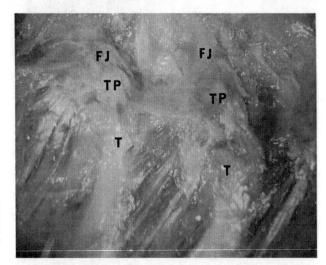

FIGURE 33N. Exposure of the tubercle (*T*) and neck of the rib adjoining the transverse process (*TP*) and lateral margin of the facet joint capsule (*FJ*) for the limited costotransversotomy approach.

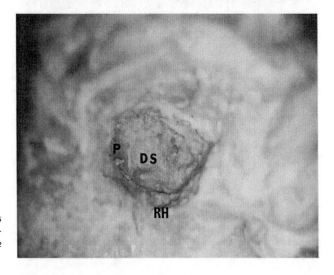

FIGURE 33O. The transverse process has been removed using the high-speed bur down to the disc space (*DS*). *RH*, rib head; *P*, pedicle.

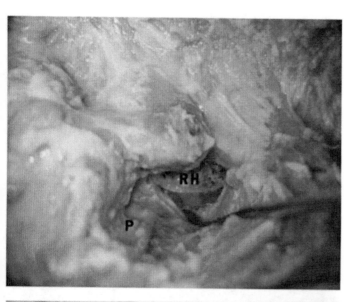

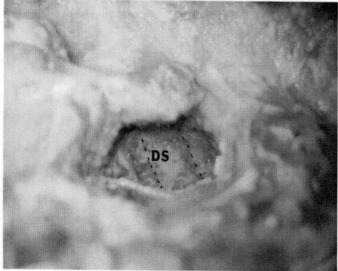

FIGURE 33P. (1) Progressive removal of the rib head (*RH*) pleura (*P*). (2) Down to the disc space (*DS*).

7. The intercostal nerve is traced medially and the intervertebral foramen is clearly defined (Fig. 33Q). Care is taken to preserve and protect the segmental artery. The intercostal nerve exits the intervertebral foramen through its rostral half; the intervertebral disc lies adjacent to the caudal portion of the foramen. The intercostal artery travels along the vertebral body and comes to lie above the nerve in the intercostal groove.

8. The caudal portion of the pedicle directly above the disc space of interest and the cephalad portion of the pedicle directly below are identified by defining the margins of the foramen with a blunt nerve hook. A small portion of each pedicle can then be removed utilizing a high-speed bur to widen the working space. Just enough of the adjoining pedicles are resected so that the lateral aspects of the spinal canal above and below the disc space of interest are adequately exposed.

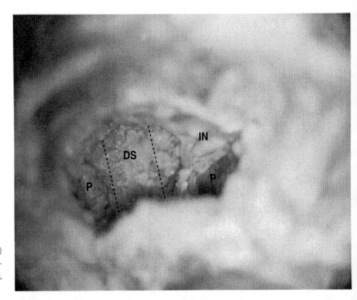

FIGURE 33Q. The intercostal nerve (*IN*) is traced medially and the intervertebral foramen defined. *P*, pedicles; *DS*, disc space

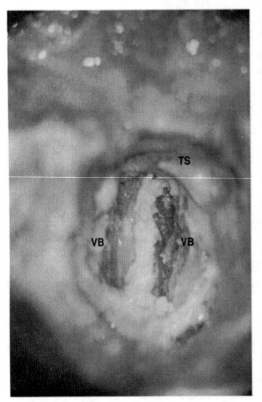

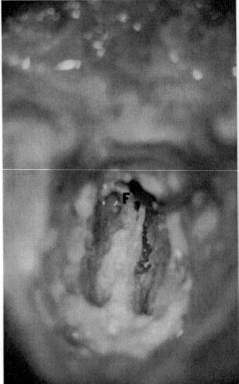

FIGURE 33R. A hollow space has been created beneath a posteriorly protruded fragment to allow its progressive displacement away from the thecal sac (*TS*).

FIGURE 33S. A displaced fragment (*F*) is retrieved back into the empty disc space.

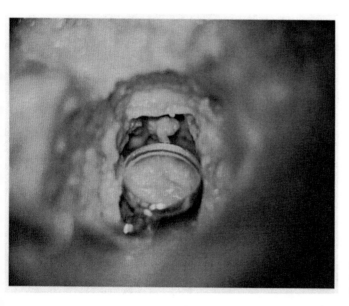

FIGURE 33T. A small mirror is used to verify adequate thecal sac decompression.

9. The disc protrusion is excised approximately 1 cm ventral to the spinal canal utilizing curettes, rongeurs, and, if calcified, a high-speed bur. This discal removal should include degenerative nuclear and annular material as well as the contiguous cartilaginous end plates.

10. Using a high-speed bur, it may be necessary, beneath an elongated and more posteriorly protruded fragment, to remove a few millimeters of the adjoining vertebral bodies to create a hollow space into which the displaced material can be progressively withdrawn away from the dural sac (thereby avoiding even the slightest distortion or manipulation of the thecal contents) (Fig. 33R). At this stage, it is possible in some cases to dissect across the base of a firm protrusion such that it can now be removed nearly intact; in others, it is necessary to retrieve the displaced material in smaller fragments (Fig. 33S). The amount of vertebral bone resected in this maneuver is insufficient to compromise the stability of the spinal column as the lamina and facet joints remain undisturbed.

11. Following removal of the most posterior and central aspects of the protruded disc (responsible for the actual spinal canal compromise), a small mirror or endoscope can be used to inspect the ventral aspects of the canal to confirm the adequacy of the decompression (Fig. 33T). The major advantage of this approach over the transpedicular one is that there is better visualization of the anterior aspects of the thecal sac, especially centrally.

12. The wound is closed in layers.

Remember:

These key concepts are important for successful thoracic disc decompression.

1. Adequate exposure with minimal removal of bony and ligamentous structures to prevent destabilization.
2. Adequate decompression of thecal sac and foraminal contents by complete extirpation of displaced disc material or osteophytes.
3. Negligible spinal cord manipulation or retraction.

4. Minimal manipulation of the intercostal nerve.

5. Preservation of radicular thoracic cord vascular supply.

6. Absolute avoidance of the pleural space and its contents.

References

1. Ahlgren BD, Herkowitz HN: A modified posterolateral approach to the thoracic spine. J Spinal Disord 8(1):69–75, 1995.
2. Alexander GL: Neurological complications of spinal tuberculosis. Proc R Soc Med 39:730, 1946.
3. Capener M: The evolution of lateral rhachotomy. J Bone Joint Surg 36B:173–179, 1954.
4. Carson J, Gumpert J, Jefferson A: Diagnosis and treatment of thoracic intervertebral disc protrusion. J Neurol Neurosurg Psychiatry 34:68–71, 1971.
5. Dietze DD, Fessler RG: Thoracic disc herniations. Neurosurg Clin N Am 4(1):75–90, 1993.
6. Dott NM: Skeletal traction and anterior decompression of the management of Potts paraplegia. Edinb Med J 54:620, 1947.
7. Hulme A: The surgical approach to thoracic intervertebral disc protrusions. J Neur Neurosurg Psychiatry 23:133–137, 1960.
8. Jefferson A: The treatment of thoracic intervertebral disc protrusion. Clin Neurol Neurosurg 78:1–9, 1975.
9. Larson SJ, Holst RA, Hemmy DC, Sances A: Lateral extra-cavitary approach to traumatic lesions of the thoracic and lumbar spine. J Neurosurg 45:628, 1976.
10. Logue V: Thoracic intervertebral disc prolapse with spinal cord compression. J Neurol Neurosurg Psychiatry 15:227, 1952.
11. LeRoux PR, Haglund MM, Harris AB: Thoracic disc disease: experience with the transpedicular approach in 20 consecutive patients. Neurosurgery 33(1):58–66, 1993.
12. Maiman DJ, Larson SJ, Luck E, Lel-Ghatit A: Lateral extra-cavitary approach to the spine for thoracic disc herniation: report of 23 cases. Neurosurgery 14:178–182, 1984.
13. Menard V: 82 ETUDE Pratique Sur le Mal de Pott. Paris, Maison CE, 1900.
14. Pasztor E, Benoist G: Modified pediculofacetectomy in ventral compression of the thoracic spinal cord. Neuro-Orthopaedics 8:97, 1990.
15. Patterson RH, Arbit E: A surgical approach to the pedicle to protruded thoracic disc. J Neurosurg 48:768–772, 1978.
16. Rogers MA, Crockard HA: Clin Orthop Relat Res 300:70–78, 1994.
17. Sekhar LN, Jennetta TJ: Thoracic disc herniation: operative approaches and results. Neurosurgery 12:303–305, 1983.
18. Simpson JM, Silveri CP, Simeone FA, Balderston RA: Thoracic disc herniations: re-evaluation of the posterior approach using a modified costo-transversectomy. Spine 18(13):1872–1877, 1993.
19. Stillerman CB, Weiss MH: Clin Neurosurg 38:325–352, 1992.
20. Walker AE: A History of Neurological Surgery. London, Bailliere, Tindall and Cox, 1951.
21. Hawk WA: Spinal compression caused by ecchondrosis of the intervertebral fibrocartilage. Brain 59:204, 1936.

Posterior Approach to the Lower Lumbar Spine

1. Bleeding from lumbar spinal surgery is best minimized by proper positioning of the patient to prevent abdominal pressure that increases spinal venous pressure. A variety of frames exist that allow proper positioning with the abdomen hanging free. Position the patient on a conventional operating table prone on the horseshoe-shaped Pheasant cushion with separate shoulder posts. Put the patient's iliac crest line at the angle on the cushion and at the break in the table. Put the table in flexion and level the back by raising the head. Pad the knees with foam rubber and the shins and anterior borders of the feet with pillows. Flex the knees with the padded 60-degree wooden wedge. Always check the pulses and use TED stockings. Adequate decompression of the abdomen and free excursion of the chest is the objective. Use a frame that allows a free abdomen and good chest expansion while still allowing some flexion and extension of the table. The shoulder posts allow full chest expansion. Position the upper arms at no more than 90 degrees to the trunk and pad the ulnar notch to prevent ulnar neuropraxia.

2. For the operative approach itself, make the incision to dermis only. Inject 1:500,000 epinephrine in saline through the dermal incision into subcutaneous tissue. Then make a straight incision to the bone of the spinous process. Use of hemostats or electrocoagulation is a matter of choice, and digital pressure on the wound edge by the assistants is important. Clear the spinous process with the cutting cautery. If the technique of Cobb elevation of the spinous process is used, start the subperiosteal dissection with the small Cobb elevator. The medium-sized Cobb is then used for subperiosteal dissection of tissue off the lamina.

3. Remember that the tip of the spinous process has a bulbous configuration; the elevator must first be directed with the cutting edge dorsally to go under the edge of the bulbous tip (Fig. 34A). Cut to bone, then with the cutting edge turned ventrally sweep out across the lamina (Fig. 34B). The potentially troublesome artery at the tip of the spinous process should be controlled in the dissection; it usually enters the cephalad third of the spinous process, and this can be avoided with a deep midline cut and careful subperiosteal dissection.

4. Pack with 4 × 8 gauze after adequately sweeping the tissue off each lamina to the facet joints with the medium-sized Cobb (Fig. 34C). Remove the packing, irrigate, and retract on the lamina with two medium Cobb elevators. Cut the intervening soft tissue from the interspinous tissue with the cautery (Figs. 34D, 34E); the broadest Cobb elevator then sweeps the material in the inner laminar area laterally to the facet joints (Fig. 34E).

5. Insert a small, self-retaining retractor or, for maximum retraction, use the Taylor retractor of appropriate depth placed outside the facet joint by the finger tip. Then use roller gauze fashioned into a sling around the surgeon's foot and tied over the handle of the Taylor retractor; this allows stay retraction of the area between the facet joints. Irrigate and visualize the interlaminar areas at each level. Various self-retaining claw retractors can be used.

6. Expose and identify the sacrum as early as possible. Test motion at each spinous process with a Lewin clamp. Tap on each lamina to find the dull sound of the sacrum and look at the preoperative anteroposterior (AP) X-ray for aid in cases of sacralization of L5. Make a definite identification and obtain an X-ray.

7. Three-dimensional thinking is most important in realizing the location of anterior structures when looking at the posterior spine. For example, when determining the location of the pedicle and the intervertebral disc in relation to the interlaminar area, remember that the L5–S1 intervertebral disc is at the level of the interlaminar space and the pedicle is caudad to the disc and under the S1 lamina. As one progresses in a cephalad direction, the disc space proportionately is in a more cephalad position than the interlaminar space. Therefore, exposure of the L2–L3 disc space requires significant removal of the second lumbar lamina, as this disc is in a more cephalad position compared with the interlaminar space. The facet joint is the important landmark for identification of spinal structures at the initial level of the spinal dissection. After identification of the facet joint, remember that the superior articular process is anterolateral to the inferior articular process. The joint capsule itself is a glistening structure with horizontal striations. By identifying the facet joints, the location of the transverse process is known. The transverse process projects laterally and slightly caudally from the *base* of the superior articular process. The pedicle is immediately anterior to the

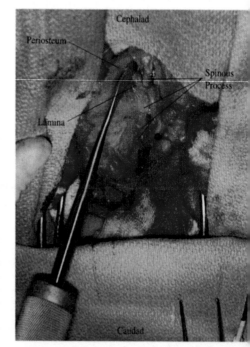

FIGURE 34A. For exposure of the lumbar spine with Cobb elevators, begin on the tip of the spinous process with the smallest Cobb to cut to bone and remove the dense attachments to the tip of the spinous process. Progressing laterally around the bulbous end of the spinous process, turn the elevator face up to allow dissection under the bulbous tip to the bone of the lamina in a subperiosteal plane. By cutting directly to bone in the midline, bleeding from the artery to the caudal tip of the process can be avoided. Electrocautery may be used to cut to the subperiosteal plane under the bulbous tip.

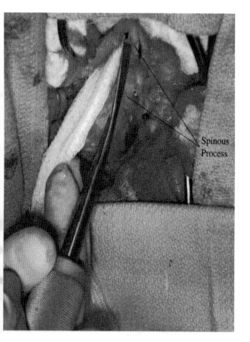

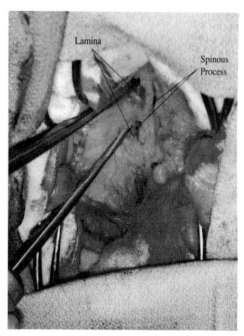

FIGURE 34B. Sweep out on the lamina subperiosteally, removing the soft tissue.

FIGURE 34D. Remove the sponges and insert two elevators, retracting the soft tissue laterally.

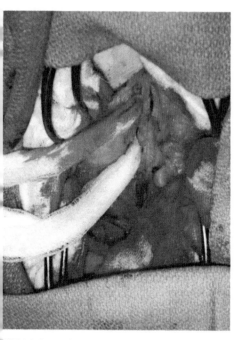

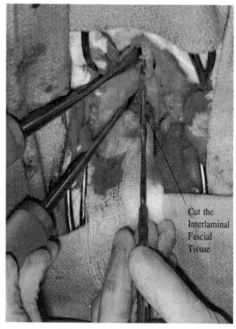

FIGURE 34C. Repeat the process at each level and pack with 4 × 8 sponges.

FIGURE 34E. Cut the remaining soft tissue in the interlaminar area with the electrocautery or #15 blade. Then sweep with the broadest Cobb in the interlaminar area out laterally to the level of the facet joints. Repack each level with a 4 × 8 sponge.

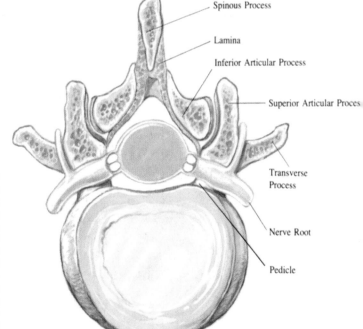

FIGURE 34F. A transverse plane section of the lumbar neuromotor segment emphasizing the orientation of the transverse process, superior articular process, and pedicle as a three-prong structure. The facet joint is seen as the roof of the lateral recess. The nerve exits below the pedicle at each level. The nerve branches into a dorsal primary ramus that innervates from one to three facet joints at adjoining spinal levels. The ventral primary ramus is responsible for limb function and sensation.

base of the superior articular process. The transverse process forms the third branch of this triplaned three-pronged structure made up of the superior articular process in the parasagittal plane, the pedicle projecting anteriorly in the transverse plane, and the transverse process projecting laterally in the coronal plane (Figs. 34F, 34G, 34H, 34I).

8. The projection of the tube of the pedicle on the dorsal elements is found at a point formed by a line bisecting the transverse process in the coronal plane and a perpendicular line just lateral to the superior articular process in the parasagittal plane.

FIGURE 34G. The initial identifying structure in the exposure of the spine is the spinous process. The laminae are next anteriorly after following the lamina laterally; the second important identifying structure is the facet joint. Three-dimensional thinking is vital to accurate spinal surgery and requires the ability to orient the intercanal structures from visualization of the posterior elements. With the facet joint identified, locate the transverse process immediately caudad and lateral to the facet. The transverse process can be exposed without dangerous plunging in the intertransverse area.

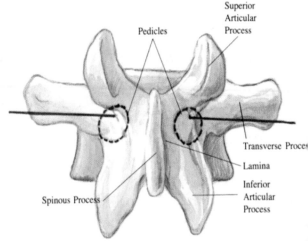

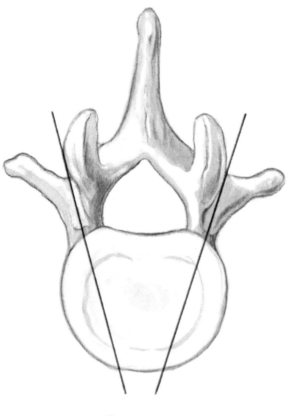

FIGURE 34H. The key to intracanal anatomy is the pedicle. With identification of the facet and the transverse process, locate the pedicle. Usually the center of the pedicle is at a point formed by the intersection of three lines, one line bisecting the midtransverse plane of the transverse process, and another parasagittal line at the lateral margin of the superior articular process. The last line in the transverse of the pedicle is approximately 20 degrees from the vertical. This last angle becomes slightly more obtuse lower in the lumbar spine. Therefore, an instrument may be passed through the posterior elements, down the tube of the pedicle into the vertebral body, by locating the projection of the pedicle on the posterior elements.

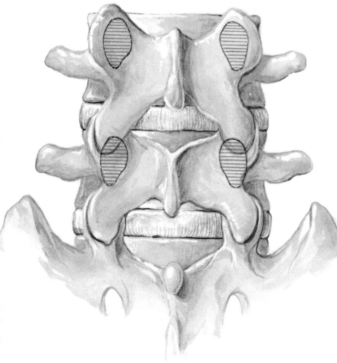

FIGURE 34I. The key to intracanal anatomy is to locate the pedicle. Identify the pedicle, and the location of the disc and nerve root can be reasonably accurately predicted. Immediately cephalad within 1 cm of the pedicle is the intervertebral disc. Immediately caudad to the pedicle is the exiting nerve root. Do not do extensive probing in the medial pedicular area, as the pedicular plexus will bleed. Location of the disc relative after the posterior structures is important. Remember, as one progresses cephalad in the lumbar spine, the disc is further cephalad relative to the interlaminar space. Therefore, the L5–S1 disc is approximately at the level of the interlaminar space between L5 and S1. The L2–L3 disc space is well cephalad under the lamina of L2 rather than at the level of interlaminar space between L2 and L3. The ligamentum flavum covers the interlaminar area. Shaded areas indicate the pedicle.

From this point the direction is approximately 20 degrees from the midline angled from lateral to medial. This is the usual orientation of the pedicle (Figs. 34G, 34H). The angle of the pedicle decreases as one proceeds cephalad in the spine, and the tube of the pedicle becomes more elliptical. For procedures in which the pedicle is opened, such as a vertebral body biopsy or the fixation of the vertebral body with a screw, the tube of the pedicle is entered with a slow-moving drill, using the landmarks presented above.

9. For an approach to the transverse process, as for an intertransverse fusion, locate the transverse process just caudal to the base of the superior articular process. Extend the electrocautery cutting of the facet joint capsule down to the base of the transverse process.

10. With a Cobb elevator, dissect the capsule and ligamentous incisions out among the transverse process, using a rotary motion, not a deep pressing scraping motion. It is very important to remember that vascular structures are just beneath the tip of the transverse process. Fracture of the transverse process or an inadvertent slip off the tip of a transverse process can produce significant bleeding and penetration into the retroperitoneal space. In many patients the transverse process is thin and easily broken. For any exposure for fusion of the intertransverse area, remember that the shallow gutter beneath the facet and at the base of the transverse process is an important area that should be cleaned of soft tissue for placement of bone graft. After elevating soft tissue

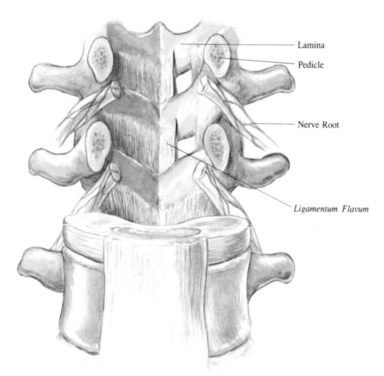

Lamina

Pedicle

Nerve Root

Ligamentum Flavum

FIGURE 34J. The ligamentum flavum inserts approximately midway under the cephalad lamina and inserts on the cephalad edge of the caudad lamina. This underview of the posterior elements from the intervertebral canal demonstrates the ligamentum flavum and its insertion on the lamina. The ligamentum flavum is the principal stabilizing ligament of the posterior elements. Prediction of spinal stability often depends on integrity of the posterior soft tissue column, specifically the ligamentum flavum. With a vertical laminar fracture, the principal function of the ligamentum flavum is maintained. By contrast, with a displaced horizontal laminar fracture of the slice variety, integrity of the ligamentum flavum is disrupted. The ligamentum flavum is thinner in the midline. It can be opened in the midline by passing a Penfield dissector under this midline portion and cutting onto the dissector. The two halves of the ligament can be opened by retracting each laterally. This midline cleft is useful in passing the laminar wires for segmental fixation.

off transverse processes, a plane between each transverse process is developed by sweeping the intertransverse material laterally to the transverse process tips.

Caution: Elevate this intertransverse material superficial to the coronal plane of the transverse processes. Do not plunge anterior to the transverse processes. Bleeding may be encountered and the retroperitoneal space may be entered. Again, once the facet joint is located, the transverse process can be located.

11. The third area of interest is the anatomy of the ligamentum flavum. The ligamentum flavum has a superficial and a deep portion. Cut the lateral edge of the superficial ligamentum flavum medial to the facet joint with a knife. Remove the superficial portion in the interlaminar space from lateral to medial with a curette. The ligamentum flavum covers the inner laminar area at each level, attached to the rim of the lower lamina and extending cephalad through approximately 50% of the undersurface of the superior lamina (Fig. 34J). Use the Kerrison to make a laminotomy in the superior lamina. The dura is protected by the ligamentum flavum for about half of the upper lamina.

12. Cut an arc-shaped incision medially in the ligamentum flavum with a knife down to the innermost layers until the blue can be seen through the fibers. Open the last fibers with the knife handle. Insert a cottonoid under the lateral leaf of ligamentum flavum and remove it with a large Kerrison.

The ligamentum flavum is thinner in the midline. After a total laminectomy, the intact exposed ligamentum flavum is opened in the midline by passing a Penfield dissector under the ligamentum flavum caudad to cephalad and cutting with a knife longitudinally in the midline. Then insert the cottonoid laterally and resect the ligamentum flavum medial to lateral on both sides. The full extent of the ligamentum flavum must be understood to make a full exposure. The ligamentum flavum extends onto the medial aspect of the facet joint itself and to the pedicle in the lateral recess of the spinal canal (Fig. 34K).

13. The ligamentum flavum forms a major portion of the soft tissue of the lateral recess (Figs. 34L, 34M, 34N, 34O). This recess is the groove traversed by the nerve root as it exits around the pedicle to the intervertebral foramen. After resection of the

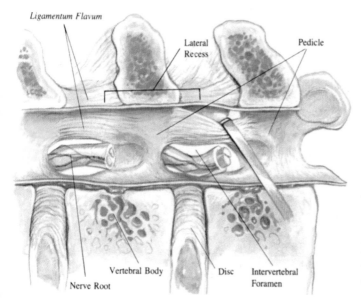

Ligamentum Flavum

Lateral
Recess

Pedicle

Vertebral Body

Nerve Root

Disc

Intervertebral
Foramen

FIGURE 34K. The parasagittal view of the spinal canal, demonstrating the anterolateral insertions of the ligamentum flavum. The ligamentum flavum inserts into the medial facet joint capsule and the pedicle at the interlaminar area. This horizontal shelf of ligamentum flavum comprises a major soft tissue component of the lateral recess, and is resected with the angled Kerrison rongeur from the opposite side of the table for a full lateral decompression and exposure.

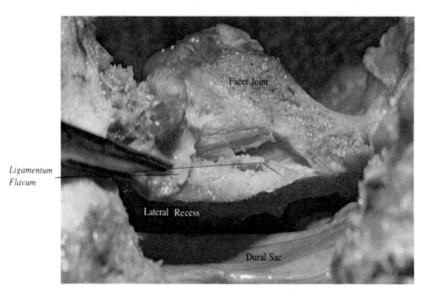

Ligamentum
Flavum

FIGURE 34L. The lateral recess as visualized across the spinal canal shows the important role of the ligamentum flavum as it sweeps down the undersurface of the lamina to insert on the pedicle and facet joint. It is a significant soft tissue component of the lateral recess.

more medial horizontal aspect of the ligamentum flavum, the lateral vertical portion of the ligamentum flavum in the lateral recess can be excised with a 40-degree angled Kerrison. The dura and root must be well retracted medially and protected.

14. In an entirely different way of retracting the ligamentum flavum, the ligamentum flavum can be cut from the bone laterally, reflected medially, sutured to the

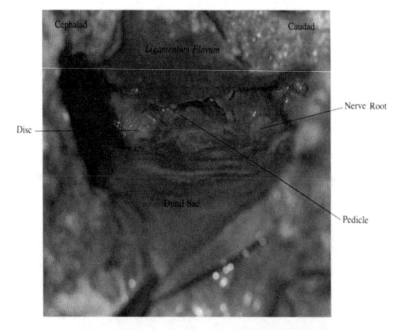

FIGURE 34M. The pedicle, disc space, and nerve root under the horizontal shelf of the ligamentum flavum in the lateral recess.

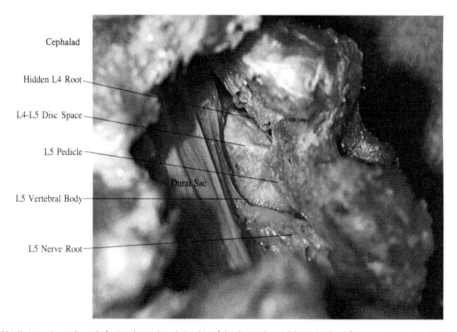

Cephalad

Hidden L4 Root

L4-L5 Disc Space

L5 Pedicle

Dural Sac

L5 Vertebral Body

L5 Nerve Root

FIGURE 34N. A specimen cleaned of veins shows the relationship of the disc to the pedicle as visualized from a partial hemilaminectomy. The nerve root exits around the pedicle and the disc space is immediately cephalad to the pedicle.

interspinous ligament during the case, and laid back over the dura afterward, preserving its dural covering capability although obviously compromising its mechanical function. Start on the leading edge of the lower lamina. Cut the ligamentum flavum off the bone with a curette. Progress around lateral cephalad until dura is identified and insert

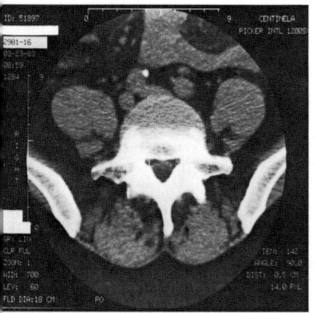

FIGURE 340. The lateral recess as visualized by computer-assisted tomography (CAT) scan. The lateral recess height is measured from the undersurface of the superior facet to the floor of the canal at the superior edge of the pedicle.

a cottonoid. The cephalad attachment is cut off the bone with a long 90-degree angled curette between the cephalad lamina and the ligamentum.

15. The key to the anatomy and the key point of reference inside the spinal canal is the pedicle (Fig. 34N). Locate the pedicle with a probe. The nerve root exits caudally around the pedicle and any retraction in a medial direction from the pedicle will be retracting the nerve root (Figs. 34I, 34J). Less than 1 cm cephalad to the pedicle is the intervertebral disc. Identify the pedicle, then approach the disc. Two cottonoids are introduced simultaneously lateral to the dura at the level of the disc, one packed cephalad, the other packed caudad. Use dural dissectors to clear the disc of fat and veins. Three cottonoid patties are placed: one cephalad, one caudad, and one laterally in the IVF. Insert a nerve root retractor on the surface of the disc to retract the dura in a medial direction.

Caution: The venous drainage in the area of the pedicle is often profuse. Excessive probing of this area will produce unnecessary venous bleeding.

Caution: Beware of a hidden fold of dura over the disc. The retractor should be held parallel to the angle of the nerve root and pressure maintained only for a minimum amount of time.

Remember:

The key to intracanal anatomy is the location of the pedicle. With the pedicle identified the disc is just cephalad, the root is medial, and the intervertebral foramen is caudad.

16. Orientation of facet joints is also critical in understanding the anatomy of the canal. Coronally oriented facet joints are common in the lower lumbar spine. The large medial overhang of a coronal facet can be very deceptive when identifying the floor of the spinal canal (Figs. 34P, 34Q). Many degenerate facets in this area have a biplane configuration with both parasagittal and coronal faces in the same articular facet. For

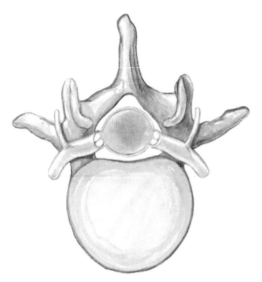

FIGURE 34P. The facet joints often assume a biplanar direction in the significant sagittal and coronal aspect of the facet. The coronal portion of the facet produces a roof to the lateral recess and contributes to compromise of space in that area.

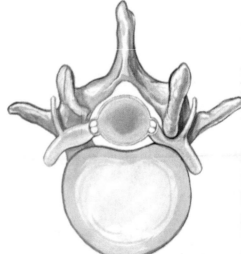

FIGURE 34Q. Malalignment of the facets, facet joint trophism, and unilateral rotational damage to the articular facet not only interfere with the basic biomechanical function of the neuromotor segment, but also, with hypertrophy and degenerative change, may contribute to nerve root canal stenosis.

a full decompression, any medial overhang of facet should be removed to the parasagittal level of the medial wall of the pedicle.

17. An important aspect of approaching the lumbar spine is to have proper depth perception thinking, that is, to be able to identify posterior structures and to locate very necessary anterior structures in relation to these posterior structures. Always reading X-rays through the film posterior to anterior helps train one to see through posterior elements to anterior structures when in surgery. When reading a lumbar spine film for lumbar fractures, we stress this progression of identification of structures from posterior to anterior at each level of the lumbar spine (Fig. 34R). Therefore, begin with the

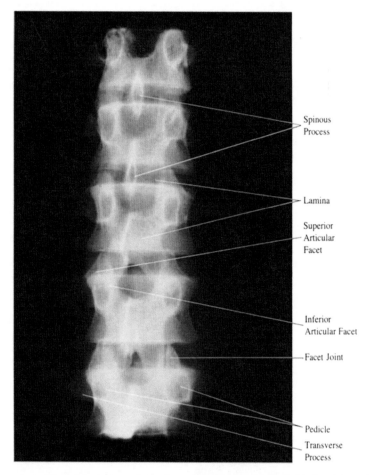

Spinous Process

Lamina

Superior Articular Facet

Inferior Articular Facet

Facet Joint

Pedicle

Transverse Process

FIGURE 34R. For traumatic conditions of the lumbar and thoracic spine, it is critically important to identify each structure on the anteroposterior (AP) X-ray film. The vast majority of posterior element fractures can be clearly identified with plane X-rays beginning with the more posterior structures and progressing anteriorly. This depth perception-type thinking is important in understanding spinal anatomy. We stress the beginning with the spinous process, and comment on the presence of fractures, spread, or rotation of the processes. The lamina is frequently difficult to see, superimposed on the rest of the spine, but laminar pathology should be identified.

Next, progress to the level of the facet joints and the pars interarticularis. Comment should be made about the spread of facet joints, integrity of articular process, and possible fractures through the pars interarticularis. The next level is the transverse process. Is it split vertically, ripped off, or damaged? Next, the pedicles: are they spread in relation to the level above and below or do they exhibit fracture lines? Next consider the posterior body wall. Spread of the pedicles indicates that there is an interruption in the posterior body wall. The lateral X-ray is often used to assess the anterior column, and oblique X-rays aid in identification of the facet and pars interarticularis area.

spinous processes and comment on the presence of fractures, and spread or rotation of the processes. The laminae are frequently difficult to see superimposed on the rest of the spine but laminar pathology should be identified. Differentiating a vertical laminar fracture from a horizontal one is of maximum clinical importance. Then proceed to the level of facet joints and pars interarticularis. Comment about spread of facet joints, about integrity of articular processes and possible fracture through the para interarticularis. The next level is the transverse process. Are these split transversely or vertically? Are they intact? Then consider the pedicles: are they spread in relation to the level above and below or do they exhibit fracture lines? Next observe the posterior body wall. The spread of the pedicles indicates that there is an interruption of the posterior body wall. Is the posterior body wall intact? Use the lateral X-ray for better definition of the anterior column. Is the bony anterior column intact, meaning the vertebral end plates and vertebral body wall? Posterior and anterior longitudinal ligaments are included with the annulus and the disc in the soft tissue anterior column. Anatomy of the lumbar spine should be divided into soft tissue posterior elements, bony posterior elements, soft tissue anterior elements, and bony anterior elements. Ligamentum flavum, interspinous ligament, and interlaminar ligament are included in the posterior column soft tissues.

18. Closure: Use a mattress suture with a large needle and absorbable suture. The lower limb of the mattress suture is to the bottom of the paraspinous musculature through the interspinous area, the upper limb through the fascia only. Follow with subcutaneous and skin closure.

Remember:

1. The first landmark is the facet joints.
2. The second landmark is the ligamentum flavum.
3. The third landmark is the pedicle.

Reference

1. Magerl F: Clinical application of the thoracolumbar junction and the lumbar spine. In Mears D (ed): External Skeletal Fixation. Baltimore, Williams & Wilkins, 1980.

Acknowledgment

Special thanks to the late Dr. Homer Pheasant for assistance with this chapter.

Lumbar Laminotomy, Foraminotomy, Root Decompression, and Discectomy in the Lateral Position

35

Michael L. J. Apuzzo

The major objective in surgery of herniated lumbar discs is decompression of the involved nerve root or roots and cauda equina with restitution of the normal anatomical disposition of elements of the cauda equina within the spinal and root canals. Minimal manipulation of neural elements is imperative, as an anatomical environment that will preclude recurrent root entrapment at the operated region is provided.

The lateral position provides a physiologic placement of the patient with maximum exposure of lateral elements of the main lumbar dural tube and nerve roots. At the same time, it provides a postural substrate that offers maximum exposure of the intralaminar space, ligamentum flavum, and interbody spaces in the region without risk of increased intraabdominal or intrathoracic pressure and secondary distension of the epidural venous complex.

1. Essentials of positioning. Following the induction of adequate general anesthesia, position the patient so that, with respect to the lateral position, his painful extremity is placed superiorly. In initiating positioning, we have found that the surgeon and three assistants are the optimum number to effect this maneuver with ease. The proposed level of operation is placed at the midpoint for flexion of the operating table and the patient's back is moved to the lateral table edge closest to the surgeon. The table is then fully flexed and the inferior lower extremity is flexed at the hip and knee, with the knee supported by a padded kidney rest inserted at the break point. The superior extremity is fully extended and supported medially by two pillows, one at the level of the thigh and the other at the level of the leg. At this time several bands of 3-inch cloth adhesive tape are run from one lateral runner of the operating table to the other to maintain the pelvis in a flexed position. These maneuvers accomplish the following: (1) the lumbar curve is straightened and largely reversed, (2) the ligamentum flavum at the operative level as well as the intralaminar space is distracted, (3) the nerve root sheaths at the superior aspect of the canal are disposed and lengthened to allow for optimum

289

exposure and visualization of the lateral recess of the spinal canal, and (4) the interbody space is distracted posteriorly and superolaterally so that adequate evacuation and visualization within the interspace may be accomplished.

The inferior axilla is supported on an axillary roll. The upper limb is supported either in a cradle or on a pillowed Mayo stand. The patient's thorax is made parallel with the floor by manipulation of the reverse Trendelenburg setting of the operating table. The table is then side-tilted away from the surgeon so that the lumbar region is turned approximately 15 to 20 degrees from the vertical plane.

2. The lumbodorsal region is appropriately prepped and then marked with a soft pen. Initially the posterosuperior iliac spines are identified and marked. The first interspace palpable superior to a line drawn between these spines is the L5–S1 intraspinous space. This is identified and an appropriate mark for level is made. To assist with identification of the appropriate operative level, a perpendicular line is drawn from the iliac crest to the midline, and the relationship of this line to the L4–L5 interspace is judged according to anteroposterior (AP) lumbosacral spine films. Rather than using X-ray identification of the proper level, we have found it efficacious to identify the sacrum and the L5–S1 level in all cases before embarking on decompression of the L4–L5 region. At higher levels X-ray identification has been used in the operating room.

For the purposes of this discussion, a L5–S1 exposure for decompression of the S1 nerve root and excision of the herniated nucleus pulposis at the L5–S1 level are described. An incision is marked 1 cm superior and lateral to the spines of L5 and S1. The length of this mark is variable according to the physique of the given patient. Infiltration is undertaken in the subperiosteal and paraspinous muscular planes at both the L5 and S1 levels with a solution of 0.5% xylocaine with epinephrine. Approximately 5 to 7 mL of this solution is used at each level. The subcutaneous tissues are then infiltrated with a similar solution in the region of the marking for the incision. We use a draping system that incorporates three towels, one at the superior, one at the inferior, and one at the medial surface of the field. A 3M Steridrape is then placed over the three towels and marked area with a cuff fashioned on the lateral field that acts as an anchor for the secondary laporotomy drapes which will follow.

After draping, the surgeon has the option of either sitting or standing during the operative procedure. The scrub nurse positions herself or himself to the right in the case of a right-handed surgeon and the assistant is positioned to the left. A Mayo stand is placed between the surgeon and the nurse with a secondary table at his or her side to augment the essential instrumentation for each portion of the case as it evolves. A French suction apparatus is positioned on the surgeon's left and a blunt-tipped bipolar coagulating forceps is placed on the surgeon's right for easy access (Fig. 35A).

3. Incision and laminar exposure. With incision of the cutaneous and subcutaneous spaces, the lumbodorsal fascia is identified approximately 1 cm parallel to the spines of L5 and S1. Bleeding at the cutaneous margins is controlled with Michel clips, which also prevent the displacement of the Steri-drape from the wound edge. The spines of L5 and S1 are identified by palpation and an incision is made parallel to these spines in the lumbodorsal fascia to expose the paraspinous muscular groups (Fig. 35B). The assistant introduces a hand Meyerding retractor and the surgeon, using a 20-mm Hoen periosteal elevator, develops a subperiosteal plane at the level of the spine of S1 and develops this plane inferiorly along the spine to the level of the lamina. Once the lamina is appreciated, the periosteal instrument is rotated in position and appropriately utilized so that the subperiosteal plane can be developed laterally to the level of the facet joint. The assistant introduces gauze sponges to assist in the dissection of the paraspinous musculature (Fig. 35C). Attention is then turned to the L5 spine where a similar dissection is undertaken, before which Mayo scissors are employed to incise the multifidus rotator that separates the two spines in a muscular band. This dissection being completed, the gauze packings are removed; the hand Meyerding retractor is introduced laterally to the level of the facet joint and palpation is undertaken. The sacrum is iden-

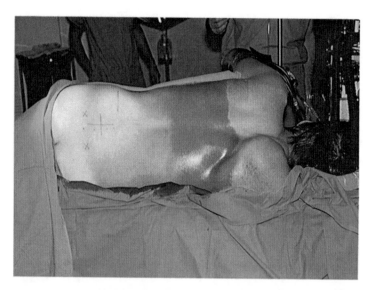

FIGURE 35A. The lateral position for lumbar disc surgery provides a physiologic placement of the patient with maximum exposure of lateral elements of the dural sac and nerve roots. The lateral position offers maximum exposure of the intralaminar space, ligamentum flavum, and interbody spaces in the region. There is no risk of increased intraabdominal or intrathoracic pressure with its secondary distension of epidural veins with the lateral decubitus position. It is a comfortable position for the surgeon either sitting or standing and provides excellent visualization for teaching. The operative level is placed at the midpoint for flexion of the operating table and the patient's back is moved to the lateral edge of the table. The lower leg is flexed and padded. The upper leg is fully extended, supported on two pillows.

The patient is stabilized in this position with rolls of tape. The inferior axilla is supported with an axillary roll. The upper limb is in a cradle. The patient's thoracic spine is made parallel with the floor by manipulation of the reverse Trendelenburg setting on the operating table. The table is then tilted away from the surgeon so that the lumbar region is turned approximately 15–20 degrees from the vertical plane. In summary, the position allows (1) straightening and reversal of the lumbar curve; (2) distraction of the inner laminar space and ligamentum flavum; (3) maximum visualization of the lateral recess of the spinal canal; and (4) distraction of the inner body space posteriorly and superolaterally so that adequate evacuation and visualization within the inner space may be accomplished.

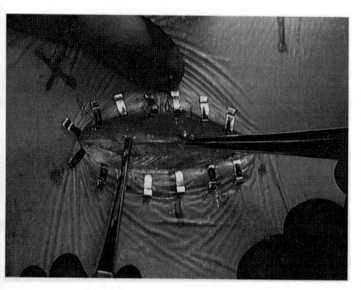

FIGURE 35B. Incise the skin and subcutaneous tissue in the midline. Michel clips are placed on the cutaneous margins of the wound. Incise the lumbar and dorsal fascia parallel to the spinous processes of L5–S1 and expose the lamina and interlaminar areas with periosteal elevators. Expose subperiosteally the lamina at the involved levels. Expose the interlaminar area as much as seen in Figures 34I–34M. The Taylor retractor inserted outside of the facet joint or the self-retaining Hoen retractor provides adequate retraction of the paraspinous musculature.

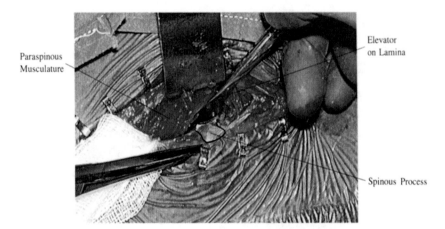

Paraspinous Musculature

Elevator on Lamina

Spinous Process

FIGURE 35C. Exposure of the ligamentum flavum is carried out by first making an incision in the lateral aspect of the inner laminar area in the soft tissue between the facet and pars. Sweep lateral to medial with a curette clearing the superficial ligamentum flavum. The stretched horizontal fibers in this position of the ligamentum flavum are easily identified by their texture and yellow color. The cephalad extent and attachment of the ligamentum flavum is dissected with a curette under the lamina of the cephalad vertebra. The caudad portion of this lamina is removed with a rongeur in fashioning the laminotomy. This removal of bone is continued laterally with the an-gled Kerrison punches until a suitable-sized laminotomy is performed. All bony exposure should be carried out before division of the ligamentum flavum, as much done as necessary for exposure. The standard ligamentum flavum removal is carried out by first making a medial cephalad-to-caudad incision in the ligamentum flavum down through its fibers until the bluish tinge of dura is seen. The last fibers of ligamentum flavum may be entered with the handle of the knife, dura pushed away, and cottonoid introduced laterally, allowing resection of the ligamentum flavum without damage to the dura.

tified as well as the lamina of L5. Retraction of the paraspinous musculature is then maintained with a Hoen self-retaining retractor. To position this instrument optimally, initially the spinous component of the retractor system is placed at the midline; next, the muscle retracting blade is placed over the hand Meyerding retractor and that retractor is removed; finally, the handle of the retractor system is attached to both blades and retraction is effected. Removal of retained muscle may then be undertaken with a pituitary rongeur.

4. Laminotomy, partial facetectomy, and foraminotomy. A 4-mm bone curette is then used under the inferior edge of the lamina of L5 to establish the plane between the leading edge of that lamina and the ligamentum flavum. As has been noted, the lateral position places the ligamentum flavum in a fully stretched position so that it is readily appreciated with a maximum visualization of the interlaminar space. Following development of the natural plane of cleavage between the ventral surface of the L5 lamina and ligamentum flavum, a laminotomy is fashioned utilizing a Leksell rongeur. We then favor employment of 45-degree angled bone punches of 3-, 5-, and 7-mm sizes with reduced depth of footplates to accomplish further superior and lateral extension of the laminotomy opening. If there is encroachment by a hypertrophied or a sizable facet joint, the medial aspect of this joint is appropriately trimmed with either a Leksell rongeur or a combination of bone curettes and angled bone punches.

Optimum exposure of the ligamentum flavum having been gained, this structure is then incised medially parallel to the spine with a #15 blade scalpel. A small cottonoid pledget is then introduced into the epidural space and the ligamentum flavum is excised with the # 15 blade, with appropriate manipulation of the cottonoid in the epidural space to protect underlying dura during the course of this maneuver. Incision is initially made along the margin of the S1 lamina, secondarily along the margin of the L5 lam-

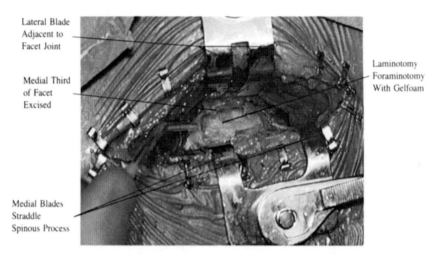

Lateral Blade
Adjacent to
Facet Joint

Medial Third
of Facet
Excised

Laminotomy
Foraminotomy
With Gelfoam

Medial Blades
Straddle
Spinous Process

FIGURE 35D. The ligamentum flavum has been resected and the laminotomy formed. Exposure of the lateral recess and lateral component of the spinal canal with entry into the root canal is imperative and is one of the primary surgical maneuvers in reducing unnecessary retraction on the nerve root during decompression and evacuation of the inner body space. This access is acquired by utilizing the angled bone punches and curettes. Cottonoids protect the dura and nerve root from the angled instruments during this lateral decompression.

ina. The ligamentum flavum is then reflected laterally and excised either with a large bone punch or by transverse incision at the region of the facet joint (Fig. 35D). *The operative procedure from the stage of excision of the ligamentum flavum onward is potentially enhanced by the employment of the operating microscope at either 6× or 10× setting with a 250- or 275-mm lens.*

With excision of the ligamentum flavum, superior and lateral bony removal is undertaken. It is important to stress that, in the course of root decompression and disc excision by this technique, *exposure of the lateral recess and lateral component of the spinal canal with entry into the root canal is imperative and is one of the primary surgical maneuvers in reducing unnecessary retraction on the root during decompression and evacuation of the interbody space.* This bony access is acquired utilizing a combination of angled bone punches initiated superiorly and laterally that are augmented by bone curettes. Important in the overall technique is the introduction of soft cottonoids before the placement of bone-cutting instruments to reduce the possibility of a dural tear or neural injury. In the event that there is considerable dorsal displacement of neural elements, it is inadvisable to introduce foot-plated instruments into the bony recess, and under these circumstances either sharp curettes or a high-speed air drill should be employed to effect appropriate bony exposure (Fig. 35E).

5. Root, fragment identification, and removal. *The ultimate goal of bony exposure before removal of a free fragment or exploration of the interspace is complete visualization of the lateral aspect of the main dural tube, the shoulder, axilla, and a minimum of 2 cm of the appropriate nerve root.* With lateral disc herniation most often there will be dorsal median displacement of the nerve root, and with the attainment of exposure of the lateral recess of the spinal canal the fragment of disc material will readily be appreciated. At this time cottonoids may be placed superior to the shoulder of the nerve root and distal and lateral on the nerve root to displace this structure slightly medially and enhance exposure of the lateral recess region. Dissection of epidural fat and/or adhesions in the region is undertaken with either a blunt-tipped or fine-tipped bipolar coagulating forceps and either a #7 French or a #5 French Frazier suction apparatus. If normal anatomical planes are obscured, it is imperative that magnification of vision be

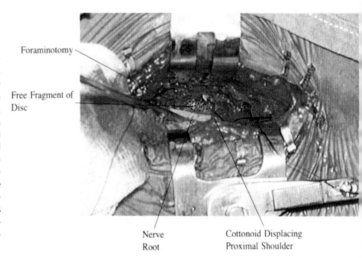

FIGURE 35E. The ultimate goal of bony exposure before removal of free fragments or exploration of the inner space is complete visualization of the lateral aspect of the main dural tube, the shoulder, axilla, and a minimum of 2 cm of appropriate nerve root. All adhesions must be carefully removed with a dural dissector before evacuation of a lateral free fragment. Cottonoids are placed superior to the shoulder of the nerve and distal-lateral to the nerve root to displace this structure slightly medially and enhance exposure of the lateral recessed region.

employed. For ultimate visualization we consider the operating microscope to be far superior to the customary headlight and loupes because of the intensity of illumination provided with the microscopic light source as opposed to the standard headlight systems as well as the versatility of magnification offered. For minimization of trauma to the root it is imperative to effect separation of adhesions particularly from the ventral surface of the root before extraction of a fragment from this interface. In particular, for lateral disc protrusions a retractor is seldom necessary to mobilize the nerve root for visualization of the disc fragment and maintenance of proper exposure for interspace exploration (Fig. 35F). Therefore, with proper placement of cottonoids the fragment is further exposed and its dorsal component freed of any epidural venous complex with bipolar coagulating forceps. A cruciate incision is then made over the fibrotic tissues and a small pituitary rongeur or Rhoton forceps is utilized to gently tease the fragment from the spinal canal. With excision of the fragment there is considerable relaxation of

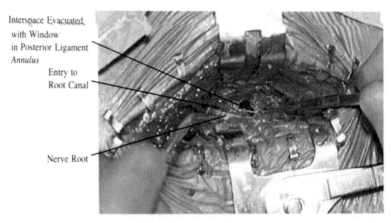

FIGURE 35F. A cruciate incision is made over the disc space and bulging disc material and a small pituitary rongeur is utilized to remove the fragment from the canal. The annulus is incised with a #11 blade and the contents removed with a pituitary rongeur. Remove the disc material that is soft and degenerated and lacks resistance to excision. Beware of penetrating the anterior annulus into the retroperitoneal space.

neural elements in the area. In the event that a fragment is not appreciated and adequate lateral bony excision and visualization have been gained, it is advisable to use angled instruments, such as an eye muscle hook or a Frazier dural guide, to explore both dorsally and ventrally along the nerve root as well as ventrally in the spinal canal in the region of the root axilla and shoulder. The fragment and/or herniation will readily be identified at this time.

Another maneuver of some value is the introduction of normal saline into the interbody space; this may be accomplished by employing a #20 spinal needle and a Luerlock syringe. A normal interspace will accept little more than 0.5 mL saline, whereas a degenerated interspace will readily accept saline solution without difficulty. With introduction of the saline it is possible to identify a region of tear in the annulus by the egress of fluid and aid in the identification of a disc fragment.

6. Disc excision. With removal of the fragment and/or identification of the interspace a window is fashioned through the posterior longitudinal ligament and annulus fibrosis with a #11 blade, with care being taken to ensure that the inferior and superior edges of the window are on the inferior and superior margins of the bodies involved and that in the course of a lateral extention of the window opening no injury is incurred by the superior nerve root in the area, which is passing laterally in the region of the pedicle. With proper execution of this maneuver one may then set the stage for complete visualization into the interspace. At this time a small pituitary rongeur is introduced into the interspace and evacuation of disc material commences. It has been our practice to remove only that disc material which is softened, degenerated, and lacks resistance to excision. We consider that the Scoville cartilage curettes are essential for proper evacuation of the interspace and, therefore, we use combinations of straight, 45-degree, and 90-degree angled curettes in effecting our exploration and excision of degenerated disc material. Following the development of a dead space in the central portion of the interspace the curettes are introduced to free degenerated material into the central portion of the dead space and then under direct vision this debris is removed. It is apparent that as more excision is undertaken it is necessary to use the 45-degree and 90-degree angled curettes to bring the disc material into the central portion of the interspace for removal by the pituitary rongeur. It is obvious that care must be taken in evacuation of the interspace to avoid transgressing the anterior annulus and entering the retroperitoneal space. Provided that the dorsal openings in the annulus and posterior longitudinal ligament are adequate, the evacuation can be accomplished under direct vision, thereby reducing the possibility of such an event (Fig. 35G). Following removal of the degenerated disc material the interspace may be inspected both by direct vision and by palpation with blunt instruments. We have used angled endoscopy

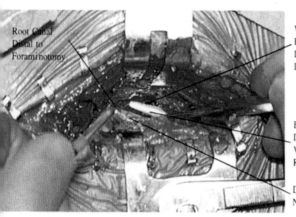

Root Canal Distal to Foraminotomy

Window in Posterior Longitudinal Ligament

Blade of Dural Guide in Ventral Root Canal

Decompressed Nerve Root

FIGURE 35G. Foraminotomy is completed using angled bone punches and/or curettes. At completion a minimum of 2–2.5 cm of nerve root is completely visualized. Exploration is undertaken with the eye muscle hooks dorsally and ventrally and down the root canal followed by Frazer's dural guide dorsally and ventrally down the root canal to ensure there is no further fracture of disc material or bone encroachment or compromise in the area. The exploration is completed ventrally in the spinal canal as well.

instruments to inspect the margins of removal of disc material from within the interspace. The interspace is then irrigated copiously with Bacitracin solution (50,000 units in 500 mL normal saline).

7. Foraminotomy completion, final exploration. Attention is once again turned to the root area, the displacing cottonoids are removed, and the foraminotomy is completed using angled bone punches and/or curettes. At completion of the procedure a minimum of 2 to 2.5 cm of nerve root is completely visualized. Finally, exploration is undertaken with eye muscle hooks dorsally and ventrally down the root canal, followed by a Frazier dural guide dorsally and ventrally down the root canal to assure that there is no further fragment of disc material or bony encroachment or compromise in the area. Exploration is then undertaken ventrally in the spinal canal in the superior and inferior plane, initially with eye muscle hooks and secondarily with the Frazier dural guide once again to ensure freedom from encroachment of any retained disc material. Copious irrigation is then undertaken with Bacitracin, and a pledget of Bacitracin-soaked gelfoam is placed in the foraminotomy laminotomy opening.

8. Closure is then accomplished in layers with meticulous hemostasis to ensure a minimal presence of blood in the muscular layer, which is a source of irritation and postoperative spasm. Care is taken to ensure a secure closure, particularly at the level of the lumbodorsal fascia.

Remember:

1. Obtain adequate bony exposure. This is required particularly in the lateral spinal recess and region of the facet joint. Care should be taken whenever possible to preserve the normal anatomical substrate.
2. Minimize handling and manipulation of the involved nerve root or nerve roots. Obtain adequate lateral exposure in the spinal canal at the lateral recess region with reduction of retraction of the involved nerve roots and gentle displacement of the same by appropriate placement of cottonoids.
3. Reduce the biomechanical impact of the surgery. Remove only what is estimated to be degenerated components of interspace material.
4. Dissection with the operating microscope is at times imperative to assure proper handling of neural elements and optimum appreciation of dissection planes.
5. Perform an adequate foraminotomy for decompression of the root with exploration of all ventral surfaces in the region with angled instruments.
6. Encourage early mobilization during the postoperative period. This action is important to reduce spasm and functional limitation as well as to build the patient's confidence in relation to his own capabilities to activity.

Microscopic Lumbar Discectomy

Microscopic lumbar discectomy is an ideal way to remove a disc fragment. Indications include the following:

1. Morbidity of sufficient severity and duration to warrant operative intervention.
2. Presence of radicular leg pain, intensity of leg pain greater than 50% over back pain, with the pain distribution preferably over the course of a radicular nerve.
3. Neurologic deficit and motor sensory reflex loss, enabling the surgeon to establish which nerve is involved.
4. Studies should indicate an anatomical lesion that corresponds to the patient's symptoms. That anatomical lesion should be in a location that corresponds to the symptoms and is usually a herniated disc, extruded disc fragment, sequestered disc fragment, or a segmental localized lateral recess stenosis.

Our decompressive technique uses microscopic operative techniques to achieve three aims:

1. Remove the obstruction from the canal and the disc fragment from the nerve.
2. Visualize the nerve and blood vessels to provide better protection for both.
3. Cause as little injury as possible to normal structures through better visualization, better lighting, and better exposure.

We are confident that removal of a source of persistent radiculopathy, such as an extruded disc fragment, in conjunction with an excellent postoperative rehabilitation program, offers the potential to return the patient to full activity.

With the patient's studies on the X-ray view box in the operating room, after induction of general anesthesia, the patient is placed on the Andrews frame. The skin is prepped, and two or three needles are inserted in a paraspinous position. A lateral X-ray is taken (Fig. 36A). Using the needles and the position of the disc as a guide, the skin incision is placed over the disc space. Usually, this is from the midportion of the disc space, approximately 2 cm caudally. After the X-ray is taken, the needles are removed and lines are drawn on the skin perpendicular to the spine with a marking pen to indicate the location of the pins. Full prepping and draping is carried out. The skin

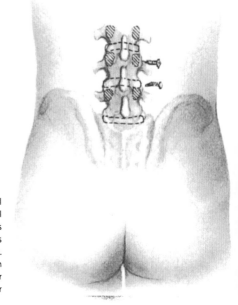

FIGURE 36A. Place two needles lateral to the spine at the approximate level of the disc space. The spinous process is not used as the marker because its relationship to the disc space varies. For an operation on the disc, the skin incision is best placed directly over the disc from the center of the disc for 2 cm caudal.

incision is made using the marking pen lines to put the incision over the disc space. Then a Cobb elevator approximately the width of the skin incision is placed into the wound, and dissection is carried gently through the subcutaneous fat to the fascia at the spinous process. The Cobb stretches the lumbodorsal fascia over the edge of the spinous process, and the fascial incision is made on the lateral edge of the bulbous tip of the spinous process. Holding the fascia with the Cobb with one hand, use the Bovie or knife to incise the fascia. Make a generous fascial incision and place the Cobb elevator into the wound onto the undersurface of the spinous process. With the curve of the blade facing medially, using gentle dissection, sweep out laterally. A lateral-facing Cobb may be inserted to pull laterally. Palpation of the cephalad and caudal lamina allows the gentle sweeping of the muscles off the interlaminar area. Holding the muscle back, place the Williams blade-point retractor. The spike is placed in the interspinous space and the blade length touches the facet capsule. Open the retractor, exposing the interlaminar area. With the retractor in place, place the Kocher in the interlaminar area (Fig. 36B). There is no vigorous exposure of the area. Palpation alone allows determining the cephalad lamina and the caudal lamina. Then, obtain a final X ray that indicates the appropriate interlaminar area. Remember that the interlaminar area is caudal to the disc space that is to be exposed. The Kocher should be caudal to the skin marks used to indicate the disc space and caudal to the disc space on the X-ray. After return of the interlaminar marking X-ray, the microscope is brought in and the Kocher removed under direct vision. The microscope is used from the time the second X-ray is taken. We use a large pituitary to gently remove any soft tissue over the interlaminar area. The superficial ligamentum flavum is exposed.

Incise the superficial ligamentum flavum laterally and dissect it medially or cut it free from the caudal lamina and dissect caudal to cephalad. The deep ligamentum flavum is exposed (Fig. 36C). We handle the deep ligamentum flavum in one of three ways. One method is to make a longitudinal incision in the lateral third of the ligamentum

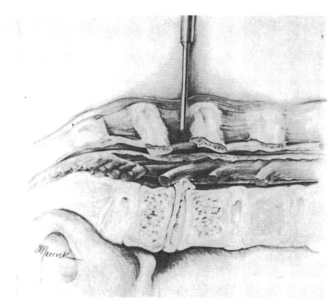

FIGURE 36B. Three-dimensional thinking is important. You must understand the relationship of the spinous process, the lamina, the interlaminar area, the facet joints, and the transverse processes to the disc space. The interlaminar area leads to the disc space. The second X-ray is taken with the Kocher in the interlaminar area.

flavum. Then, protecting the nerve with the Penfield 4, resect the lateral third of the ligamentum flavum with the Kerrison. A more common method is to use a small cutting acorn bur and do a laminotomy of the cephalad lamina to the insertion of the ligamentum flavum. The laminotomy can be small and in the cephalad lateral corner to expose the lateral ligamentum flavum. Use a curette to detach the cephalad insertion of the ligamentum flavum. Use a nerve hook to free up the ligamentum flavum and to dissect it cephalad to caudal. The nerve hook can hold the ligamentum flavum up and allow removal with the Kerrison to begin.

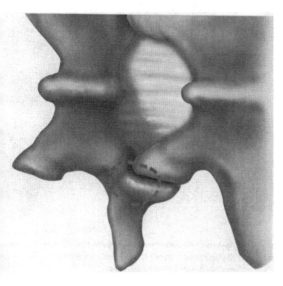

FIGURE 36C. The exposed right-side interlaminar area with the view of the pedicle superimposed. The superficial layer of the ligamentum flavum can be removed by gently cutting the attachment of the superficial ligament to the facet joint capsule and dissecting this medially with the curette. This maneuver exposes the yellow longitudinal fibers of the deep ligamentum flavum. The dashed line indicates the pedicle.

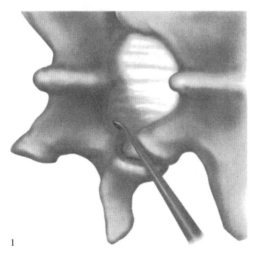

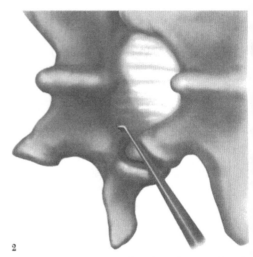

1

2

FIGURE 36D. A straight (1) and then an angled (2) curette are used to detach the deep ligamentum flavum from the cephalad edge of the caudal lamina. The ligamentum flavum inserts directly on the edge. The elastic nature of the ligamentum flavum allows it to shrink slightly, which helps distance it from the caudal lamina. Then, the curette detaches the ligamentum flavum laterally from the medial aspect of the facet joint capsule.

The method we prefer is to use a curette to detach the caudal attachments of the deep ligamentum flavum from the leading edge of the caudal lamina and from the lateral wall of the facet (Fig. 36D). With the Kerrison, do a small laminotomy to open the epidural space (Fig. 36E). The ligamentum flavum is removed with the Kerrison caudal to cephalad. The ligament, being elastic, shrinks up, helping the dissection. Detach it laterally and dissect it cephalad (Fig. 36F). To ensure lateral exposure, first the inferior and then the superior facet may need to be trimmed with a Kerrison (Fig. 36G).

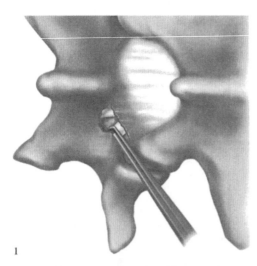

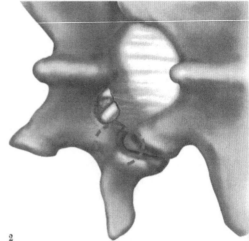

1

2

FIGURE 36E. The Kerrison may be used caudally to open the entry zone of the caudal foramina at the critical angle (1). The critical angle is the junction of the caudal lamina and the superior facet. The nerve root exits under this critical angle. Removal of bone in this area (2; *dashed line*) is usually carried out after detachment of the ligamentum flavum from the caudal edge.

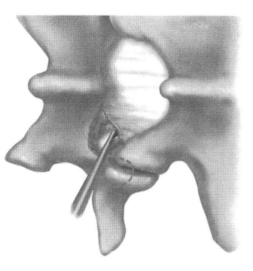

FIGURE 36F. The nerve hook or curette is used to dissect a space between the dura and the ligamentum flavum.

Gentle palpation with the dental identifies the pedicle. You should have a distinct understanding of the intracanal structures. The pedicle is the key to intracanal anatomy (Fig. 36H). When the pedicle is identified, you know that the disc space is less than 1 cm cephalad. The traversing nerve root is immediately medial and the exiting foramen is caudal to the pedicle. The foramen below is caudal to the pedicle; the foramen above is cephalad to the pedicle. The exiting nerve root of that segment is cephalad to the disc space and the pedicle. The traversing nerve root of one segment becomes the exiting root of the level below. For example, the 5th nerve root is the traversing root of the L4–L5 neuromotion segment (or level) and the exiting nerve root of the L5–S1 segment. The exiting nerve root of the L4–L5 segment is the 4th nerve root.

The ligamentum flavum attaches to the leading edge of the caudal lamina and to less than 50% of the surface of the cephalad lamina. It is not necessary to remove all

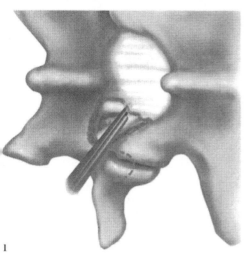

1

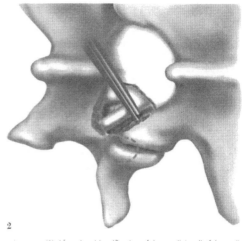

2

FIGURE 36G. The Kerrison removes the ligamentum flavum from caudal to cephalad (1). Careful definition of the space between dura and ligamentum flavum is continued. A cottonoid can be inserted into the space (2). After clear identification of the medial wall of the pedicle and the nerve, the lateral recess can also be excised.

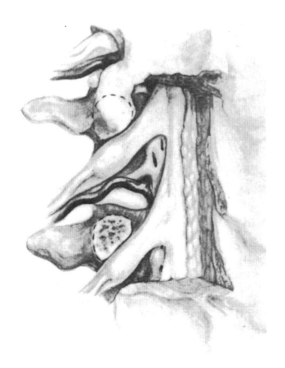

FIGURE 36H. The relationship of the pedicle to the disc space and the nerve root. Identify the pedicle in the wound with the nerve hook or dental. Knowing the pedicle, you can identify the disc less than 1 cm cephalad to the pedicle. The nerve root is immediately medial to the pedicle and the nerve root in the interlaminar area is immediately caudal to the nerve root. The transverse process is immediately lateral to the pedicle. To identify the pedicle from the transverse process, simply bisect the diameter of the transverse process; this leads directly to the pedicle. The vascular leash is caudal to the nerve root, slightly cephalad to the disc space, or over the disc space for larger exposures of the spinal canal. The vascular leash should be identified and coagulated with the bipolar. The safe zone for expo- sure for the disc is lateral to the medial wall of the pedicle and just cephalad to the pedicle. The traversing nerve root is medial and the exiting nerve root is too far cephalad. There are blood vessels in this area. You can expose and enter the disc here when the nerve root is tight, allowing an excavation of a portion of the disc.

This view shows:

1. Location of the safe zone of disc entry
2. The medial border of the pedicle
3. The traversing nerve root
4. The exiting nerve root

At L4–L5, for example, #1 is the L4–L5 disc space, #2 the L5 pedicle, #3 the 5th root, and #4 the 4th root.

the ligamentum flavum when excising an extruded disc fragment. The amount of ligamentum flavum removed is determined by the surgeon's ability to adequately assess the retractability of the nerve after fragment removal as well as his or her ability to identify the nerve and fragment before removal. When there is an element of lateral recess stenosis and a significant portion of the medial aspect of the facet is removed, then more of the ligamentum flavum should be resected. An assessment of preoperative studies should be the best indication of how large the laminotomy and medial facetectomy should be. Remove enough bone to safely expose the nerve.

With identification of the pedicle, a safe zone to enter the disc is immediately cephalad to the pedicle and lateral to the medial wall of the pedicle. The traversing nerve root will not be located lateral to the medial wall of the pedicle. This method allows a lateral exposure of the disc. When the nerve root is very tight and cannot be retracted, use one of the following five approaches.

1. Go lateral. Identify the medial wall of the pedicle; go cephalad and lateral to the medial wall of the pedicle. Remove the lateral ligamentum flavum (Fig. 36I). When removing lateral portions of the ligamentum flavum, dissect a plane directly on the undersurface of the ligamentum flavum to be removed. In cases of an axillary fragment, the nerve root may be pushed laterally under the ligamentum flavum and in danger of injury unless the Kerrison punches only the ligamentum flavum. Expose the disc laterally and puncture the disc with a micro-Penfield 4 (Fig. 36J). When it is obvious that

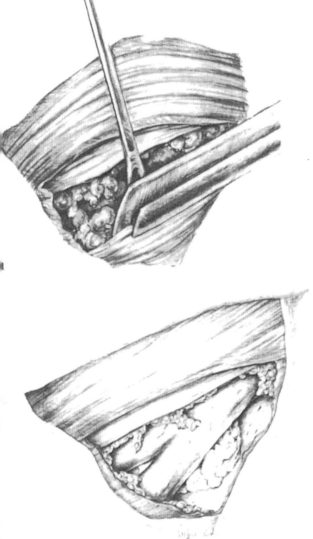

FIGURE 36I. (1) When exposure is needed lateral to the nerve root, the Penfield 4 is inserted under the lateral leaf of the ligamentum flavum. Between this lateral leaf of the ligamentum flavum and the dural sac, gently retract the dura away from the lateral leaf of the ligamentum flavum. This step allows insertion of the small 40-degree-angle Kerrison rongeur to remove the lateral leaf of the ligamentum flavum. (2) The nerve is exposed and the ligamentum flavum partially resected.

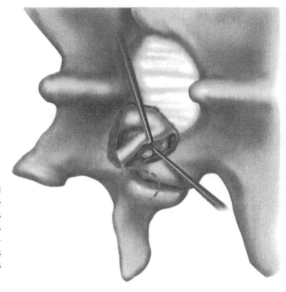

FIGURE 36J. After removal of the lateral leaf of the ligamentum flavum, the nerve root is well visualized as well as the suggestion of nuclear fragments under the root. Gently insert the Penfield 4 lateral to the nerve root. Assess the tension in the nerve root and its ability to be retracted.

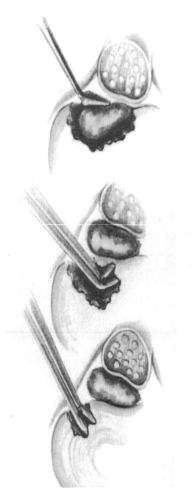

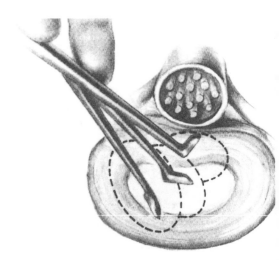

FIGURE 36K. The down-pushing Scovall curettes can be used to work disc material from under the nerve root down into the disc space, allowing safer removal of disc material lateral to the nerve root (1). By creating space in the disc space with disc removal, a fragment can be worked into the disc space to allow removal lateral to the nerve root (2); this is particularly important for large fragments medial to the nerve root, because under such circumstances retraction of the nerve root against the fragment can produce significant nerve root damage.

you have punctured the disc, not the nerve, expand the hole in the annulus with a regular Penfield 4 or make a small cruciate incision with a #15 blade. Remove disc material with a micro-pituitary while protecting the nerve with the microsucker retractor. Then insert the down-pushing Epstein curette under the annulus. Push down with the Epstein curette and attempt to push disc material down into the disc space to remove the disc material laterally (Fig. 36K). Keep the Epstein under the annulus or posterior longitudinal ligament. Use the right-angled Shuler or Frazier or the dental to go between the nerve and the annulus, and push down on the posterior longitudinal ligament to push the disc fragment into the disc space.

2. Check the axilla (Fig. 36L). Often a large, extruded axillary fragment can be removed very early in the approach before there is any attempt at retracting the nerve root. Exposure of the axilla usually requires doing a limited laminotomy of the caudal lamina. We do not significantly retract the nerve root until the fragment has been removed.

3. Remove more of the lateral recess stenosis out to the medial wall of the pedicle.

4. Remove bone at the critical angle, which is the junction of the caudal lamina and the superior facet, doing an entry-zone foraminotomy of the traversing nerve root.

5. The fifth tactic is to do a laminotomy of the cephalad lamina up to the insertion of the ligamentum flavum and remove the cephalad-most insertion ligamentum flavum. Approach the nerve root from the cephalad-most aspect of the interlaminar area at the shoulder of the nerve root and palpate the back of the body above. Often

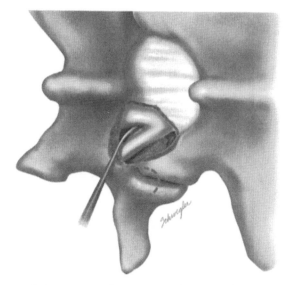

FIGURE 36L. If the tension is too great in the nerve root to allow any manipulation of the root, the surgeon must undertake the following steps:

1. Check the axilla. Often a large fragment can be removed from the axilla without first attempting to expose the nerve root. Retraction of the nerve root against a large axillary fragment can produce nerve root damage.

2. Go lateral. In this lateral area, by removal of the lateral leaf of ligamentum flavum in a small portion of the medial aspect of the superior facet, the disc can be exposed and the fragment removed.

3. Remove a small portion of bone over the critical angle. The critical angle is the junction of the caudal lamina and the superior facet. It is the entry zone to the exiting foramina below the pedicle.

4. Expose the shoulder of the root. Remove an additional amount of ligamentum flavum and caudal portion or the cephalad lamina and expose the disc and floor of the canal cephalad to the nerve root. The tight nerve root may be more retractable in a more cephalad position than it is caudally in an area where the nerve root is tighter as it attempts to exit around the pedicle.

the nerve root can be manipulated slightly more easily from this more cephalad position than from a more caudal position that is closer to the pedicle that the nerve root is exiting around.

With a large, extruded, more central lesion producing cauda equina compromise, several unusual steps may be necessary, such as first decompressing the opposite sides, then removing the fragment after a large laminotomy on its more prominent side.

After identification of a free fragment, isolate it with the microsucker retractor and a regular Penfield 4 (Fig. 36M). Use a nerve hook to remove the fragment; then expose the disc space; identify the hole in the annulus of the disc space; go into the disc

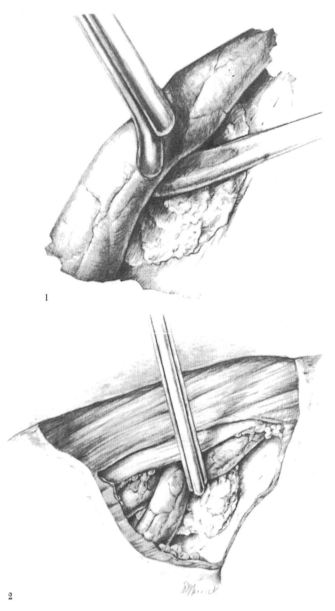

1

2

FIGURE 36M. Whether from this lateral position or a much more medial position in a less critical situation, the Penfield 4 is inserted with the right hand (1) and the Williams microsucker retractor is inserted with the left hand (2).

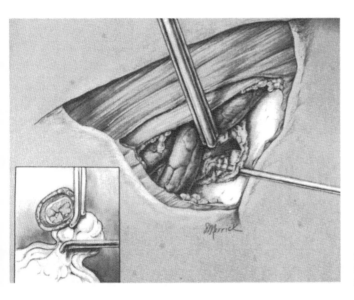

FIGURE 36N. The microsucker retractor is used to gently retract and elevate the nerve root, allowing disc removal.

space with the micro-pituitary; and remove any other loose pieces of disc material. Beware of overpenetration into the disc space; try to go only to the depth of the joint on the pituitary. Use the nerve hook to bring fragments to the annulotomy (Fig. 36N). We use the shortened Frazier and the dental to explore the spinal canal cephalad, then caudal, in the axilla and in the foramina to find any other loose pieces. When the fragment is under the posterior longitudinal ligament, we use the micro-Penfield 4 to puncture the posterior longitudinal ligament. Expand the hole with a regular Penfield 4 and identify the disc contents before making a small cruciate incision with a #15 blade to facilitate exposure of the disc material. We do not do a large annulectomy or incision of the annulus or a radical debridement or curetting of the disc space. We do only what is necessary to remove loose fragments of intervertebral disc and to accomplish the ultimate objective, which is freeing the nerve root. Retractability and lack of tension in the nerve root are the key to the success of the surgery and mark the end of the operation. Do a final exploration of the back of the vertebral body above and below, the foramen above and below, the axilla, and the disc hole. Gently palpate the undersurface of the nerve for an adherent fragment. When the nerve root is free and easily retractable, with no obstruction and no nerve root tension, then adequate decompression has been achieved. Obtain hemostasis, and follow with irrigation and closure. This surgery can be done as an outpatient procedure with special precautions set up or with 1- to 2-day hospital stay. Prophylactic antibiotics are continued for 24 hours.

Keep the wound dry for 10 days after the surgery. The usual restrictions involve not driving and not lifting anything heavier than a coffee cup for 3 to 4 weeks. We begin the postoperative trunk stabilization rehabilitation program between 2 and 4 weeks after the surgery and start over with the initial stages of the trunk stabilization program. We encourage patients to walk as much as is comfortable, as often as possible, from the time they wake up from the surgery.

Use of the microscope definitely provides better lighting and better visibility. The technique of using the scope and getting used to moving the scope around for a proper view of the interlaminar area allows the surgeon to better accomplish the objective of the operation. Virtually any operation medial to the medial wall of the pedicle can be done effectively through the scope with excellent lighting and visibility. By moving the scope around and positioning it and looking into the interlaminar area from several different angles, visibility of the interlaminar area and its contents should be enhanced. Techniques of exploration of the interlaminar area are enhanced by the microscope.

The autofocus and zoom lenses enhance visibility. We often use the drill under the scope. The drill can be used to perform the medial facetectomy or limited laminotomy with great effectiveness. Understanding the anatomy, palpating the back of the body above and the back of the body below, exploring the axilla, and palpating the exiting foramina are all techniques necessary for disc excision. Adequate care must be taken with draping of the scope to prevent its contamination. Once these techniques are understood, the risk of infection should be lower with the small incision and smaller exposure. The small incision is simply a result of not needing a larger incision for effective removal of a herniated disc.

otal En Bloc Spondylectomy: A New Surgical Technique for Malignant Vertebral Tumors

Norio Kawahara • *Katsuro Tomita* • *Hiroyuki Tsuchiya*

Conventionally, because of the difficulty in surgical approach and the anatomical proximity of the major vessels to the involved vertebra(e), curettage and resection of vertebral tumors have been commonly practiced, including removal of the malignant tissue in a piecemeal fashion. The disadvantages of these conventional approaches are clear, including a high possibility of tumor cell contamination of the surrounding structures and difficult identification of a demarcation zone separating neoplastic tissue from healthy tissue. These factors may contribute to incomplete resection of the tumor as well as recurrence of the spinal malignant neoplasm.[1,2]

To reduce local recurrence as much as possible and to increase survival rate, we have developed a new surgical technique of spondylectomy (vertebrectomy) termed total en bloc spondylectomy (TES).[1-5] Using this technique, we were able to excise the tumor mass with a wide or narrow margin, but sometimes with an minimal intralesional margin in the pedicle.

Indications for Total En Bloc Spondylectomy

The TES operation was designed primarily for patients who met the following criteria: a primary malignant tumor, aggressive benign tumor, or solitary metastasis that did not spread into or invade adjacent visceral organs, showed little or no adhesion to the vena cava or aorta, and did not show multiple metastases. A contiguous involvement of three or fewer vertebrae represented a relative indication for the TES operation.

The indications for surgical treatment of spinal metastases are neurologic deficit, intractable pain, and spinal instability. The oncologic factors to be considered include the success of treatment of the primary tumor, whether the metastases are solitary and localized, if the metastases are limited and can be controlled, and if there is a life expectancy of at least 12 months.

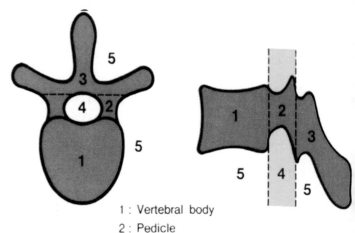

FIGURE 37A. Definitions of anatomical sites of the vertebra. (From Tomita N, et al: Int Orthop 18:292, 1994.)

1 : Vertebral body
2 : Pedicle
3 : Lamina, Spinal process
4 : Epidural space
5 : Paraspinal area

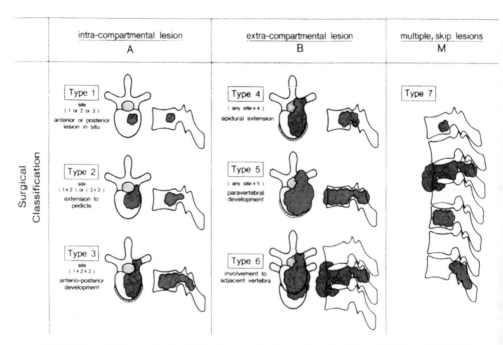

FIGURE 37B. Schematic diagram of surgical classification of vertebral tumors. (From Tomita N, et al: Int Orthop 18:292, 1994.)

To provide a more informative staging, a new surgical classification was devised that incorporated a description of the affected anatomical site and the extent of the tumor. The anatomical site of the neoplasm was classified as follows: (1) vertebral body, (2) the pedicle, (3) the lamina and spinous process, (4) spinal canal (epidural space), and (5) paravertebral area (Fig. 37A). The numbers used to denote the anatomical sites reflect the common sequence of tumor progression. The number of anatomical sites is also related to the surgical classification as described here. Using the anatomical and surgical classification, the new surgical classification of vertebral tumors was designed (Fig. 37B). The classification concept was modified from the surgical staging system of Enneking and coworkers.[6] For instance, type 3 lesion in our classification involves the vertebral body (anatomical site 1), the pedicle (anatomical site 1), and the lamina (anatomical site 3). We considered type 1, 2, and 3 lesions as intracompartmental and types 4, 5, and 6, as extracompartmental. Type 7 tumor is a multiple skip lesion. The TES operation is recommended for type 2, 3, 4, and 5 lesions, relatively indicated for type 1 and 6 lesions, and not recommended or contraindicated for type 7 lesions.

Surgical Technique

The TES technique consists of two steps: en bloc resection of the posterior element and en bloc resection of the anterior column. The following is a description of each step.

Step 1: En Bloc Laminectomy (En Bloc Resection of the Whole Posterior Element of the Vertebra)

1. Exposure

The patient is placed prone over the Relton–Hall four-poster frame to avoid compression to the vena cava. A straight vertical midline incision is made over the spinous processes and is extended three vertebrae above and below the involved segment(s). The paraspinal muscles are dissected from the spinous processes and the laminae, and then retracted laterally. If the patient underwent posterior route biopsy, the tracts are carefully resected in a manner similar to that used in a limb-salvaging procedure. After a careful dissection of the area around the facet joints, a large articulated spinal retractor is applied. By spreading the retractor and detaching the muscles around the facet joints, a wider exposure is obtained. The operative field must be wide enough on both sides to allow dissection under the surface of the transverse processes. In the thoracic spine, the ribs on the affected level are transected 3 to 4 cm lateral to the costotransverse joint, and the pleura is bluntly separated from the vertebra (Fig. 37C).

To expose the superior articular process of the uppermost vertebra, the spinous and the inferior articular processes of the neighboring vertebra are osteotomized and removed with dissection of the attached soft tissues, including the ligamentum flavum.

2. Introduction of the T-Saw Guide

To make an exit for the T-saw guide through the nerve root canal, the soft tissue attached to the inferior aspect of the pars interarticularis is dissected and removed, using utmost care so as not to damage the corresponding nerve root. A C-curved malleable T-saw guide is then introduced through the intervertebral foramen in a cephalocaudal direction. In this procedure, the tip of the T-saw guide should be introduced along the medial cortex of the lamina and the pedicle so as not to injure the spinal cord and the nerve root (Fig. 37D). After passing the T-saw guide, its tip at the exit of the nerve root canal can be found beneath the inferior border of the pars interarticularis. In the next step, a threadwire saw (T-saw; flexible multifilament threadwire

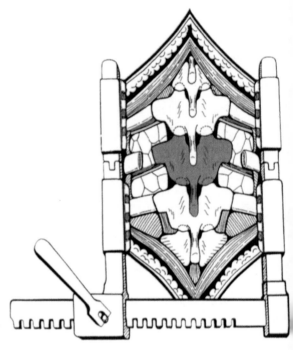

FIGURE 37C. Operative schema of the posterior exposure.

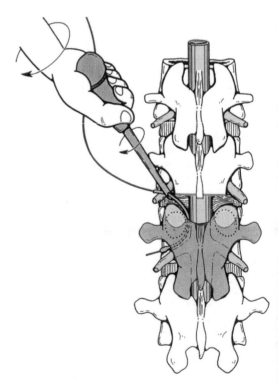

FIGURE 37D. Operative schema of introducing the T-saw guide.

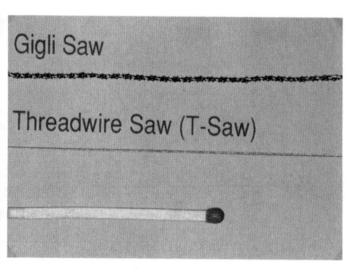

FIGURE 37E. Photograph of the thread-wire saw (T-saw) compared with a Gigli saw and a match.

saw, 0.54 mm in diameter[7]; Fig. 37E) is passed through the hole in the wire guide and is clamped with a T-saw holder at each end. The T-saw guide is removed, and tension on the T-saw is maintained. When two or three vertebrae are resected, the T-saw is inserted into a thin polyethylene catheter (T-saw catheter) and both are passed under the lamina. This procedure is also applied to the contralateral side.

3. Cutting the Pedicles and Resection of the Posterior Element

While tension is maintained, the T-saw is placed beneath the superior articular and transverse processes with a specially designed T-saw manipulator. With this procedure, the T-saw placed around the lamina is wrapped around the pedicle. With a reciprocating motion of the T-saw, the pedicles are cut and then the whole posterior element of the spine (the spinous process, the superior and inferior articular processes, the transverse process, and the pedicle) is removed in one piece (Fig. 37F). The cut surface of the pedicle is sealed with bone wax to reduce bleeding and to minimize contamination by tumor cells. To maintain stability after segmental resection of the anterior column, a temporary posterior instrumentation is performed (Fig. 37G). When one vertebra is resected, segmental fixation at two above and two below is recomended. However, if two or three vertebrae are resected, more than two above and two below segmental fixation is mandatory.

Step 2: En Bloc Corpectomy (Resection of the Anterior Column of the Vertebra)

1. Blunt Dissection Around the Vertebral Body

At the beginning of the second step, the segmental arteries must be identified bilaterally. The spinal branch of the segmental artery, which runs along the nerve root, is ligated and divided. This procedure exposes the segmental artery, which appears just lateral to the cut edge of the pedicle. In the thoracic spine, the nerve root is cut on the side from which the affected vertebra is removed. The blunt dissection is done on both sides through the plane between the pleura (or the iliopsoas muscle) and the vertebral body. Usually, the lateral aspect of the body is easily dissected with a curved vertebral spatula. Then, the segmental artery should be dissected from the vertebral body. By continuing dissection of both lateral sides of the vertebral body anteriorly, the aorta is carefully dissected posteriorly from the anterior aspect of the vertebral

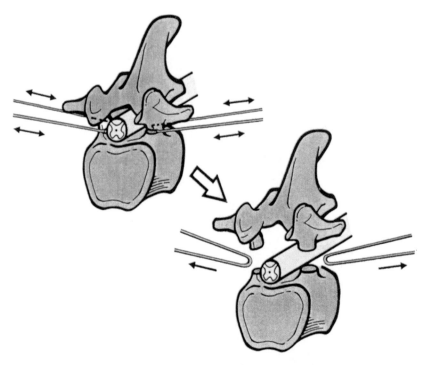

FIGURE 37F. Operative schema of the pediclotomy.

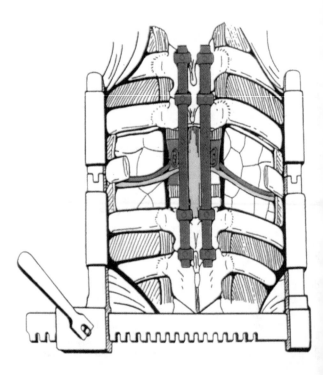

FIGURE 37G. Operative schema of setting the posterior instrumentation.

body with a spatula and the surgeon's fingers (Fig. 37H1, 37H2). When the surgeon's fingertips meet anterior to the vertebral body, a series of spatulas, starting from the smallest size, are inserted sequentially to extend the dissection. A pair of the largest spatulas is kept in the dissection site to prevent the surrounding tissues and organs from iatrogenic injury and to make the surgical field wide enough for manipulating the anterior column.

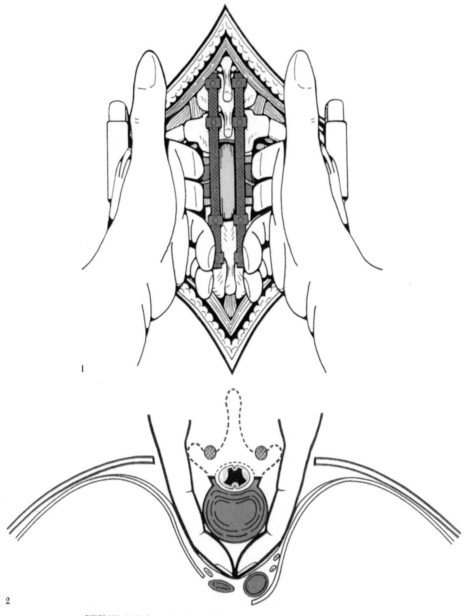

FIGURE 37H. (1, 2) Operative schema of anterior dissection around the vertebral body.

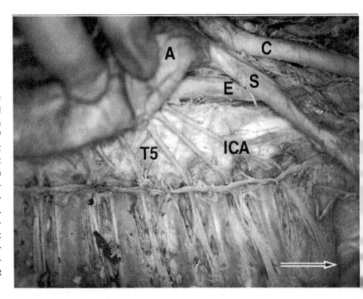

FIGURE 37I. Topographic view of the aortic arch and posterior intercostal arteries at the upper thoracic spine on the right side in the cadaveric study.[8] The highest aortic arch level was at T3–T4, and the subsequent thoracic aorta descends in direct contact with the vertebrae at T5 or below. The second to fourth posterior intercostal arteries originate from the aorta at T5. *C,* common carotid artery; *S,* subclavian artery; *E,* esophagus; *A,* aortic arch; *T5,* T5 vertebral body; *ICA,* intercostal artery. *Arrow* indicates the cranial direction. (From Kawahara N, et al: Spine 21(12):1402, 1996.)

2. Vascular Anatomy Around the Vertebral Body

It is important to understand vascular anatomy around the vertebral body.[8] The first four segmental (posterior intercostal) arteries commonly run directly upward apart from the vertebral column and turn more transversely over the costovertebral joint (Fig. 37I). The azygos vein cephalad to T4 ascends away from the vertebral column (Fig. 37J). This anatomical specificity in the upper thoracic area indicates that there is a decreased chance of critical damage to these vessels during isolation of the affected vertebral body and paired discs posteriorly in total en bloc spondylectomy.

At spinal levels caudal to T4, the thoracic and abdominal aorta descends downward in direct contact with the anterior vertebral column. Obviously, it is true that surgeons

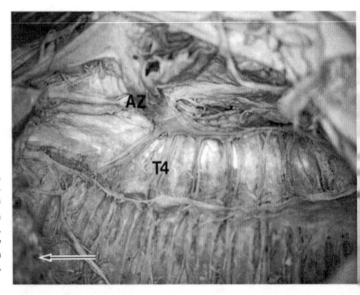

FIGURE 37J. Photograph shows the azygos vein ascending in the upper thoracic spine in the cadaveric study.[8] The azygos vein directly contacts with the thoracic vertebrae at T4 or below. *AZ,* azygos vein; *T4,* T4 vertebra. *Arrow* indicates the cranial direction. (From Kawahara N, et al: Spine 21(12):1403, 1996.)

must be extremely careful not to violate the vessel but they can usually make sure of the aortic pulsation at their fingertips and thus the retraction of the aorta anteriorly from the affected vertebral body is relatively undemanding, technically speaking.

In the cases of our cadavor reseach,[8] the segmental artery to the vertebra had some variations: 48 of 348 segmental arteries in 17 subjects originated from intercostal arteries adjacent to the corresponding level, not from the thoracic aorta: 38 variants were identified at T4 or more cephalad and 10 at T5 or caudal. Adachi observed that 88 (9%) of all 977 intercostal arteries did not originate from the thoracic aorta (n = 48): 28 of 88 variations were at T5 or caudal (Fig. 37K).[9] Adachi concluded that, in Japanese, approximately 4% of thoracic segmental arteries do not originate directly from the thoracic aorta, and 8% of the vertebrae lack a segmental artery in the middle to lower thoracic spinal levels.[9] This anatomical variation must be kept in mind when no segmental arteries are identified around the affected vertebral bodies during total en bloc spondylectomy.

In the lumbar spine between L1 and L4, the lumbar artery consistently arose from the abdominal aorta at each corresponding spinal level bilaterally in our cadaver series.[8] The first and second lumbar arteries arising on each side of the posterior aortic midline display essentially horizontal segmental distribution, whereas those from L3 and L4 levels run vertically downward behind the aorta and then horizontally up to the intervertebral foramina. Variations in origins and distribution can occur and should be anticipated. In 63 cadavers, Adachi observed that 5 (1%) variants in a total of 498 lumbar arteries had been recorded between L1 and L4 that did not arise from the abdominal aorta.[9] Based on anterior scoliosis surgery, Winter et al.[10] reported that the number of lumbar arteries may vary: four in 70% to 74% of the clinical cases, three in 20% to 22%, and five in 5% to 7% of their cases. Variations include a conjoined form of lumbar artery distributing two segments simultaneously, and the collateral branched from the lumbar artery at neighboring levels.

The muscle fibers of the medial crus of the lumbar diaphragm originated most frequently and firmly from the L2–L3 disc levels bilaterally, and the second lumbar artery ran dorsally to the medial crus (Fig. 37L). This important portion of the diaphragm must be separated posteriorly before the isolation and excision of vertebral tumors. In total en bloc spondylectomy attempted to this level, it is thus very important to

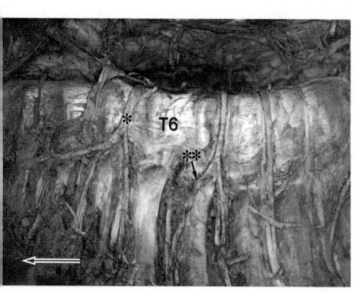

FIGURE 37K. Variations in intercostal arteries in the cadaveric study.[8] The left second, third, and fourth intercostal arteries branch from the fifth intercostal artery (*) anterior to the head of the fifth rib. The left sixth intercostal artery (**) branches as a variant seventh intercostal artery. *T6,* T6 vertebra. *Arrow* indicates the cranial direction. (From Kawahara N, et al: Spine 21(12):1404, 1996.)

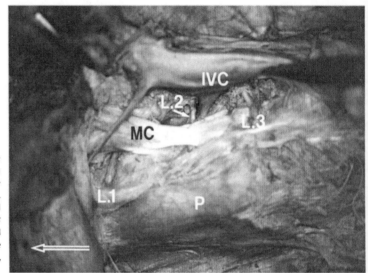

FIGURE 37L. Right medial crus of the lumbar diaphragm and surrounding vessels in the cadaveric study.[8] The medial crus originates at L2–L3. *IVC*, inferior vena cava; *MC*, right medial crus; *P*, psoas muscle. *L.1*, *L.2*, and *L.3* indicate the first, second, and third lumbar arteries. *Arrow* indicates the cranial direction. (From Kawahara N, et al: Spine 21(12):1404, 1996.)

separate the medial crus from its vertebral origin, followed by the exploration of the second lumbar artery from L2 involved with malignancy. At this spinal level, however, the aorta pulsates very strongly with decreased risk of injury if it is carefully retracted forward. The inferior vena cava ascends anterior to the medial crura of the diaphragm, primar-ily on the right. Additionally, great care must be taken because the azygos and hemiazygos veins are dorsal and cephalad to the medial crura of the diaphragm, especially in the case with an L1 vertebral tumor. Attention must also be paid not to injure the inferior vena cava posteriorly because it ascends in direct contact with the vertebral column at L3 and L4, the same as actual for aortic bifurcation as well as venous confluence at L4 and L5 (Fig. 37M).

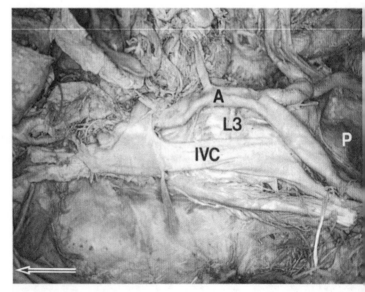

FIGURE 37M. Major vessels in the lumbar spine in the cadaveric study.[8] The inferior vena cava ascends in tight contact with the vertebrae in conjunction with lordosis. *A*, aorta; *IVC*, inferior vena cava; *P*, promontrium; *L3*, L3 vertebra. *Arrow* indicates the cranial direction. (From Kawahara N, et al: Spine 21(12):1404, 1996.)

3. Passage of the T-Saw

T-Saws are inserted at the proximal and distal cutting levels of the vertebral bodies, where grooves are made along the desired cutting line using a V-notched osteotome after confirmation of the disc levels with needles.

4. Dissection of the Spinal Cord and Removal of the Vertebra

Using a cord spatula, the spinal cord is mobilized from the surrounding venous plexus and the ligamentous tissue. The teeth-cord protector, which has teeth on both edges to prevent the T-saw from slipping, is then applied. The anterior column of the vertebra is cut by the T-saw, together with the anterior and posterior longitudinal ligaments (Fig. 37N). After cutting the anterior column, the mobility of the vertebra is again checked to ensure a complete corpectomy.

The freed anterior column is rotated around the spinal cord and removed carefully to avoid injury to the spinal cord. With this procedure, a complete anterior and posterior decompression of the spinal cord (circumspinal decompression) and total en bloc resection of the vertebral tumor are achieved (Fig. 37O).

5. Anterior Reconstruction and Posterior Instrumentation

Bleeding, mainly from the venous plexus within the spinal canal, should be exhaustively arrested. An anchor hole on the cut end of the remaining vertebra is made on each side to seat the graft. A vertebral spacer, such as autograft, fresh and/or frozen allograft, apatite-wollastonite glass ceramic prosthesis (Lederle, Tokyo, Japan), and a titanium mesh cylinder (MOSS-Miami, DePuy Motech, Warsaw, IN), is properly inserted to the anchor holes within the remaining healthy vertebrae. After checking the appropriate position of the vertebral spacer radiographically, the posterior instrumentation is adjusted to slightly compress the inserted vertebral spacer. If two or three vertebrae are resected, application of the connector device between the posterior rods and anterior spacer is recommended (Fig. 37P1–37P3). Finally, a Bard Marlex mesh (Bard, Billerica, MA, USA) covers the entire anterior and posterior reconstructed areas to establish the compartment for suppressing bleeding.

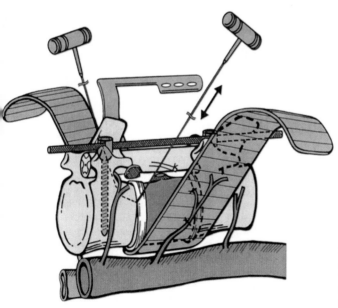

FIGURE 37N. Operative schemes for cutting the anterior column. A pair of the spatulas is kept around the affected vertebral body to prevent the surrounding tissues and organs from iatrogenic injury and to make the surgical field wide enough for manipulating the anterior column. The anterior column of the vertebra is cut by the T-saw, together with the anterior and posterior longitudinal ligaments. The teeth-cord protector, which has teeth on both edges to prevent the T-saw from slipping, is then applied.

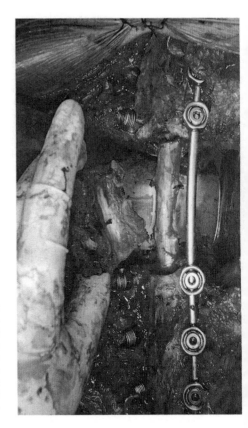

FIGURE 370. Photograph of the en bloc corpectomy. The freed anterior column is rotated around the spinal cord and removed carefully to avoid injury to the spinal cord. With this procedure, a complete anterior and posterior decompression of the spinal cord (circumspinal decompression) and total en bloc resection of the vertebral tumor are achieved.

6. Postoperative Management

Suction draining is preferred for 2 to 3 days after surgery, and the patient is allowed to start walking 1 week after surgery. The patient wears a thoracolumbosacral orthosis for 2 to 3 months until the bony union or incorporation of the artificial vertebral prosthesis is attained.

Case Study

A 58-year-old man was hospitalized because of severe back pain and paraparesis. Eight years before admission, the patient was diagnosed with thyroid cancer, which was treated with thyroidectomy. Imaging workup showed a tumor growth throughout the entire T6 vertebra as well as the epidural space of T5 and T6 (Fig. 37Q). Examination of a biopsy material confirmed the lesion to be a metastatic thyroid cancer. Total en bloc spondylectomy was performed at the T5 and T6 vertebrae (Fig. 37R). Anterior reconstruction was carried out using a titanium mesh cylinder, containing autogenous iliac cancellous chip bones. A MOSS Miami screw and rod arrangement was performed posteriorly between T2 and T9 levels. A pair of DLT bars of the Cotrel–Dubousset construct allowed the titanium mesh cylinder to be securely positioned. Radiographs did not show any loosening of the implants anteriorly and posteriorly at 2.5-year follow-up (Fig. 37S1, 37S2). The patient has been well for the past 3 postoperative years.

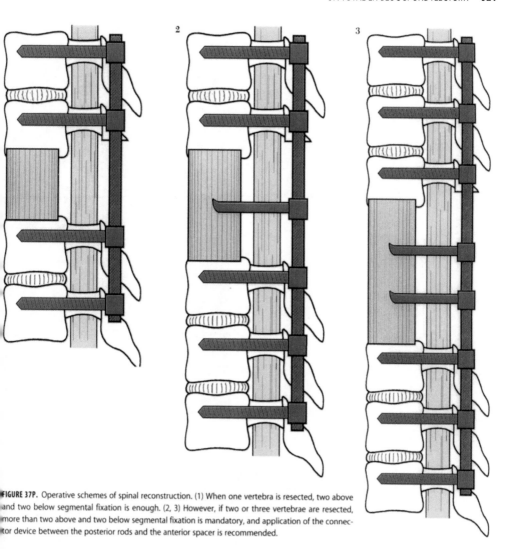

FIGURE 37P. Operative schemes of spinal reconstruction. (1) When one vertebra is resected, two above and two below segmental fixation is enough. (2, 3) However, if two or three vertebrae are resected, more than two above and two below segmental fixation is mandatory, and application of the connector device between the posterior rods and the anterior spacer is recommended.

Discussion

The ring-shaped bony structure of the vertebra, containing the spinal cord, hinders a wide surgical margin. Other obstacles exist, such as the thin surrounding soft tissues, major vessels, and visceral organs neighboring the involved vertebra. Thus, most operations are amenable to curettage or piecemeal resection. However, the intralesional procedure apparently leads to incomplete resection and to definite contamination by tumor cells.

Roy-Camille et al.,[11,12] Stener,[13–15] Stener and Johnson,[16] Sundaresan et al.,[17] and Boriani et al.[18,19] have described total spondylectomy for improving local curability, with excellent clinical results. In contrast, our procedure involves peripheral manipulation, except for the pedicle, and the lesion is removed en bloc. The TES technique minimizes the risk of contamination compared with that described by these authors.

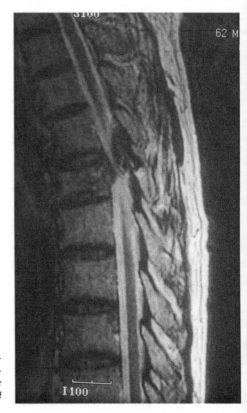

FIGURE 37Q. The T$_2$-weighted magnetic resonance imaging of the patient with solitary thyroid cancer metastasis, showing compression of the cord at T5 and T6 levels.

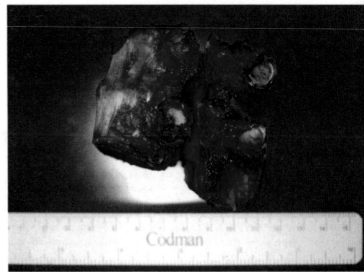

FIGURE 37R. Photograph of the resected specimen of the T5 and T6 vertebrae.

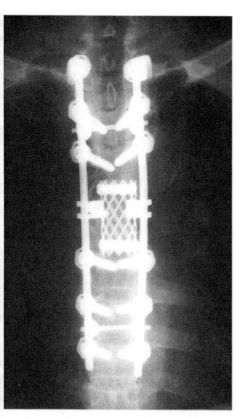 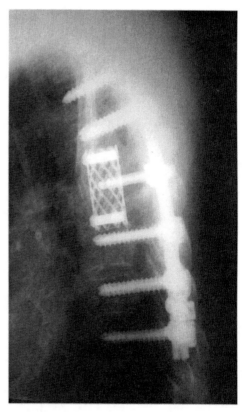

FIGURE 37S. Radiograph taken 2.5 years after surgery without instrumentation failure posteriorly. (1) Anteroposterior view. (2) Lateral view.

The major risks in TES operation include (1) mechanical damage to the adjacent neural structures during the excision of the pedicles; (2) possible contamination by tumor cells during pediculotomy; (3) injury of the major vessels during blunt dissection of the anterior aspect of the vertebral body; (4) disturbance of spinal cord circulation at the level of surgery; and (5) excessive bleeding from the internal vertebral vein and epidural venous plexus during the second step of surgery. To reduce the risk of nerve root and spinal cord damage, we designed the T-saw.[7] It is made of multifilament twisted stainless steel wires and has a smooth surface to cut hard bony materials with minimal damage to the surrounding soft tissues. If the T-saw is properly passed into the nerve root canal and pulled posteriorly, it should not damage the nerve root. It is obvious that resection of the vertebra in one piece without cutting a certain point of the ring-shaped bony structure is impossible because of the encasement of the spinal cord within the vertebra. The pedicle is the best site for this purpose since (1) it is the narrowest portion connecting the posterior element with the anterior part so that the intralesional cut surface will minimize the chance of contamination to a great extent, and (2) the spinal cord and the nerve root can be freed easily atraumatically. Pediculotomy is thus justified from the anatomical standpoint. However, the pedicle does not always serve as a safe point for cutting, particularly when it is involved with the malignant process. Under such circumstances, the ipsilateral side of the lamina and contralateral part of the pedicle are cut together. These cutting levels may be considered separately in each case.

Blunt dissection of the anterior part of the vertebral body is another risky maneuver in the TES operation. The anatomical relationship between the vertebra, major vessels, and the visceral organs should be well acknowledged.[8] Based on anatomical studies on cadavers, TES is less likely to damage the thoracic aorta between T1 and T4. However, the artery must be carefully retracted anteriorly in areas caudal to T5 before manipulation of the affected vertebra(e). For a lesion at L1 and L2, the diaphragm and the first two lumbar arteries should be treated with utmost care. Possible circulatory compromise after the ligation of the radicular artery is another concern. In the cat model, the authors[3] found that ligation of the Adamkiewicz artery reduced spinal cord blood flow by approximately 81% of the control value, and this decrementation did not affect spinal cord evoked potentials. Abundant arterial network around the dura mater and the spinal cord may completely compensate for the ligation of one or two radicular arteries. Actually, there has been no neurologic degradation in all 60 patients in our series who underwent TES. Bleeding from the epidural venous plexus is often profuse. Hemostasis of tamponade in the epidural space using Oxycell cotton, Aviten, or fibrin glue is mandatory. In addition to hypotensive anesthesia (systolic blood pressure, 60–80 mmHg), exhaustive management to arrest bleeding must be followed.

Roy-Camille et al.[11,12] suggested that the origin of the iliopsoas and iliac muscles from the lumbar spine make one-stage posterior total spondylectomy unfeasible. They also stressed the close proximity of major abdominal vessels to the anterior vertebral column in the lumbar spine, which enhances the risk in a patient with increased lumbar lordosis. For this reason, they recommended a two-stage operation to resect malignant vertebral neoplasms occurring between L2 and L4. Stener reported total spondylectomy through a single-stage posterior approach for tumors at L3 or cephalad but denied the indication of this procedure at L4.[15] Stener advocated combined anteroposterior approach for a tumor at L4 based on the following reasons: the close contact of major vessels, especially the inferior vena cava with the L4 vertebral body, and interference by the iliac crest in accessing L4–L5 and L5 posteriorly. The authors[1–4] agree with these two anatomical annoyances pointed out by Stener[15] but, for a case with an iliac wing positioned rather distal, they do not always disagree with single-stage posterior total en bloc spondylectomy for a solitary L4 vertebral tumor. For a tumor involving the L5 vertebra, it is undoubtedly necessary to use a two-stage anteroposterior approach because of the additional difficulty of managing the common iliac and iliolumbar arteries and veins as well as the lumbosacral neural plexus.

A wide surgical margin or at least a minimal margin is achievable around the affected vertebra(e) when the lesion is intracompartmental (type 1, 2, or 3), particularly when the healthy part of the lamina or pedicle is cut. For a vertebral tumor extending into the spinal canal (type 4) or one invading the paravertebral areas (type 5), a marginal margin may be possible when the lesion is well encapsulated with a fibrous reactive membrane. In type 6 lesions, it is possible to obtain a wide margin at the proximal and caudal osteotomized sites of the vertebrae, but paravertebral tumor sometimes adheres to or invades surrounding soft tissues, major vessels, and visceral organs neighboring the involved vertebra. In such a instance, anterior dissection followed by a posterior TES operation is indicated.

References

1. Tomita K, Kawahara N, Mizuno K, Toribatake Y, Kim SS, Baba H, Tsuchiya H: Total en bloc spondylectomy for primary malignant vertebral tumors. In: Rao RS, Deo MG, Sanghri LD, Mittra I (eds): Proceedings of the 16th International Cancer Congress. Bologna, Monduzzi Editore, 1994, pp 2409–2413.
2. Tomita K, Kawahara N, Baba H, Tsuchiya H, Fujita T, Toribatake Y: Total en block spondylectomy. A new surgical technique for primary malignant vertebral tumors. Spine 22:324–333, 1997.

3. Tomita K, Toribatake Y, Kawahara N, Ohnari H, Kose H: Total en bloc spondylectomy and circumspinal decompression for solitary spinal metastasis. Paraplegia 32:36–46, 1994.

4. Tomita K, Kawahara N, Baba H, Tsuchiya H, Nagata S, Toribatake Y: Total en bloc spondylectomy for solitary spinal metastasis. Int Orthop 18:291–298, 1994.

5. Kawahara N, Tomita K, Fujita T, Maruo S, Otsuka S, Kinoshita G: Osteosarcoma of the thoracolumbar spine. Total en bloc spondylectomy. A case report. J Bone Joint Surg [Am] 79:453–458, 1997.

6. Enneking WF, Spanier SS, Goodmann MA: A system for the surgical staging of musculoskeletal sarcoma. Clin Orthop 153:106–120, 1980.

7. Tomita K, Kawahara N: The threadwire saw: a new device for cutting bone. J Bone Joint Surg [Am] 78:1915–1917, 1996.

8. Kawahara N, Tomita K, Baba H, Toribatake Y, Fujita T, Mizuno K, Tanaka S: Cadaveric vascular anatomy for total en bloc spondylectomy in malignant vertebral tumors. Spine 21:1401–1407, 1996.

9. Adachi B: Das Arteriensystem der Japaner. Kyoto, Maruzen, 1928, pp 1–10.

10. Winter RB, Denis F, Lonstein JL, Caramella J: Techniques of surgery: anatomy of thoracic intercostal and lumbar arteries. In: Lonstein JL, Bradford DS, Winter RB, Ogilvie JW (eds): Moe's Textbook of Scoliosis and Other Spinal Deformities, 3rd edn. Philadelphia, Saunders, 1994, pp 1.

11. Roy-Camille R, Mazel CH, Saillant G, Lapresle PH: Treatment of malignant tumor of the spine with posterior instrumentation. In: Sundaresan N, Schmidek HH, Schiller AL, Rosenthal DI (eds): Tumor of the Spine. Philadelphia, Saunders, 1990, pp 473–487.

12. Roy-Camille R, Saillant G, Bisserie M, Judet TH, Hautefort E, Mamoudy P: Resection vertebrale totale dans la chirurgie tumorale au niveau du rachis dorsal par voie posterieure pure. Rev Chir Orthop 67:421–430, 1981.

13. Stener B: Total spondylectomy in chondrosarcoma arising from the seventh thoracic vertebra. J Bone Joint Surg [Br] 53:288–295, 1971.

14. Stener B: Complete removal of vertebrae for extirpation of tumors. Clin Orthop 245:72–82, 1989.

15. Stener B: Technique of complete spondylectomy in the thoracic and lumbar spine. In: Sundaresan N, Schmidek HH, Schiller AL, Rosenthal DI (eds): Tumor of the Spine. Philadelphia, Saunders, 1990, pp 432–437.

16. Stener B, Johnsen OE: Complete removal of three vertebrae for giant-cell tumour. J Bone Joint Surg [Br] 53:278–287, 1971.

17. Sundaresan N, Rosen G, Huvos AG, Krol G: Combined treatment of osteosarcoma of the spine. Neurosurgery 23:714–719, 1988.

18. Boriani S, Biagini R, De Lure F, Di Fiore M, Gamberini G, Zanoni A: Vertebrectomia lombare per neoplasia ossea: tecnica chirurgica. Chir Organi Mov 79:163–173, 1994.

19. Boriani S, Chevalley F, Weinstein JN, et al. Chordoma of the spine above the sacrum. Treatment and outcome in 21 cases. Spine 21:1569–1577, 1996.

38A

Bilateral Paraspinous Lumbosacral Approach

Robert G. Watkins III • Robert G. Watkins IV

The most commonly used approaches to this area are the direct paraspinous muscle-splitting incision and the more lateral approach, which elevates and dissects under the lumbosacral muscle (Fig. 38A). The muscle-splitting incision affords not only alar transverse exposure for fusions but also excellent exposure for laminectomy.[1,2] The more lateral approach removes a bicortical portion of the posterior superior iliac spine, attempts to preserve muscle and fascial integrity, and allows excellent exposure of the tips of the transverse processes to the facet joints.[3,4] There is probably no great advantage to preserving the denervated muscle with the more lateral approach. We recommend the more lateral approach for alar transverse fusion and the muscle-splitting incision when laminectomy and root exploration are needed in addition to fusion.

1. Position the patient prone on the table with an appropriate operating frame.

2. After adequate prepping and draping, make a curved paraspinous incision approximately three fingerbreadths from the midline, L4 to S2 (Fig. 38B).

3 Cut through skin and subcutaneous tissue to the lumbar fascia. The posterior superior iliac spine is in the inferior portion of the wound. Palpate the transverse process of L5 and L4. Remove the fascial insertions on the iliac crest and reflect medially with a s mall sliver of bone (Fig. 38C).

4. With an elevator, dissect subperiosteally both the inner and outer tables of the posterior iliac crest to a depth of 2 to 3 cm.

5. Osteotomize the ilium with an osteotome, beginning at the medial portion of the posterosuperior iliac spine not involving the sacral iliac joint and extending approximately 5 to 6 cm on the iliac crest.

Caution: The clunial nerves will be in the lateral aspect of the wound and must be avoided. A safe margin of error is approximately one handbreadth lateral to the posterosuperior iliac spine.[1]

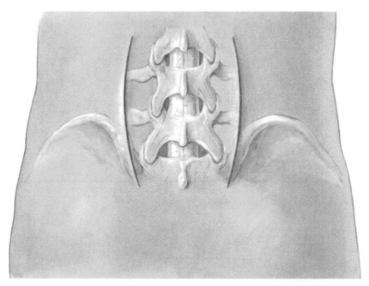

FIGURE 38A. The skin incisions on the bilateral paraspinous approach to the lower lumbar spine may be one of two types: (1) a lateral incision three fingerbreadths from the midline designed to include the iliac crest in the wound while the iliac crest is removed and dissection performed under the paraspinous musculature from lateral to medial; (2) a more medial paraspinous approach designed for muscle splitting and direct approach to the facet joint and transverse processes without including the iliac crest through that incision. A midline incision may be used for a bilateral paraspinous fusion. The incision must be long to allow adequate lateral retraction to help develop the incision in the lumbodorsal fascia and lateral approach to the paraspinous musculature.

6. Remove the bicorticate iliac spine graft. The incision in the paraspinous fascia is extended cephalad on the lateral border facet to the proximal level of the L4 transverse process. Medially, the interlaminar areas can be exposed for a canal decompression or a laminectomy (Fig. 38D).

7. Dissect under the fascia through the muscle with a finger or blunt instrument and sweep the muscle tissue from lateral to medial off the transverse processes. Dissect bluntly until the exact location of the transverse process is identified, then dissect with an elevator the muscle and fascial tissue from the transverse process.

8. Identify the L5–S1 facet joint. Lateral to this is the alar of the sacrum; cephalad to this is the transverse process of L5 (Figs. 38E, 38F).

Caution: Beware of the first posterior sacral foramen and its vessels. Avoid this by staying cephalad in the area of the ala of the sacrum.

9. Elevate the soft tissue from the dorsal surface of the transverse process of L5, the ala of the sacrum, and the L5–S1 facet joint. If L4 is to be fused, the same exposure should apply to the L4 transverse process and the L4–L5 joint.

Caution: Beware of the vessels between the transverse process of L5 and the ala of the sacrum. Avoid breaking the transverse process and causing bleeding anterior to the intertransverse muscles. The spinal nerves are anterior in the retroperitoneal space. Penetration of the retroperitoneal space in this area is possible.

10. Use a Hibbs or self-retaining Gelpi-type retractor to open the wound. Do not expose areas not to be fused. For fusions in this area, be sure the so-called gutter

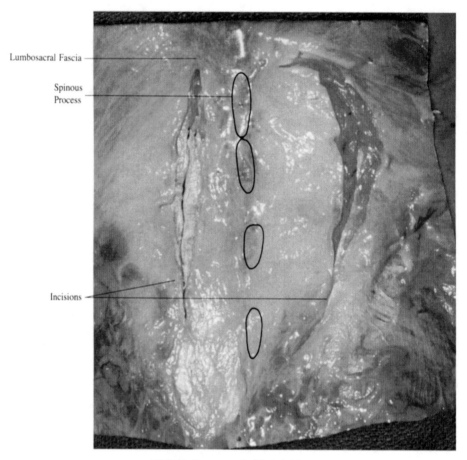

Lumbosacral Fascia

Spinous
Process

Incisions

FIGURE 38B. The paravertebral fascia incisions.

between the base of the transverse process and the base of the superior articular process is completely cleaned of soft tissue.

11. Closure: Reapproximate the lumbar fascia to the fascial tissue in the area of the removed posterosuperior iliac spine.

Laminectomy and Root Exploration Combined with Fusion

1. The approach is essentially as described above with a curved incision made through the lumbar fascia.

Open the fascia and dissect with your finger directly through the muscle to the transverse process of L5. Palpate the L5–S1 facet and ala of the sacrum.

2. With the periosteal elevator, remove the muscle attachments to the posterior elements in this area and expose the bone of the lamina, facet joint, and transverse process. Use a self-retaining Gelpi retractor to expose the posterior elements. No attempt is made to expose the spinous process tips.

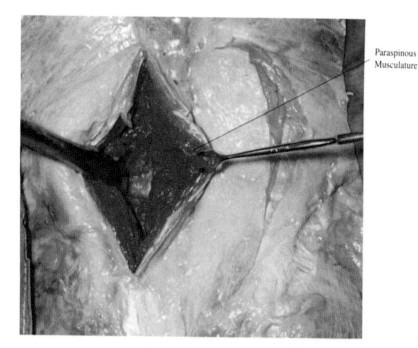

Paraspinous
Musculature

FIGURE 38C. The more medial paraspinous muscle-splitting incision. Open the fascia and dissect with your finger directly through the muscle to identify the L5–S1 facet, the ala of the sacrum lateral to that facet, and the L4–L5 joint cephalad. Remove the muscle attachments to the facets and transverse processes from L4 to the sacrum.

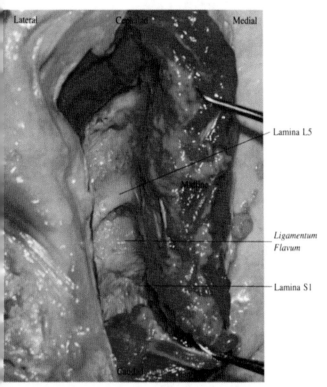

Lateral Cephalad Medial

Lamina L5

Midline

Ligamentum Flavum

Lamina S1

Caudad

FIGURE 38D. If a decompression is to be done, dissect more medially and clear the laminae of soft tissue.

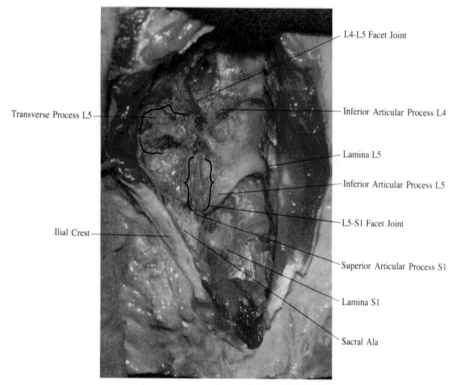

Transverse Process L5

Ilial Crest

L4-L5 Facet Joint

Inferior Articular Process L4

Lamina L5

Inferior Articular Process L5

L5-S1 Facet Joint

Superior Articular Process S1

Lamina S1

Sacral Ala

FIGURE 38E. Identify the L5–S1 facet. Lateral to this facet is the ala of the sacrum, and cephalad to this is the transverse process of L5. Beware of the first posterior sacral foramen and its vessel. Avoid this by staying cephalad at the level of the ala of the sacrum. Elevate the soft tissue from the dorsal surfaces of the transverse processes of L5, the ala of the sacrum, and the L5-S1 facet. Beware of the vessels between the transverse processes of L5 and the ala of the sacrum. Avoid breaking the transverse process. Spinal nerves are anterior in the retroperitoneal space and must be protected.

4. Removal of the lamina and canal exploration should proceed as described in Chapters 34 and 35.

5. A separate fascial incision should be made over the outer table of the iliac crest for the fusion. Remove the periosteum from the outer table, split the outer table, and obtain the graft.

6. Closure: Resuture the lumbar fascia and close the skin.

Midline Skin Incision

1. Often bilateral alar transverse fusions are done through a midline incision. Also, exposure of the ala of the sacrum may be needed for hook insertion for Harrington instrumentation. A sufficient longitudinal skin incision is required to allow full exposure under the skin and subcutaneous tissue.

2. When the pathology does not require a midline fascial incision, the same curved-type paraspinous fascial incision described above can be made bilaterally for the alar transverse fusion in combination with the midline skin and subcutaneous incision.

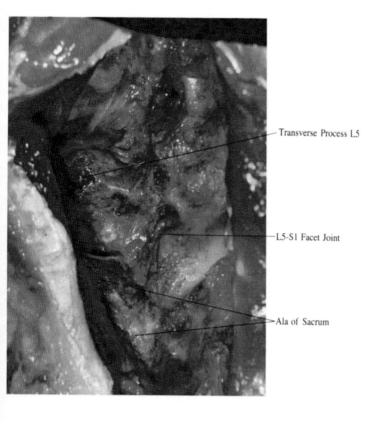

Transverse Process L5

L5-S1 Facet Joint

Ala of Sacrum

FIGURE 38F. A better view of the ala of the sacrum. For the more lateral approach, remove the medial 5–6 cm of the iliac crest using an osteotome. *Caution:* The clunial nerves will be in the lateral aspect of the wound and must be avoided. The safe margin of error is approximately one handbreadth lateral to the posterosuperior iliac spine. Removal of the posterosuperior iliac spine improves visualization. Then continue the exposure of the transverse processes, facets, and ala of the sacrum.

3. For pathology that requires a midline fascial incision such as a total laminectomy or Harrington instrumentation, cut directly to the spinous process and use a periosteal elevator to clean the muscle tissue from medial to lateral off the spinous processes, lamina, and dorsal surface of the sacrum. Muscle and fascia must be elevated medial to lateral out to the tips of the transverse processes. Bleeding is often encountered underneath the large amount of laterally retracted muscle and fascia and subcutaneous tissue.

4. Identify the transverse process of the 5th lumbar vertebrae. Locate this by identifying the L4–L5 facet. Use the base of the superior articular process of L5 to find the transverse process of L5. For the deepest L5 with partial sacralization of the transverse process of L5, the intertransverse space caudad to the transverse process of L5 may be minimal.

5. Identify the L5–S1 facet joint and the superior articular process of S1. The ala of the sacrum is much like a transverse process of S1 and is lateral and caudad to the superior articular process of S1.

Caution: Beware of the dorsal foramen of S1 and its accompanying vessels.

6. Dissect with a periosteal elevator laterally from the superior articular process of S1 to the ala of the sacrum. Verification by X-ray is very difficult, as in many cases the projection of the ala is on the anterior surface of the sacrum.

7. Remove the fascial attachments to the edge of the ala anteriorly and posteriorly with a periosteal elevator. Beware of bleeding in the intertransverse area between L5 and the ala. Packing of these areas when bleeding starts is often of greater benefit than excessive electrocautery. The retroperitoneal space and 5th lumbar nerve root are anterior to the structures and should not be violated in the approach.

8. With identification of the L5–S1 facet, the transverse process of L5, and the ala of the sacrum, any necessary procedure in this area can be completed.

9. Closure: Allow muscle layers to fall together; close fascia, subcutaneous tissue, and skin.

Remember:

1. Position the fascial incision so as to allow full retraction and proper exposure under the lumbar fascia.
2. Use finger palpation to identify the important structures, that is, transverse process of L5, L5–S1 facet joint, and ala of the sacrum.
3. Removal of a bicorticate posterosuperior iliac spine enhances exposure.
4. Use packing with hemostatic material when possible to control bleeding.
5. Avoid fracture and damage to the transverse process.
6. Expose the transverse process but beware of vessels and spinal nerves anterior to the intertransverse musculature.

Lateral Approach to the Disc

Robert G. Watkins III • *Robert G. Watkins IV*

1. The patient is positioned on a standard operating frame.

2. A skin incision is made two fingerbreadths lateral to the spinous process after lateral skin marking needles are aligned over the transverse processes of the involved segment. For L4–L5, the needle markers are aligned over the transverse process at L4 and the transverse process at L5. An incision is made from the transverse process to transverse process, two fingerbreadths off the spinous process (Fig. 38G).

3. The incision is carried through the skin subcutaneous tissue. The fascia is opened enough to admit an index finger that dissects down in a muscle-splitting dissection to the cephalad transverse processes. A Penfield 1 instrument is used to identify the transverse processes, or a small Cobb elevator is used to identify the transverse processes, but the vigorous muscle dissection is not carried out at this point. The finger also palpates medially on the cephalad transverse process to the area of the pars interarticularis, just cephalad to the facet joint. The Penfield 1 is rested on the more cephalad transverse process, and the McCulloch blade-spike retractor is placed. The blade is placed laterally against the soft tissue; then, the spike is placed medially just dorsal to the pars interarticularis. It is not hooked under the pars interarticularis.

4. Opening the retractor, the transverse process is visualized and a lateral film is obtained with a needle on the transverse process (Fig. 38H).

5. The Bovie and curette are used to dissect the soft tissue off the pars interarticularis, the base of the transverse process.

6. It is important to see the bone of the pars interarticularis. Too often the dissection is carried out too laterally. The transverse process is cleared off, but the actual location of the pedicle is more medial, and too much time is wasted in a more lateral position. Identify the pars and follow the bone of the transverse process back to the dorsal surface of the pedicle. At this point there are times when a portion of the cephalad facet joint, or cephalad lateral portion of the inferior facet, must be removed with the Kerrison to provide proper exposure of the intertransverse area. For better

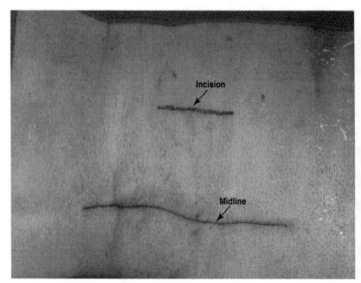

FIGURE 38G. An incision is made from the transverse process to transverse process, two fingerbreadths off the spinous process.

exposure, laterally, retract the muscle off the intertransverse ligament and hold it with the lateral blade retractor (Fig. 38H).

7. Using a straight curette and an angled curette, the intertransverse ligament is detached from the cephalad transverse process, the dorsal surface of the pedicle, and the lateral surface of the pars interarticularis. This ligament is identified, hooked with a blunt nerve hook, pulled laterally, and freed up with the small Kerrison under direct visualization.

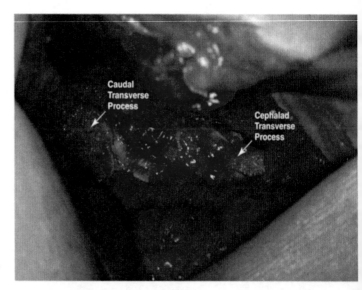

FIGURE 38H. Identify the two transverse processes.

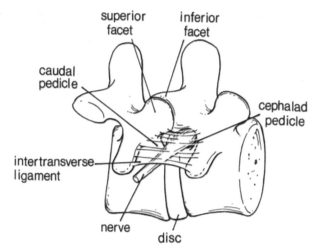

FIGURE 38I. Identify the nerve as it exits around and just caudal to the cephalad pedicle.

Caution: Distinguishing the ligament from the nerve is sometimes difficult. Proceed carefully.

8. Identify the nerve as it exits around and just caudal to the cephalad pedicle (Fig. 38I).

9. Use the Penfield 4 to gently palpate cephalad to the nerve, starting at the medial wall of the pedicle and progressing laterally. Beware of bleeding in this area.

10. Identify the caudal aspect of the nerve and use the microsucker retractor to retract the nerve cephalad. Using the Penfield 4, identify the disc caudal to the nerve. Beware; the dorsal ganglion of the nerve may feel like a disc fragment under the nerve. Carefully identify the nerve and the disc (Fig. 38J).

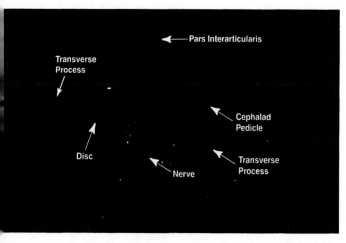

FIGURE 38J. Carefully identify the nerve and the disc.

Remember:

1. Identify the cephalad transverse process.
2. Identify pars interarticularis to stay medially.
3. The pedicle is the key landmark.
4. Laterally retract the intertransverse ligament.

References

1. Wiltse LL: The paraspinal muscle splitting approach to the lumbar spine. Clin Orthop 91:48–57, 1973.
2. Wiltse LL, Bateman JG, Hutchinson RH, Nelson WE: Paraspinal muscle approach to the lumbar spine. J Bone Joint Surg 50A:919, 1963.
3. Watkins MD: Posterior lateral fusion of the lumbar and lumbosacral spine. J Bone Joint Surg 34A:1014–1016, 1953.
4. Watkins MD: Posterior lateral fusion in pseudoarthrosis in posterior element defects of the lumbar spine. Clin Orthop 35:80, 1964.

Laparoscopic Approach to the L3–L4 and L4–L5 Intervertebral Discs

Namir Katkhouda • *Sanjay Ghosh* • *Srinath Samudrala*

Step 1: Positioning

The patient must be positioned to accommodate the laparoscopic surgeon (LS) at the patient's head and to the patient's right, the camera assistant (CA) to the patient's left, the spine surgeon (SS) at the patient's feet and to the right, and the anesthesiologist (A). The operating theater must allow for appropriate placement of television monitors, fluoroscopy monitors, and a c-arm.[1,2] The patient must be adequately secured to the table so that the steep Trendelenburg position may be used to assist with the exposure. The patient's arms should be folded over the chest to allow fluoroscopic visualization of the spine (Fig. 39A).

Step 2: Trocar Placement

A Veress needle is placed in the umbilicus (A) and the peritoneal cavity is insufflated to 15 mmHg pressure. A 10-mm trocar is then placed into the umbilicus (A), and the laparoscopic camera is placed into this port (Fig. 39B). Two other 10-mm trocars are placed at the level of the anterosuperior iliac spines just lateral to the rectus abdominis muscles (B, C). These ports allow the laparoscopic surgeon (S) to perform the dissection with the left hand through port C and the right hand through port B. The procedure will eventually require the placement of a 5-mm port to the left of the camera to assist with retraction of the transverse mesocolon (D). A final 18-mm port is then placed in the suprapubic area to accommodate the spinal instrumentation (E). The position of the ports in the axial plane can be modified to adapt for various levels of disc dissection.[3,4]

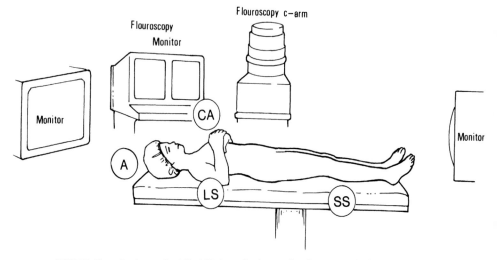

FIGURE 39A. The patient's arms should be folded over the chest to allow fluoroscopic visualization of the spine.

Step 3: Exposure of the Pelvic Brim

The patient is placed in steep Trendelenburg to allow the small bowel to fall out of the pelvis and away from the target site. This exposure is difficult if not impossible to achieve if the small bowel is distended. The patient should therefore have a bowel preparation preoperatively, which may involve a full liquid diet 2 days before surgery and a colon preparation the night before surgery.

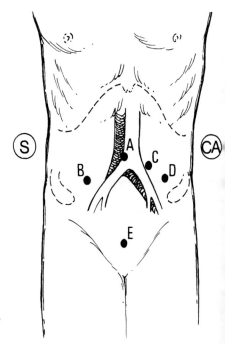

FIGURE 39B. Port positions for trocar placement.

Step 4: Retraction of the Sigmoid Colon

The sigmoid colon is then elevated with the mesocolon to expose the sacral promontory. Staples can be placed to secure the pericolic fat to the anterolateral abdominal wall to keep the sigmoid colon out of the field. Care must be taken to ensure that the pericolic fat alone is stapled.[5]

Step 5: Dissection Through the Peritoneum

The aorta and inferior vena cava can be visualized through the peritoneum. The ureters can also be visualized lateral to the lumbar vertebral bodies overlying the psoas muscles. The ureters are lateral to the disc space and can generally be avoided during the approach to the intervertebral disc space.

The peritoneum is incised using sharp dissection (Fig. 39C). At this point, only ligatures and pressure should be used to control bleeding. Monopolar electrocautery in this area may lead to injury of the hypogastric plexus of the sympathetic nerves, causing the complication of retrograde ejaculation in men.[6,7]

Step 6: Mobilization of the Left Illiac Artery and Vein

The aortic bifurcation is identified (Figs. 39D, 39E). In the crotch of the bifurcation lies the middle sacral artery. This vessel is ligated with vascular clips and divided, which

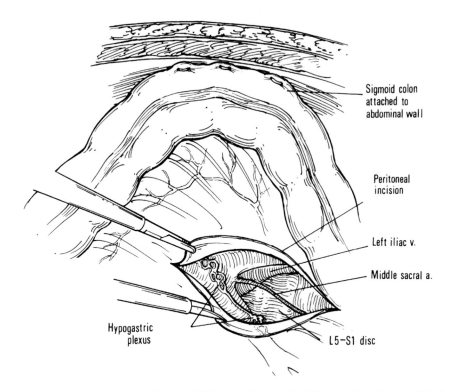

Sigmoid colon
attached to
abdominal wall

Peritoneal
incision

Left iliac v.

Middle sacral a.

Hypogastric
plexus

L5–S1 disc

FIGURE 39C. The peritoneum is incised using sharp dissection. Only ligatures and pressure should be used at this point to control bleeding. Electrocautery in this area may lead to injury of the hypogastric plexus.

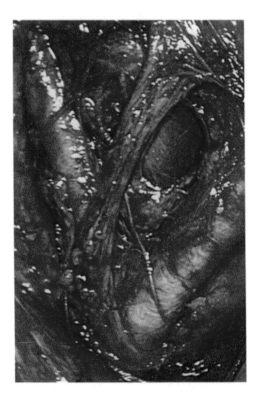

FIGURE 39D. Intraoperative view of the superior hypogastric plexus, left and right iliac arteries, and the left iliac vein.

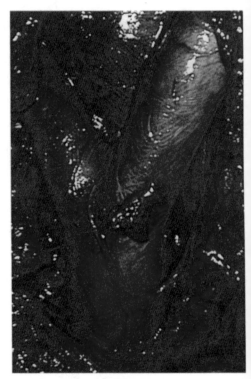

FIGURE 39E. Dissection of the aortic bifurcation and left iliac vein after the superior hypogastric plexus has been bluntly dissected laterally.

allows mobilization of the left iliac artery. A vessel loop should be placed around the left iliac artery and gently retracted to the left (Figs. 39F).

Medial to the left iliac artery lies the left iliac vein. Arising from this large vein is the iliolumbar vein. The iliolumbar vein must be isolated and divided to allow the mobilization of the left iliac vein. This step requires particular care. A tear in the iliolumbar vein is equivalent to an injury to the iliac vein and can prompt rapid conversion to an open procedure.[8,9]

Step 7: Identification of the L4–L5 Intervertebral Disc Space

After the left iliac artery and iliac vein are mobilized, gentle retraction may be placed on these vessels to expose the L4–L5 intervertebral disc space (Fig. 39G). The left iliac artery is mobilized to the patient's left and the left iliac vein is mobilized to the patient's right. It is also possible to retract both the iliac vein and artery together to the patient's right side once the iliolumbar vein is divided. This maneuver also provides exposure of the L4–L5 disc space.

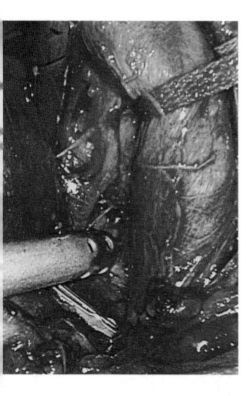

FIGURE 39F. Laparoscopic view of the L4–L5 intervertebral disc space with a vessel loop about the left iliac artery, a vessel clip on the iliolumbar vein, and the left iliac vein pushed laterally (see Fig. 39G).

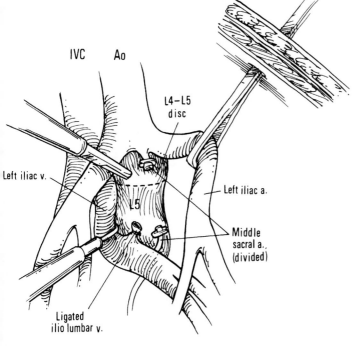

IVC   Ao

L4–L5 disc

Left iliac v.

Left iliac a.

L5

Middle sacral a. (divided)

Ligated ilio lumbar v.

FIGURE 39G. After the iliac artery and the iliac vein are mobilized, gentle retraction may be placed on these vessels to expose the L4–L5 intervertebral disc space. The left iliac artery is mobilized to the patient's left, and the left iliac vein is mobilized to the patient's right. *IVC*, inferior vena cava.

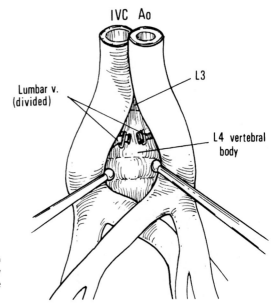

FIGURE 39H. The inferior vena cava (*IVC*) can be gently retracted away from the aorta (*Ao*) to reveal the L3–L4 intervertebral disc space.

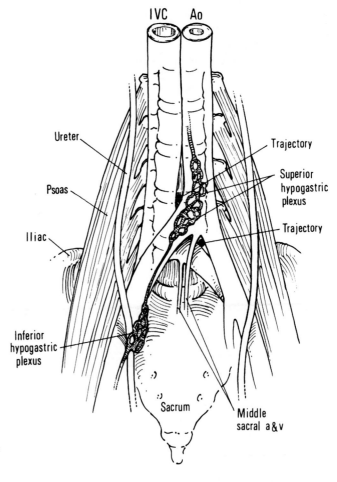

FIGURE 39I. The trajectory of the two approaches.

Step 8: Mobilization of the Aorta and Vena Cava

The peritoneum overlying the aorta and vena cava is identified. Gentle dissection identifies the space between these two vessels. The lumbar vein, which drains into the inferior vena cava and courses behind the aorta, can be isolated. This vein should be divided.[9,10]

Step 9: Identification of the L3–L4 Intervertebral Disc Space

The inferior vena cava can then be gently retracted away from the aorta to reveal the L3–L4 intervertebral disc space. The vena cava is retracted to the patient's right, and the aorta is retracted to the patient's left (Fig. 39H). Both great vessels can also be retracted together to the patient's right if the mobilization of the aorta and inferior vena cava is adequate.[11–13]

Figure 39I shows the trajectory of the two approaches. The L4–L5 intervertebral space is approached between the left iliac artery and vein after the middle sacral artery and the iliolumbar vein are divided. The L3–L4 disc space is approached between the aorta and inferior vena cava after the corresponding lumbar vein is divided.

Remember:

1. The superior hypogastric plexus lies over the aorta and vertebral bodies in the retroperitoneal space. Monopolar electrocautery should be avoided during this portion of the dissection.
2. Identify and ligate the middle sacral artery before mobilizing the left iliac artery.
3. Identify and ligate the iliolumbar vein before retracting the left iliac vein.
4. Dissect and ligate the lumbar vein draining into the inferior vena cava before separating the vena cava from the aorta.
5. These large arteries and veins must be protected during each step of spinal instrumentation.
6. An injury to the iliac vessels should lead to prompt conversion to an open procedure so that repair of the injured vessel can be performed.
7. The retroperitoneum should be closed at the end of the procedure.

References

1. Katkhouda N: Advanced Laparoscopic Surgery: Techniques and Tips. Philadelphia: Saunders, 1998, pp 157–163.
2. Cloyd DW, Obenchain TG, Savin M: Transperitoneal laparoscopic approach to lumbar discectomy. Surg Laparosc Endosc 5(2):85–89, 1995.
3. Regan JJ, McAfee PC, Guyer RD, Aronoff RG: Laparoscopic fusion of the lumbar spine in a multicenter series of the first 34 consecutive patients. Surg Laparosc Endosc 6(6):459–468, 1996.
4. Obenchain TG: Laparoscopic lumbar discectomy: case report. J Laparoendosc Surg 1(3):145–149, 1991.
5. Mahvi DM, Zdeblick TA: A prospective study of laparoscopic spinal fusion. Technique and operative complications. Ann Surg 224(1):85–90, 1996.
6. Olsen D, McCord D, Law M: Laparoscopic discectomy with anterior interbody fusion of L5–S1. Surg Endosc 10(12):1158–1163, 1996.
7. Maun RA: Laparoscopic L5–S1 diskectomy: a cost-effective, minimally invasive general surgery-neurosurgery team alternative to laminectomy. Am Surg 62(6):516–517, 1996.

8. Obenchain TG, Cloyd D: Laparoscopic lumbar discectomy: description of transperitoneal and retroperitoneal techniques. Neurosurg Clin N Am 7(1):77–85, 1996.
9. Slotman GJ, Stein SC: Laparoscopic L5–S1 diskectomy: a cost-effective, minimally invasive general surgery-neurosurgery team alternative to laminectomy. Am Surg 62(1):64–68, 1996.
10. Slotman GJ, Stein SC: Laparoscopic lumbar diskectomy: preliminary report of a minimally invasive anterior approach to the herniated L5–S1 disk. Surg Laparosc Endosc 5(5):363–369, 1995.
11. Mathews HH, Evans MT, Molligan HJ, Long BH: Laparoscopic discectomy with anterior lumbar interbody fusion. A preliminary review. Spine 20(16):1797–1802, 1995.
12. McAfee PC, Regan JR, Zdeblick T, Zuckerman J, Picetti GD, Heim S, Geis WP, Fedder IL: The incidence of complications in endoscopic anterior thoracolumbar spinal reconstructive surgery. A prospective multicenter study comprising the first 100 consecutive cases. Spine 20(14):1624–1632, 1995.
13. Zelko JR, Misko J, Swanstrom L, Pennings J, Kenyon T: Laparoscopic lumbar diskectomy. Am J Surg 169(5):496–498, 1995.

Transperitoneal Laparoscopic Approach to L5–S1

Salvador A. Brau

The patient is placed in the supine position on a Jackson table with an inflatable bag under the lumbar spine in case extension becomes necessary during the procedure. Shoulder supports should be placed, and straps applied across the thighs and chest to prevent the patient from slipping when placed in the deep Trendelenburg position. The table itself needs to be rigged so the maximum Trendelenburg position can be achieved. This positioning is very important so that the bowel can be kept away from the target area by using gravity rather than retractors. In addition, this position places the L5–S1 disc at a better angle for performance of the discectomy. A Foley catheter and a nasogastric tube are inserted to minimize obstruction to access by either a distended bladder or stomach, and to prevent injury to the bladder from trocar insertion near the symphysis pubis.

With the patient in the moderate Trendelenburg position, a small infraumbilical incision is made and a Veress needle inserted into the peritoneal cavity. Insufflation is then carried out to 15 mmHg, and then a 10-mm trocar is inserted followed by passage of the laparoscope. Two other 10-mm trocars are then inserted under direct vision to prevent inadvertent injury to any peritoneal contents. These trocars are placed at the midclavicular line to the right and to the left of the umbilicus (Figs. 40A, 40B). Careful exploration of the peritoneal cavity is then carried out for any other obvious pathology that may interfere with the planned procedure. If adhesions are found, they are then taken down using graspers for traction and endoscissors with cautery for dissection. Adhesions need to be taken down to allow for proper mobilization of the small bowel away from the pelvis and into the upper abdomen. If the bowel should be injured in this process, repair with endoscopic stapling devices can be carried out. If endoscopic repair proves difficult, an open laparotomy is then indicated. Under these circumstances, the endoscopic approach must then aborted because of the resulting contamination by bowel contents. The procedure, however, may be completed via the anterior muscle-sparing extraperitoneal approach if so desired, assuming the

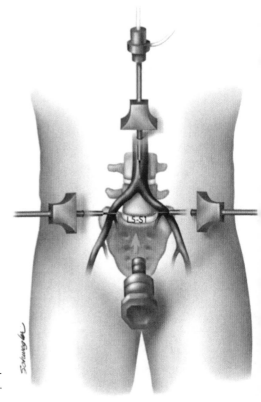

FIGURE 40A. Schematic of proper positioning of the trocars for L5–S1 fusion.

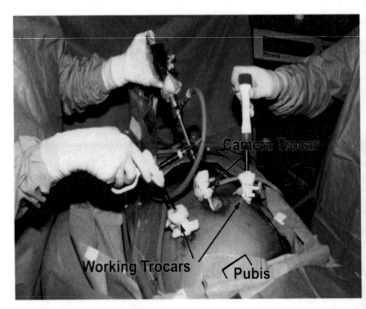

FIGURE 40B. The 10-mm upper trocars are in proper locations with instruments inserted into the peritoneal cavity.

contamination is minimal and the peritoneum is not entered during the extraperitoneal dissection.

After completion of the exploration, assuming there are no abnormal findings, the patient is placed in the deepest possible Trendelenburg position and the bowel is mobilized cephalad; this is done by first grasping the omentum with endoscopic Babcock forceps and draping it up over the stomach. The loops of small bowel are then grasped and carried cephalad to the upper abdomen to expose the sacral promontory. If the Trendelenburg position is adequate, gravity should keep these loops of bowel from obscuring the operative field for the duration of the procedure. The sigmoid colon may then need to be mobilized from its lateral peritoneal attachments using graspers and cautery and then also pushed cephalad toward the left upper quadrant. At this point, a fan retractor needs to be placed through the left trocar to hold the sigmoid colon laterally away from the sacral promontory (Fig. 40C).

The aortic bifurcation and both right and left iliac vessels as well as the right ureter can be easily identified at this point. The left ureter is not easy to visualize because it lies under and lateral to the mesocolon. Gentle poking with a blunt grasper is carried out between the iliac vessels until the sacral promontory becomes obvious. In all but the very obese patients, this landmark is easy to visualize and the poking simply serves to confirm its identification. The peritoneum overlying this area is then gently lifted and carefully incised transversely with endoscissors and without using any cautery to avoid injury to sympathetic fibers. There is an avascular plane here that allows incision of the peritoneum without any bleeding whatsoever.

Endoscopic Kittner pushers are then used to gently but firmly dissect laterally to both left and right, thus moving the sympathetic fibers away from harm and exposing the disc space. Any bleeding here should be controlled with pressure or small clips, but cautery must be avoided to prevent injury to the nerve fibers involved in the ejaculatory process in males. The middle sacral vessels are identified here and gently lifted with graspers and then clipped and transected. The cut ends are then pushed out of the way with soft blunt dissectors. Further lateral dissection is then carried out to com-

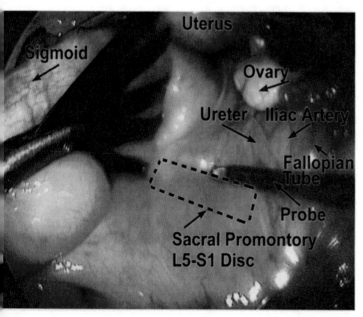

FIGURE 40C. Sacral promontory with sigmoid colon retracted to the left and iliac vessels and ureter under grasper to the right.

pletely expose the disc space. To the left, the iliac vein must be gently swept away from the anterior surface of the disc using Kittners and blunt dissectors. This dissection must be carried out very carefully because any tear or laceration of this vessel or one of its larger branches will precipitate an open laparotomy for control. Attempts to repair a possible iliac vein laceration laparoscopically can only lead to significant blood loss endangering the patient's life. Should this occur, the vessel can be repaired at laparotomy using standard vascular techniques with the spine procedure completed openly so long as the blood loss is not large enough to cause hemodynamic embarrassment.

The left iliac vein must be mobilized enough to allow insertion of a Steinmann pin into the body of L5 for retraction if necessary. The vessels on the right are not usually in contact with the disc space and exposure of the right side is therefore much easier. The vessels, however, must be clearly identified to avoid inadvertent injury. Once the disc space is completely exposed, a decision is made as to whether Steinmann pins will be necessary for retraction and adequate exposure. If needed, the pins are inserted percutaneously under direct vision as they enter the peritoneal cavity. They are guided with graspers to the midbody of L5 while the soft tissues are retracted away with soft pushers. The pins are then tapped into the vertebra with a mallet. Clear visualization is paramount here to avoid inadvertent piercing of the iliac vessels with the pins.

Once the exposure is considered acceptable, another Steinmann pin is inserted percutaneously and under direct vision at a point midway between the umbilicus and the pubis (Fig. 40D). This pin is guided into the disc, and fluoroscopy is used to document that the pin is indeed in the L5–S1 disc. In addition, this pin will help guide the placement of the working trocar through which the reaming sleeves and the distractors are inserted. These instruments need to be perpendicular to the anterior surface of the disc and parallel to the end plates of L5 and S1. By observing the angle of the pin in relation to the end plates, this working trocar can then be placed ideally to provide direct anteroposterior (AP) access to the disc space, which is done under close fluoroscopy guidance (Fig. 40E). In most cases, this location is 1 to 2 inches cephalad to the pubis. The inflatable bag is now expanded to produce extension and increase lordosis.

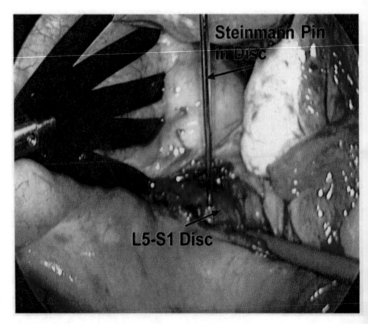

FIGURE 40D. Steinmann pin placed into disc percutaneously.

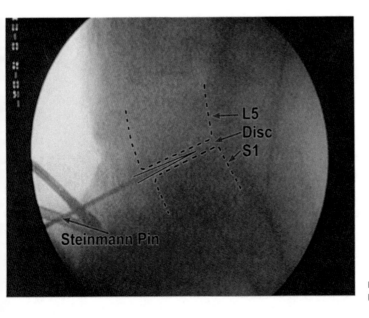

FIGURE 40E. Steinmann pin seen parallel to end plates on fluoroscopy.

Depending on the instrumentation being used, the appropriate trocar is then inserted under vision into the peritoneal cavity. Again using a Steinmann pin and fluoroscopy, the midline of the disc is identified and marked. Through this trocar (Fig. 40F) the appropriate sleeves are inserted, and through the sleeves discectomy, distraction, reaming, and insertion of the threaded devices are carried out. It is very important to carefully visualize the insertion of these sleeves until they are securely impacted into the vertebral bodies and later when they are removed (Fig. 40G). These sleeves have sharp spikes that could easily injure a vessel, and their edges could pinch off the side-

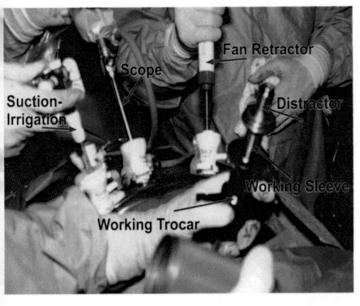

FIGURE 40F. Working trocar in the suprapubic position with distractor and sleeve inserted through it.

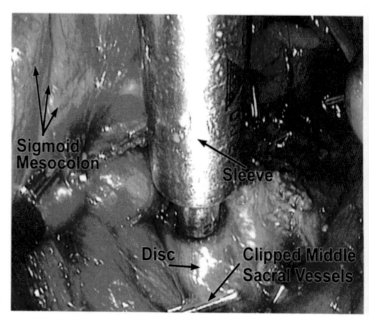

FIGURE 40G. Distractor in disc space; sleeve will pass over distractor under direct vision and anchor to vertebrae.

wall of an iliac vein, resulting in a tear followed by hemorrhage. Should this occur, immediate laparotomy is indicated.

Once the threaded devices are in place (Fig. 40H), irrigation with antibiotic solution is carried out and the operative field is inspected for hemostasis and evaluation of the vessels and other adjacent structures that may have been injured. Hemostasis is ob-

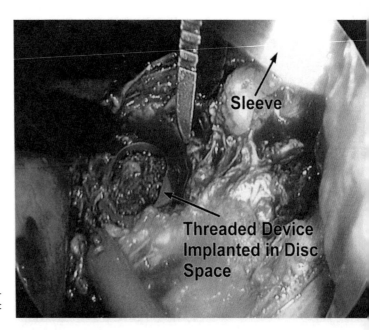

FIGURE 40H. Sleeve removed after insertion with threaded device in disc space.

tained with pressure and with endoclips applied to the bleeding area while it is being gently grasped with a blunt grasper. Use of cautery again is discouraged to avoid damage to neural structures. It is then optional to close the peritoneum over the devices. If elected, this can be done by grasping the edges of the peritoneum and approximating them while endostaples are applied to complete the closure.

The patient is then returned to a neutral position and the working trocars are removed under vision. The pneumoperitoneum is then evacuated and the camera trocar removed. The trocar sites are then closed using the surgeon's preferred method after infiltration with a local anesthetic. The nasogastric tube and Foley catheter can be removed before moving the patient to the recovery room.

Remember:

1. Rig the table so it can go into the deepest Trendelenburg position possible.
2. Avoid using cautery when exposing the disc to prevent injury to the superior hypogastric plexus (in males).
3. Try to visualize the left iliac vein, if possible; this helps prevent injury to that vessel.
4. If Steinmann pins are needed for retraction, make sure they are placed under direct vision to avoid injury to the left iliac vein.
5. If bleeding occurs from a suspected iliac vein injury, proceed with laparotomy immediately.
6. The procedure can be completed through laparotomy if such becomes necessary to control bleeding.
7. Use a Steinmann pin to determine the exact point of insertion of the working trocar.
8. Monitor closely the insertion and removal of the spiked sleeves to prevent injury to surrounding structures.
9. The entire procedure must be carefully monitored laparoscopically, even after the sleeves are in place.
10. In males use clips rather than cautery to obtain hemostasis.

Balloon-Assisted Endoscopic Retroperitoneal Gasless (BERG) Approach to the Lumbar Spine

John S. Thalgott • *John A. Ameriks* • *Frank T. Jordan* •
James M. Giuffre

1. The balloon-assisted endoscopic retroperitoneal gasless (BERG) approach is executed with one spinal surgeon, one vascular/general surgeon, and one endoscopically trained technician (Fig. 41A).

2. The patient is placed in the supine position. Following general anesthesia, the patient is draped and prepped in standard fashion and preoperative antibiotics are given. Fluoroscopy is used to find the landmarks of the appropriate lumbar level. The skin is marked identifying the level and angle of the pathologic disc interspace(s). These marks are drawn on the lateral aspect of the left abdomen, marking the angles of the disc spaces to be addressed (Fig. 41B).

3. A transverse 20-mm left flank incision is made approximately 1 cm above the left iliac crest in the midaxillary line (Fig. 41B). The dissection is taken down through the external oblique, internal oblique, and transversus muscles under direct vision to the preperitoneal fat layer using a clear-ended, laparoscopic dissecting port.

4. The retroperitoneal space is then gently insufflated with a bulb syringe and then digitally dissected into the iliac fossa to allow for balloon insertion. An undeployed elliptical-shaped preperitoneal balloon (PDB-2; Origin Medsystems, Meno Park, CA) is advanced through the incision until the entire balloon is within the retroperitoneal space (Fig. 41C).

5. A 0-degree-angle endoscope is placed through the lumen of the dissection cannula, and the balloon is expanded to an approximate volume of 1 L (Fig. 41D).

6. The endoscope is directed toward the anterior abdominal wall; this allows the identification of the peritoneal reflection on the anterior abdominal wall, at the rectus sheath above and below the line of Douglas (Fig. 41E).

7. The peritoneal reflection is used as a landmark for the anterior working/re-

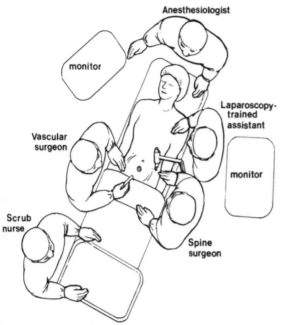

FIGURE 41A. Operating room setup and patient positioning.

traction port. The anterior working/retraction port is located lateral to the peritoneal reflection on the rectus sheath.

8. This port is formed at a level determined by the preoperative markings on the abdomen that corresponds to the interspace angulation. A 2- to 3-cm paramedian incision is made through the anterior abdominal wall and carried down through the fascia.

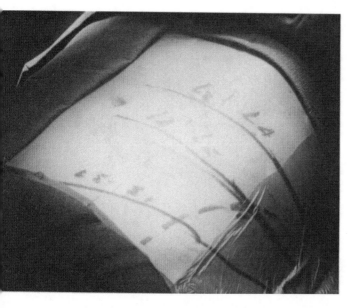

FIGURE 41B. Following fluoroscopy, the angle of disc spaces to be addressed are marked on the lateral aspect of the abdomen. The initial left flank incision is made approximately 1 cm above the iliac crest in the midaxillary line.

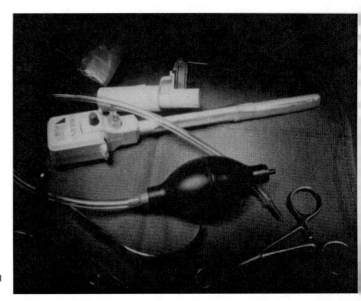

FIGURE 41C. The PDB-2 (preperitoneal dissection balloon-2).

This incision is done lateral to the peritoneal reflection and with great care to avoid the peritoneal sac; this creates the anterior working/retraction port (Fig. 41F).

9. The balloon is removed after a 1-cm malleable retractor is placed between the two ports under direct endoscopic vision. Once the retroperitoneal space has been mobilized, the next goal is the retraction of the abdominal contents.

10. Three levels of retraction are necessary to access the anterior lumbar spine. The first of these is distraction of the anterior abdominal wall, which is accomplished by the insertion of a Laprofan retractor (Origin Medsystems) into the flank port (Fig. 41G).

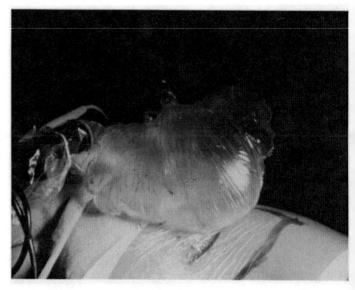

FIGURE 41D. The PDB-2 expanded to an approximate volume of 1 L.

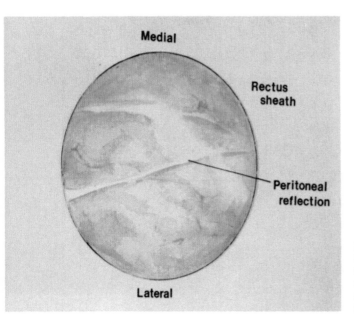

Medial

**Rectus
sheath**

**Peritoneal
reflection**

Lateral

FIGURE 41E. The endoscope is directed toward the anterior abdominal wall. Location of the peritoneal reflection marks the lateral line where the anterior working/retraction port is fashioned.

11. The Laprofan is expanded under direct endoscopic vision. Once expanded, the Laprofan is attached to a mechanical lifting arm, the Laprolift (Origin Medsystems) (Fig. 41H).

12. The abdominal wall is elevated by the Laprolift/Laprofan combination, creating the retroperitoneal space and replacing the need for gas. A flexible nonvalved port, utilized for lateral visualization and retraction, is placed directly below the legs of the fan retractor to provide a clean path for the endoscope (see Fig. 41F).

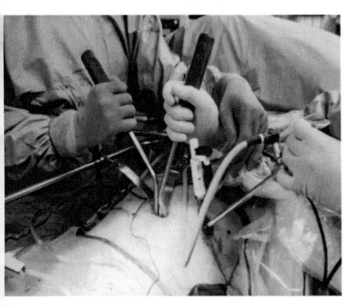

FIGURE 41F. The anterior working/ retraction port to the left, with the Laprofan/Laprolift combination retracting the abdomen to the right. The visualization/retraction port is shown below the Laprofan retractor within the initial left flank incision.

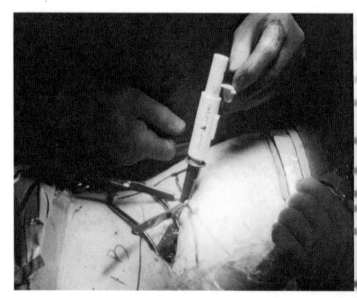

FIGURE 41G. The Laprofan retractor shown to scale with both fans extended.

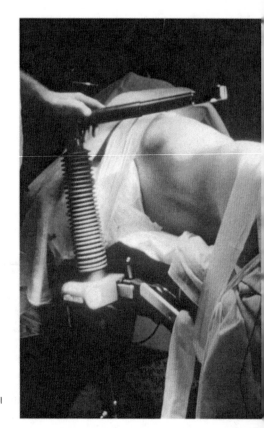

FIGURE 41H. The Laprolift mechanical arm.

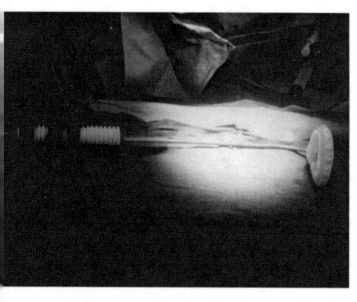

FIGURE 41I. The Helping Hand retractor.

13. The second level of retraction is necessary to displace the peritoneal contents past the midline to provide access to the lumbar spine and vascular anatomy. The Helping Hand retractor (Origin Medsystems) is inserted through the newly created lateral working port in the initial left flank incision to push the peritoneal sac and intraabdominal contents aside, creating the working space (Figs. 41I, 41J).

14. The third level of retraction in this approach is vascular. Following establishment of the operative cavity, the psoas muscle and vascular anatomy are used as reference landmarks. The psoas muscle is bluntly dissected to expose the pathologic disc space(s).

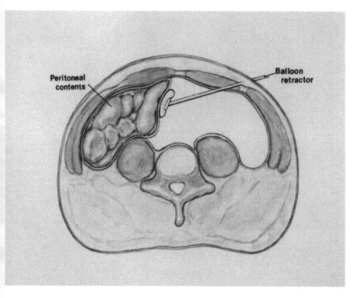

FIGURE 41J. The Helping Hand retractor is used to push the peritoneal contents laterally to expose the anterior spine.

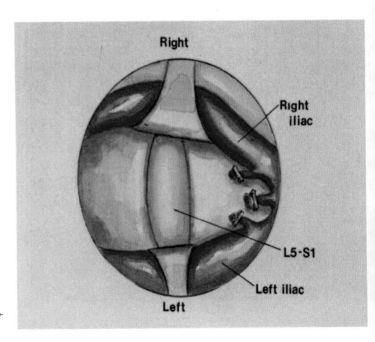

15. The L5–S1 vascular retraction begins by identifying the right iliac vein and utilizing an AO anterior vascular retractor to retract the fascia and presacral veins, thereby exposing the anterior aspect of the L5–S1 interspace. Through the visualization/retraction port, a standard vein retractor is passed and is used to retract the iliac vein

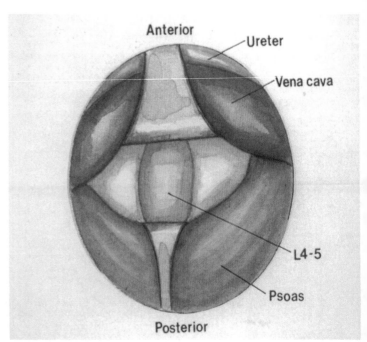

FIGURE 41L. Vascular dissection to obtain access to the L4–L5 interspace.

laterally. Once this is done, the presacral veins are ligated or cauterized with bipolar cautery. Great care must be used to in dissecting the anterior soft tissues to maintain the integrity of the presacral plexus (Fig. 41K).

16. The L4–L5 exposure is more complex. It begins by utilizing the AO anterior vessel retractor and displacing the vena cava or left iliac vein; this is placed on tension and the iliolumbar vein is identified. The iliolumbar vein is ligated using a right-angled clip and corporeal knot tying; this is generally reenforced with two specific ligatures. The posterior aspect of the iliolumbar vein can be handled with vascular clips. Once the iliolumbar vein is ligated, gentle soft dissection is used to retract the left iliac vein, exposing the L4–L5 interspace past the midline (Fig. 41L).

17. The vascular retraction for L3–L4 is performed in a similar way but does not require ligation of the iliolumbar vein.

18. Following psoas dissection and vessel retraction, a spinal needle is placed into the disc and fluoroscopy is used to confirm the operative level. The anterior working port allows for both vascular retraction and the introduction of standard spinal instruments such as dissectors, rongeurs, curettes, and endplate cutters.

19. Our experience with the BERG approach has consisted of anterior lumbar interbody fusion (ALIF).

Remember:

1. Careful delineation of retroperitoneal space from the flank incision, that is, the visualization/retraction port.
2. The PDB-2 balloon must be contained within the retroperitoneal space.
3. Visualization of the lateral reflection of the peritoneum on the rectus sheath must be identified for the anterior working port.
4. Great care must be taken to open the retroperitoneum *lateral* to the peritoneal reflection at the rectus sheath.

42

Video Endoscopic Approach to the Thoracic Spine

Salvador A. Brau

An anterior approach is optimal for many disease processes of the thoracic spine. These approaches have required a posterolateral thoracotomy to access the vertebral bodies or intervertebral disc spaces. This procedure carries with it the same known incisional morbidity of any intrathoracic procedure, making video-assisted thoracoscopic surgical techniques the clear choice in treating diseases of the thoracic spine. All patients sign a consent for video-assisted thoracoscopic surgery (VATS) of the spine with possible open thoracotomy and understand that such will be performed if VATS is unsuccessful.

All procedures should be performed under general endotracheal anesthesia with either a double lumen or Univent tube to allow for ipsilateral lung collapse and single lung ventilation. The patient is placed on a beanbag in the lateral decubitus position with the table maximally flexed to widen the intercostal spaces. The spine can be approached from either side, with the determining factor being the side to which the pathology presents. Because the spine is posterior, the patient should be rotated slightly anteriorly (20 to 30 degrees) to allow more anterior trocar placement. Placing the trocars too far posteriorly will make the visualization and work very difficult, especially when trying to identify the pedicles and the canal. A 30-degree-angle viewing scope should be used, and the surgeon and camera operator both stand on the ventral side of the patient. For proper orientation, the spine should be kept on the horizontal plane on the video monitor.

Trocar placement depends on the level of the spine to be approached, with the initial trocar inserted two levels above the affected disc space or vertebra at the anterior axillary line (Fig. 42A). Ventilation to the ipsilateral lung is stopped to allow the lung to start collapsing before entering the pleural cavity. A 10-mm horizontal skin incision is then made at the chosen site, and a hemostat is used to spread the muscles and enter the pleural cavity by gently poking into it. A finger is then inserted through this incision to check for adhesions, which if found can be cleared with finger dissection to

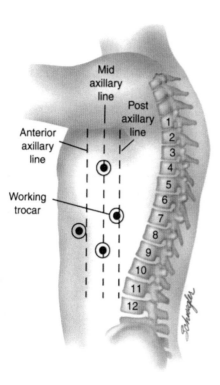

FIGURE 42A. Diagram for trocar positions at T5–T6 for pathology at T7–T8.

allow for a large enough space to insert a trocar. A 10-mm, 30-degree-angled scope is then inserted through this trocar and an initial exploratory thoracoscopy is performed. If adhesions are found, a second and third trocars are then inserted under vision to avoid lung injury. One should be two levels above and the other two levels below the original trocar and both slightly more anterior (Fig. 42B). Through these working channels, the adhesions can be taken down using graspers, cautery, and the endoscissors. Any small pleural tears can be ignored at this time as they will seal spontaneously. Larger tears to the lung and pleura may need to be repaired using standard stapling techniques.

A fan retractor is then used to help finish collapsing the lung (by gently pushing on it) and to hold it anteriorly and visualize the spine through the parietal pleura. The target level is then tentatively identified by counting the ribs. The 1st rib is not visible through the parietal pleura, but it can be palpated with a blunt grasping instrument. The appropriate rib is followed and its base identified (Fig. 42C). A long needle or pin is then inserted percutaneously into the pleural cavity and guided with a grasper into the disc space adjacent to the rib head (Fig. 42D). Radiologic confirmation is then obtained.

If no adhesions are found (as should be the case in most cases not having prior pulmonary pathology or surgery), then it is best to try to identify the site before inserting additional trocars; this will allow for more accurate placement of these ports in relation to the target. The scope itself can be used to help collapse the lung and also to push it anteriorly to visualize the spine. In some cases, a brief period of carbon dioxide insufflation with 8 to 10 cm of water pressure may be necessary to complete resorptive

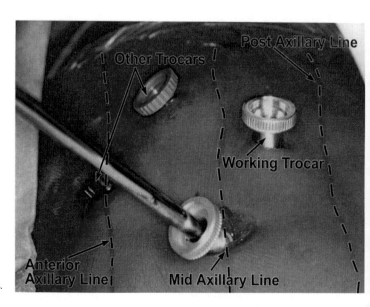

FIGURE 42B. Actual trocar positions.

atelectasis and enhance collapse of the lung. As the procedure progresses, the lung can usually be kept from crowding the field by more anterior rotation combined with either Trendelenburg or reverse Trendelenburg position, depending on the level. The fan retractor can then be removed and that port used as a working channel.

The fourth trocar, 12 mm in size, is then inserted as close to parallel to the level of the pathology as possible and more posterior than the first trocar. This trocar will be the main working channel through which the orthopedic instruments pass. This placement also provides two ports at the level of the disc or vertebral body to be approached

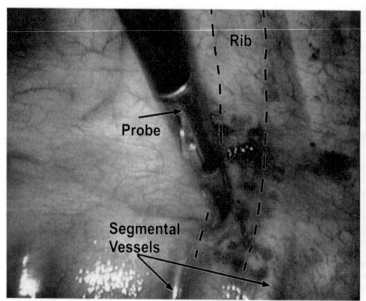

FIGURE 42C. Appropriate rib identified between segmental vessels.

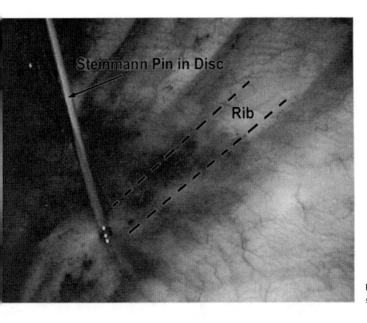

FIGURE 42D. Pin inserted into disc space for radiologic confirmation.

and will be helpful in the dissection because the scope sometimes must be passed through either the upper or lower trocars then directed to the site, taking advantage of the 30-degree angle.

Electrocautery is then used to divide the parietal pleura, starting at the base of the adjacent rib then progressing to the anterior longitudinal ligament and any surrounding soft tissues (Fig. 42E). The parietal pleura is reflected using blunt graspers and pushers until the segmental vessels lying in fat midway between the vertebral bodies are exposed caudad and cephalad to the level of the disc involved (Fig. 42F). For most

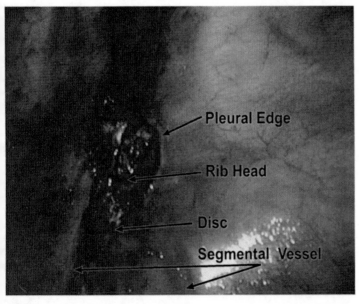

FIGURE 42E. Initial cautery dissection vertically along head of rib.

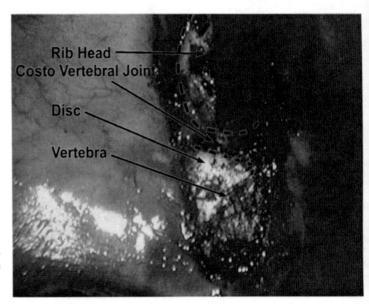

FIGURE 42F. Demonstration of costovertebral joint with dissection from rib head to vertebral body.

cases, it is not necessary to ligate these vessels, but if inflammation, tumor, or a collapsed vertebral body is present, then vessels in the area are identified and ligated early on. This step is done by gently dissecting under them and ligating with endoclips, then gently pushing them away with pushers and blunt graspers. The inflammatory mass can then be entered carefully, watching out for neovascular formation in the area. When no such pathology exists, the base of the rib, the rib head, and the disc space should then be clearly visible and ready for resection.

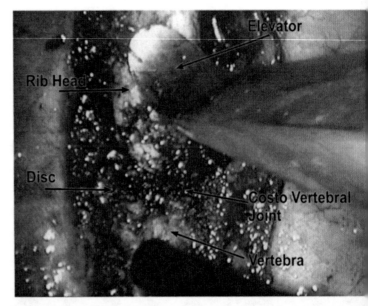

FIGURE 42G. Curved elevator initiating dissection of rib head for excision.

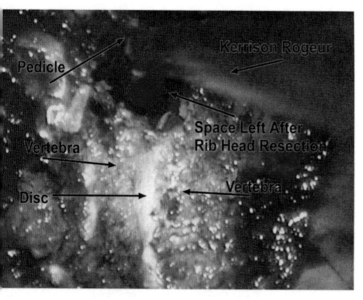

FIGURE 42H. Dissection into disc space after removal of rib head.

Standard orthopedic instruments are then introduced and resection of the rib head is carried out (Fig. 42G). In doing this, the intercostal vessels, which course along the caudal edge of the rib, may be lacerated. Endoclips and cautery are usually effective in obtaining hemostasis in this area. It is best, however, to exercise extreme care in dissecting the rib to avoid injury to these vessels, because inability to obtain control with clips and cautery may lead to an open thoracotomy. Continuous suction is necessary when cautery is used to keep visibility optimal. Resection of the rib head leads directly into the disc space where further dissection is then carried out by standard orthopedic technique. (Fig. 42H). At times the instruments may be too large to pass through the largest trocar. The trocar can then be removed and the instrument inserted directly through the chest wall (Fig. 42I).

If a multilevel discectomy for spinal deformity is attempted, additional trocars may be inserted as necessary to obtain adequate visualization and access. These trocars must be inserted under direct vision to avoid injury to the lung.

Unexplained bleeding must be investigated immediately because injury to the great vessels requires immediate open thoracotomy. Subcutaneous emphysema noted during the procedure may be a clue to a lung laceration and must also be evaluated as soon as it is observed. A small visceral pleural tear is enough to produce this and should be repaired by standard thoracoscopic technique once discovered. If no apparent cause for the emphysema is found, and it persists, then a tracheal tear due to the insertion of the double lumen tube must be suspected and the procedure may need to be aborted. Bronchoscopy then needs to be performed to further evaluate the situation, with appropriate treatment depending on the findings.

After completion of the orthopedic procedure, a single 22 French argyle chest tube is inserted through the most caudad trocar and placed adjacent to the operative site with the tip near the apex. The parietal pleura need not be closed. Copious irrigation with antibiotic solution is then carried out and hemostasis obtained as needed. The lung is then allowed to expand under direct vision to ensure that all segments are ventilating properly. The trocar sites are then closed using absorbable 2-0 sutures for the fascia and staples for the skin. The chest tube is secured with 2-0 silk and connected to underwater seal and suction.

A postoperative chest X-ray is then taken to ensure complete expansion of the lung. The chest tube is left in place until there is no air leak or until drainage is less than

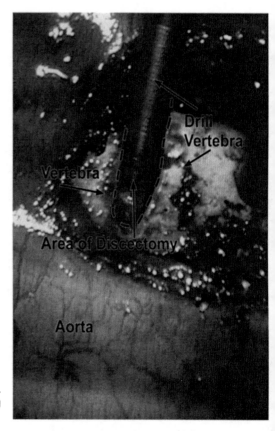

FIGURE 42I. Disc removed. Intervertebral space being prepared with drill for insertion of bone graft.

150 mL in a 24-hour period; this usually happens within 24 hours, and the chest tube is removed the day after surgery.

The advantage of the video endoscopic technique is the lessened morbidity attributable to the minimally invasive approach. Magnification and video monitoring appear to provide excellent visualization, and as a result there has been no compromise in the ability to decompress the spinal canal with no additional surgical time or risk.

Remember:

1. Rotate the patient slightly anteriorly and stop ventilation to the ipsilateral lung before initial trocar placement.
2. Insert additional trocars under direct vision.
3. After lung collapse, unexplained bleeding and subpleural emphysema must be investigated immediately.
4. Confirm level radiographically before initiating dissection.
5. Carefully dissect undersurface of the rib to avoid injury to intercostal vessels.
6. Segmental vessels need not be ligated in most cases, but should be controlled if there is any doubt that they will be in the way of the exposure.
7. Pleura need not be reapproximated at the end of the procedure.
8. Observe lung expansion before scope removal and closure of trocar sites.
9. Use the lowermost trocar site for insertion of the chest tube.
10. Do a postoperative X-ray to ensure full lung expansion.

Microendoscopic Discectomy for Lumbar Disc Herniations: Paramedian and Far Lateral Approaches

Kevin T. Foley · Maurice M. Smith · Y. Raja Rampersaud

Paramedian Approach

1. Microendoscopic discectomy (MED) can be performed under local, regional, or general anesthesia. Epidural anesthesia is preferred, because it is more comfortable for the patient than local anesthesia and avoids the side effects of general anesthesia. The anesthesiologist should place the epidural catheter while the patient is in the preoperative holding area. The catheter should be inserted in an upper lumbar or lower thoracic interspace well away from the operative field.

2. In the operating room, place the anesthetized patient in the prone position with abdomen free and spine flexed to open the interlaminar space. Position a C-arm fluoroscope to obtain lateral fluoroscopic images of the operative interspace. Check these images before prepping and draping the patient to ensure that the operative level can be visualized. A typical operating room setup is pictured in Figure 43A.

3. After the operative field has been prepped and draped, attach the flexible arm assembly to the operating table rail ipsilateral to the disc herniation; the arm will hold the tubular retractor/endoscope assembly in position, freeing the surgeon's hands. Palpate the lumbar midline and mark this line with a surgical pen. Draw a second line parallel to the midline, approximately one fingerbreadth (1.5 cm) to the side of the disc herniation. Insert a 22-gauge spinal needle into the paraspinous tissues along this paramedian line at the approximate level of the appropriate disc space. Under fluoroscopic guidance, reposition the needle until an imaginary line drawn along the needle is parallel to the vertebral endplates and bisects the disc space (Fig. 43B). At the L5–S1 interspace, where the end plates are typically divergent, the needle trajectory should be parallel to the L5 end plate. Accurate placement of the skin incision directly in line with the final surgical target (e.g., disc space) facilitates optimal use of the space within the tubular retractor; this optimizes the various trajectories attainable by the surgical instrument(s) without having to move the tubular retractor. Adhering to this principle

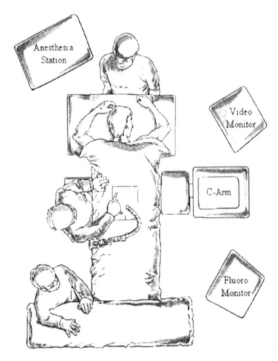

FIGURE 43A. The typical operating room setup for a microendoscopic discectomy (MED). The surgeon is positioned ipsilateral to the disc herniation. The video monitor (contralateral side) is placed in the surgeon's functional line of sight, and the fluoroscopy monitor is placed toward the foot of the patient.

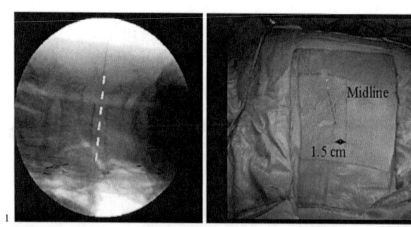

FIGURE 43B. The incision is placed along a paramedian line located 1.5 cm from the midline, ipsilateral to the side of the disc herniation. (1) Using fluoroscopy, the trajectory of a 22-gauge spinal needle should be parallel to the vertebral end plates and bisect the disc space, as illustrated. (2) It is important to ensure that the skin incision is accurately placed in line with the surgical pathology.

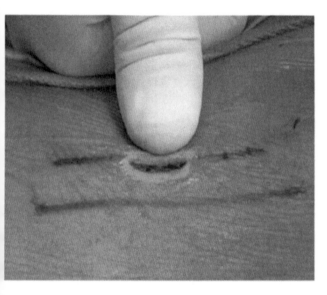

FIGURE 43C. A 15-mm longitudinal skin incision is made to the depth of the superficial subcutaneous tissue.

significantly improves the efficiency of this procedure. Withdraw the needle and make a 15-mm longitudinal incision centered at the needle puncture site. Carry the incision into the superficial subcutaneous tissues only (Fig. 43C).

4. Insert the 12-inch, 0.062-diameter guidewire through the incision under fluoroscopic guidance. Direct the guidewire toward the inferior edge of the superior lamina. Stop advancing it after the dorsal lumbar fascia has been penetrated (Fig. 43D).

5. Insert the cannulated soft tissue dilators over the guidewire and each other (Fig. 43E). After the first dilator has penetrated the dorsal lumbar fascia, remove the

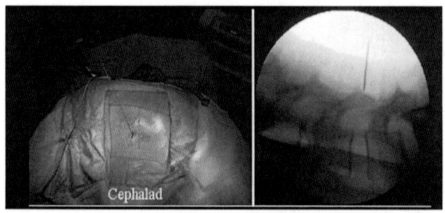

FIGURE 43D. (1) External and (2) fluoroscopic images illustrate placement of the guidewire through the dorsolumbar fascia toward the inferior laminar edge.

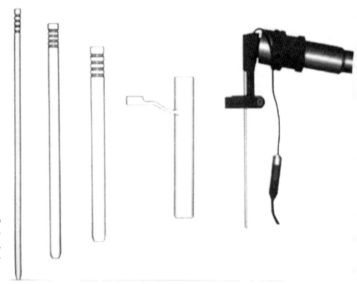

FIGURE 43E. Illustrated from *left* to *right* are the three cannulated sequential dilators (5.3 mm, 10 mm, 14.5 mm), the 16-mm tubular retractor, and the 25-degree endoscope.

guidewire and advance the dilator until it is docked on the inferior edge of the superior lamina. Confirm the positioning of the dilator in the sagittal plane using lateral fluoroscopy (Fig. 43F). It is important to obtain a true lateral image to avoid erroneous information from the bony landmarks of the contralateral side. Determine axial plane orientation by palpating the lamina with the tip of the initial dilator; it should lie just lateral to the base of the spinous process and just above the laminar edge.

6. Use the first dilator to gently dissect the soft tissue from the dorsal aspect of the laminar edge; this allows for easier identification of this important landmark. Place the second and third dilators over the first in a sequential manner, establishing an

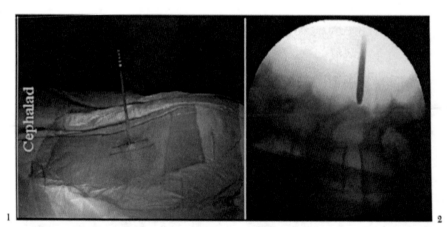

FIGURE 43F. (1) External and (2) fluoroscopic images illustrate docking of the initial dilator tip onto the inferior edge of the superior lamina. Confirmation of this important landmark is easily accomplished by "walking" the tip of a dilator in the caudal direction until the stepoff into the interlaminar space is identified and confirmed fluoroscopically.

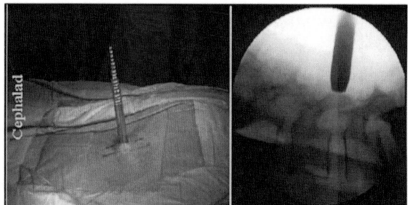

FIGURE 43G. (1) Placement of the sequential dilators with a rotating motion gently dilates the fascia and paraspinal muscles to establish the initial operative corridor to the disc space. (2) Fluoroscopy is used to confirm that each dilator is docked onto bone; this minimizes the amount of soft tissue that can enter into the tubular retractor.

operative corridor between the fibers of the lumbar paraspinous muscles, but leaving their normal spinal attachments intact (Fig. 43G).

7. Advance the tubular retractor over the third dilator, down to the lamina. Maintain downward pressure on the dilators so that they remain docked and paraspinous tissue cannot enter the retractor. Connect the tubular retractor to the flexible arm assembly to maintain its position. Confirm the position of the retractor fluoroscopically and remove the dilators (Fig. 43H).

8. Connect the endoscope to the coupler and camera, the light source, and a suction tube. White balance the endoscope. Insert the endoscope into the tubular retractor. Secure the endoscope to the retractor using the attached ring clamp. The endoscope can be positioned anywhere within the 360-degree arc of the tubular retractor (Fig. 43I) and can be advanced or withdrawn within the retractor, allowing for variable

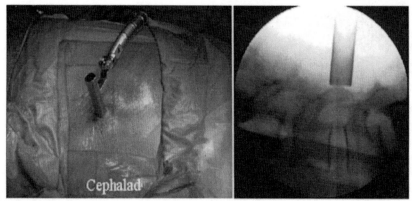

FIGURE 43H. (1) The tubular retractor is centered on the laminar edge. This position is confirmed fluoroscopically (2) and the retractor is locked in place as shown on the *left*.

magnification (Fig. 43J). Condensation on the endoscope lens is removed by attaching the aspiration port to suction. Other extraneous matter can be removed from the lens by irrigation or by removing the endoscope, wiping the lens, and reinserting it.

9. After the endoscope is inserted into the tubular retractor, orient the video image to correspond with the underlying anatomy (Fig. 43K). Medial anatomy should appear at the top of the video screen (12 o'clock), and lateral anatomy should appear at the bottom (6 o'clock). To achieve proper orientation, place a surgical instrument in a lateral anatomical position within the tubular retractor. Rotate the camera/coupler until the video image shows the instrument at the bottom of the video screen.

10. Identify the inferior edge of the superior lamina using a curette. Remove residual soft tissue overlying the lamina with a pituitary rongeur or clear soft tissue using electrocautery (a Bovie with an extended tip). Provide hemostasis with either the Bovie or the modified bipolar forceps (Fig. 43L).

11. Detach the ligamentum flavum from the undersurface of the lamina using the small, angled curette (Fig. 43M). Proceed with laminotomy or medial facetectomy using the various Kerrison punches or a modified high-speed drill, if bone work is necessary (Fig. 43N). Open the ligamentum flavum with the angled curette and remove it in piecemeal fashion with a Kerrison rongeur (Fig. 43O). In general, use the 90-degree Kerrisons when working medially or inferiorly and the 40-degree Kerrisons when working superiorly or laterally.

12. There is an initial tendency to "cone" the exposure down to the final target. Inadequate exposure restricts the already confined working space of the tubular retractor. To avoid this, it is important to complete soft tissue or bony exposure at each level before proceeding into the epidural space; this allows for optimal utilization of the available working space within the tubular retractor and improves efficiency. Further, obtain progressive hemostasis to avoid pooling of blood from above the level of interest.

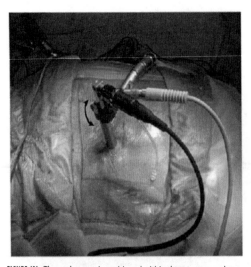

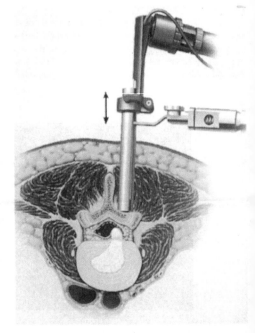

FIGURE 43I. The endoscope is positioned within the retractor and can be rotated 360 degrees around the retractor perimeter. This usage ensures optimal visualization of a given area and allows the surgeon to move the endoscope assembly if it impedes an instrument's trajectory, without having to move the entire retractor.

FIGURE 43J. Magnification of the anatomy is achieved by telescoping (*arrow*) the endoscope within the tubular retractor.

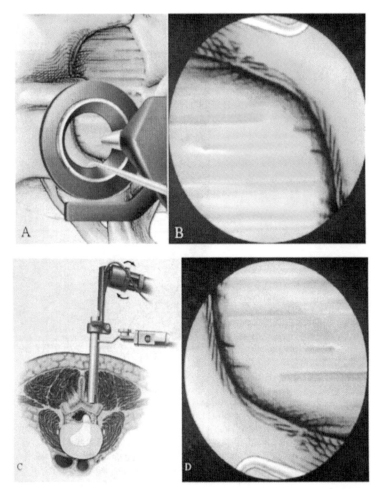

FIGURE 43K. (A, B) The initial orientation of the endoscopic picture relative to the patient's anatomy is random. The picture is oriented by placing an instrument in the lateral anatomical position of the tubular retractor. (C, D) The camera/coupler mechanism is then rotated until the image corresponds to the patient's orientation.

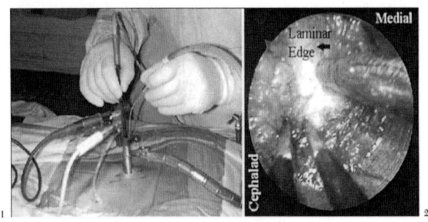

FIGURE 43L. (1) External and (2) endoscopic images illustrate the use of the bipolar cautery and suction to achieve hemostasis along the laminar edge.

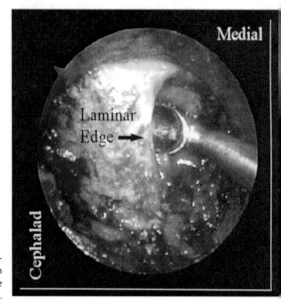

FIGURE 43M. Endoscopic image illustrates detachment of the ligamentum flavum from the undersurface of the inferior aspect of the superior lamina.

13. To operate beyond the confines of the tubular retractor, "wand" the retractor. Wanding is accomplished by loosening the flexible arm, pivoting the tubular retractor within the small skin incision, and tightening the arm. Pedicle-to-pedicle access can thus be achieved through the initial 15-mm incision (Fig. 43P). This maneuver may be necessary if the surgeon cannot access a particular surgical "target," such as a portion of the lamina, ligamentum, or disc immediately adjacent to the tip of the endoscope. If this should occur, wand the retractor to bring the target to the center of the operative

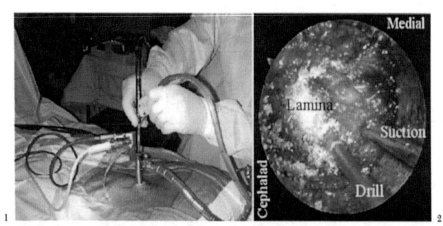

FIGURE 43N. Using standard open microsurgical techniques through the tubular retractor, bony resection is performed with the Kerrison punches or the drill. The extent of bony resection is customized to allow adequate access to the herniated disc or any migrated frag- ments. These external (1) and endoscopic images (2) illustrate the use of the MedNext drill to perform a laminotomy. The drill is commonly used in conjunction with a suction tube to minimize "spray-ing" of the endoscope lens with bone dust and blood.

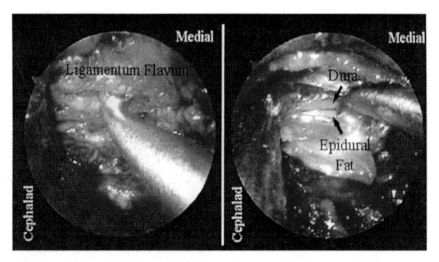

FIGURE 43O. Endoscopic images demonstrate the technique used for opening the ligamentum flavum. Alternatively, if a large enough laminotomy or lateral recess exposure is performed, the ligament can be easily detached from its cephalad bony or lateral capsular attachments. The ligament can then be partially retained as a flap or removed, if necessary.

field. As with other endoscopic procedures, centering the area of interest maximizes visualization and allows efficient instrument use within the retractor.

14. Identify the nerve root adjacent to the dural sac. Perform epidural dissection using any one or a combination of the Penfield instruments, the fine suction tip, the bipolar forceps, the modified ball-tip probe, the micronerve hook, or the 90-degree dissector. Undercut enough of the medial facet so that the lateral edge of the nerve root is exposed before retraction (Fig. 43Q). Use the pedicle as a landmark; it can be palpated with the ball-tip probe and will allow definitive identification of the nerve root if the anatomy is difficult to discern (Fig. 43R).

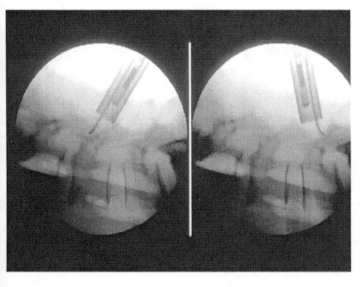

FIGURE 43P. Fluoroscopic images demonstrate the pedicle-to-pedicle access attainable by wanding (pivoting) the retractor in a cephalad or caudad direction.

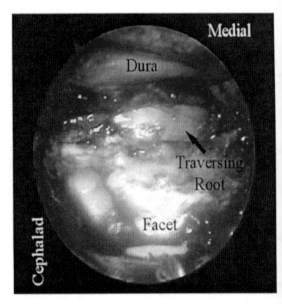

FIGURE 43Q. The lateral edge of the traversing root must be identified. Undercutting the lateral recess aids exposure of the root. The 25-degree endoscope is positioned medially, providing a "medial-to-lateral" view of the lateral recess and facet. Note that the traversing root is stretched over an underlying contained disc herniation.

15. Identify disc herniations by exploring the nerve root with the Penfield 4 or the small ball-tip probe. If necessary, retract the root medially and protect it with the modified nerve root retractor or the suction retractor. Fine cotton patties (cottonoids) can also be used to provide dural retraction. Control epidural bleeding, if encountered, using Gelfoam, cotton patties, or the bipolar forceps. Use the microscissors to divide coagulated epidural veins or tenacious epidural adhesions.

16. If required, use the microknife to perform an annulotomy, protecting the nerve root with the retractor (Fig. 43S). Remove herniated disc material with the various pituitary rongeurs in a standard fashion. Carry out intradiscal and extradiscal exploration

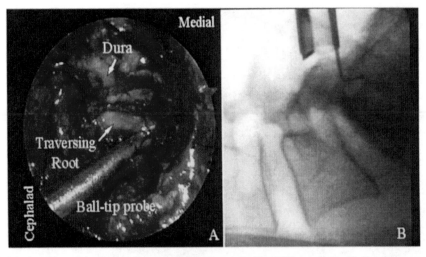

FIGURE 43R. Palpation of the caudal pedicle with the ball-tip probe as illustrated in (A) and (B) helps with identification of the nerve root when the anatomy is unclear.

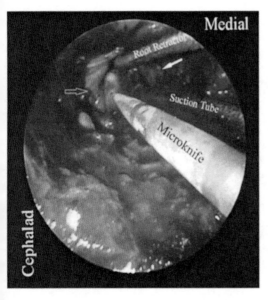

FIGURE 43S. Endoscopic image illustrating a left-sided herniated disc at L4–L5 in a patient with conjoined L4 and L5 roots. The traversing L5 root (*solid arrow*) is being retracted medially by the root retractor; the exiting L4 root (*open arrow*) can be seen at the disc level. An annulotomy was performed in the axilla of the L4 root with the microknife.

using techniques commonly used during open microdiscectomy. Finally, check the root for evidence of residual compression or retained disc fragments using various instruments (e.g., ball-tip probes, 90-degree dissector).

17. Following nerve root decompression, irrigate the wound thoroughly through the tubular retractor. Loosen the flexible arm and remove the retractor. As the retractor is withdrawn, the surgical corridor closes spontaneously as the paraspinous muscles resume their normal anatomical position (Fig. 43T). Close the fascia with a single suture. Close the subcutaneous tissues with an inverted suture. Apply sterile closure tapes and a small adhesive bandage to the skin (Fig. 43U).

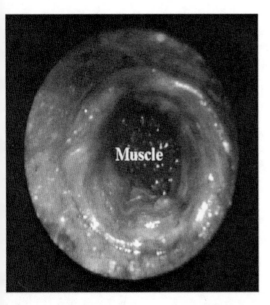

FIGURE 43T. Endoscopic image illustrates reapposition of the dilated paraspinal muscle as the tubular retractor is removed.

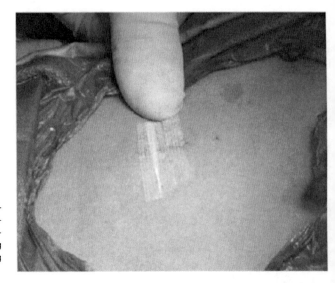

FIGURE 43U. Microendoscopic discectomy (MED) allows for effective discectomy using standard open microsurgical techniques while providing the cosmetic and muscle-sparing benefits of endoscopy.

Far Lateral Approach

1. Administration of anesthesia, positioning of the patient, and operating room setup are performed as described for the paramedian approach.

2. After the operative field has been prepped and draped, identify and mark the lumbar midline. Draw another line 4.5 to 5 cm lateral to the midline, ipsilateral to the disc herniation. Identify the level of the appropriate interspace using a 22-gauge spinal needle and the C-arm (Fig. 43V). As with the paramedian approach, an imaginary line extending along the needle should bisect the disc space. After removing the needle, center a 15-mm incision on the needle entry site and carry the incision into the subcutaneous tissues.

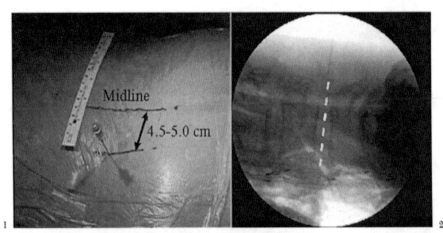

FIGURE 43V. (1) The incision for the far lateral technique is located along a paramedian line drawn 4.5 to 5 cm to the side of the disc herniation. (2) A 15-mm incision is made along this line and centered over the affected disc space.

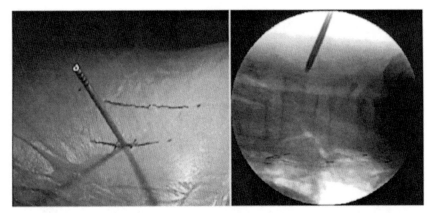

FIGURE 43W. External and fluoroscopic images illustrate placement of the initial dilator. With fluoroscopic guidance, the tip of the initial dilator is directed in a cephalad and medial direction to the junction of the base of the transverse process and the pars interarticularis.

3. Insert a K-wire through the incision and underlying lumbodorsal fascia, directing it toward the transverse process and pedicle of the superior vertebra (e.g., the L4 vertebra for a far lateral disc herniation at L4–L5). Insert the initial dilator over the K-wire, through the lumbodorsal fascia, and remove the K-wire. Dock the dilator on the base of the transverse process at its junction with the pars interarticularis. Confirm sagittal orientation of the dilator using the C-arm. Determine mediolateral orientation by palpating the bony landmarks with the tip of the dilator (Fig. 43W).

4. Insert the two sequential dilators over the initial dilator, followed by the tubular retractor. Remove the dilators from the tubular retractor and connect the retractor to the flexible arm. Insert the endoscope through the retractor and ensure proper image orientation (Fig. 43X).

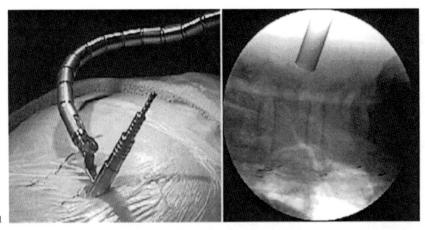

1   2

FIGURE 43X. The external image (1) demonstrates placement of the tubular retractor over the dilators. The fluoroscopic image (2) confirms the initial position of the retractor, centered at the junction of the transverse process and pars, after the dilators have been re- moved. There is a danger of inadvertently advancing the dilators or the tubular retractor into the intertransverse space. Therefore, it is imperative that these instruments are docked onto bone and that their depth is guided and confirmed fluoroscopically.

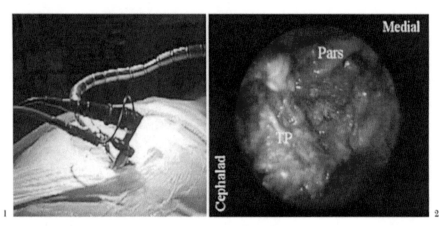

FIGURE 43Y. The endoscopic image is oriented to the patient's anatomical position (1) as previously noted. (2) Once exposed, the pars can be seen medially and the inferior edge of the transverse process (*TP*) is cephalad, running in a medial-to-lateral direction.

5. Clear residual soft tissue from the base of the transverse process and pars using a small pituitary rongeur and the electrocautery (Fig. 43Y). Coagulate the pars artery with a bipolar forceps and divide it with the microscissors. Separate soft tissue from the undersurface of the pars using the small, angled microcurette (Fig. 43ZA). This maneuver detaches the medial edge of the intertransverse ligament from the pars and allows for entry into the neuroforamen.

6. Remove bone from along the inferomedial aspect of the transverse process and most lateral aspect of the pars with an angled Kerrison rongeur (Fig. 43ZB). This maneuver opens the lateral aspect of the neuroforamen, allowing for palpation of the pedicle with the ball-tip probe and straightforward identification of the exiting nerve root as it travels around the pedicle (Fig. 43AA).

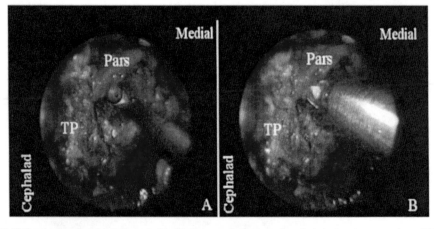

FIGURE 43Z. (A) The superior and medial attachments of the intertransverse ligament are released using a curved curette, as shown. (B) The most lateral aspect of the foramen can then be "unroofed" to allow identification of the pedicle and exiting nerve root.

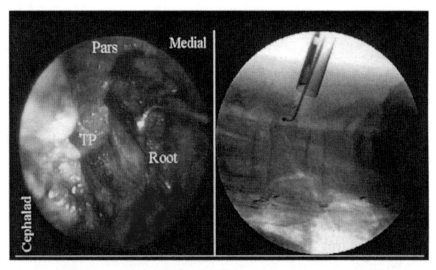

FIGURE 43AA. By definitively palpating the pedicle (fluoroscopic image), the surgeon can reliably identify the exiting root as it travels around this structure. The root can then be safely exposed, as demonstrated.

7. When the exiting nerve root has been definitively identified at the level of the pedicle, dissect laterally and inferiorly along the root, following its caudad course toward the disc by "wanding" the tubular retractor. If an overhanging articular process is encountered (secondary to coexisting facet hypertrophy), remove the lateral margin of the articular process with a Kerrison rongeur or endoscopic drill, further exposing the distal course of the root (Fig. 43BB).

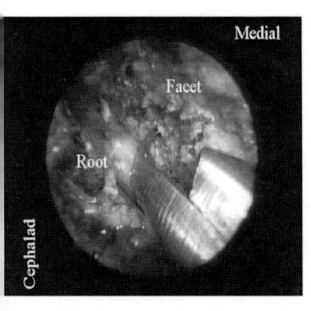

FIGURE 43BB. The root is followed by wanding the retractor in a caudal direction to the level of the disc space. If there is significant facet hypertrophy limiting access to the disc space medial to the root, resection of the lateral margin of the facet can be performed using the drill and/or the Kerrison punches.

8. Identify the dorsal root ganglion, which comprises the enlargement of the exiting nerve root just lateral and inferior to the neuroforamen. Treat this structure gently, as excessive manipulation of the dorsal root ganglion can produce significant postoperative pain.

9. Explore and decompress the root and remove herniated disc fragments (Fig. 43CCA–43CCC). If necessary, enter the interspace for further disc removal. Finally, reexplore the root to confirm that it has been fully decompressed (Fig. 43CCD).

10. Irrigate the wound, remove the tubular retractor, and close the fascia and subcutaneous tissues. Apply sterile skin closures and a small adhesive bandage.

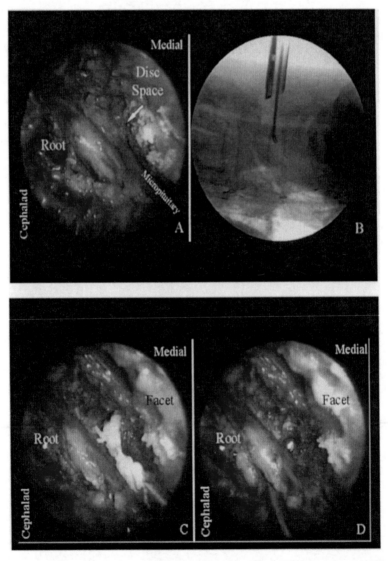

FIGURE 43CC. Discectomy and removal of any free fragments is performed under direct vision (A–C). The root is thoroughly examined to ensure decompression has been achieved (D).

Remember (for Paramedian Approach):

1. Ensure the skin incision is in line with the main surgical "target."
2. Identify (and confirm by palpation and fluoroscopy) the inferior laminar edge of the superior vertebra.
3. Obtain optimal exposure and hemostasis at each level before entering the epidural space.
4. Center your "target" by wanding the tubular retractor.
5. Definitively identify the lateral edge of the nerve root by undercutting the medial aspect of the facet and palpating the pedicle.
6. Confirm adequate decompression in all directions.

Remember (for Far Lateral Approach):

1. Skin incision is 4.5 to 5.0 cm from the midline at the level of the disc space.
2. Confirm by palpation and fluoroscopy that the initial dilator tip is at the junction of the transverse process and pars interarticularis of the superior vertebral body.
3. Identify and coagulate the pars artery at the lateral edge of the pars.
4. Remove just enough of the inferomedial aspect of the transverse process and the superolateral aspect of the pars to definitively identify the pedicle and the exiting nerve root.
5. Follow the root distally to the disc space and pathology.
6. Remove the lateral aspect of the facet, if necessary.
7. Avoid excessive manipulation of the dorsal root ganglion.

Index